The Auditory Periphery

BIOPHYSICS AND PHYSIOLOGY

The Auditory Periphery

BIOPHYSICS AND PHYSIOLOGY

PETER DALLOS

Auditory Research Laboratory (Audiology)
and Department of Electrical Engineering
Northwestern University
Evanston, Illinois

ACADEMIC PRESS New York and London 1973
A Subsidiary of Harcourt Brace Jovanovich, Publishers

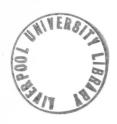

ACADEMIC PRESS, INC.
111 Fifth Avenue, New York, New York 10003

United Kingdom Edition published by
ACADEMIC PRESS, INC. (LONDON) LTD.
24/28 Oval Road, London NW1

LIBRARY OF CONGRESS CATALOG CARD NUMBER: 72-9324

PRINTED IN THE UNITED STATES OF AMERICA

To the memory of E. Ascher

Contents

Preface

My major motivation for writing this book was that a comprehensive description of the functioning of the peripheral auditory system was not available. To teach the subject one was forced to rely on journal articles, some reviews, and on some excellent but older books such as those of Stevens and Davis or Wever and Lawrence. The content of "Physiological Acoustics" (Wever and Lawrence) was closest to what I envisioned as desirable, but it was fifteen years old and, moreover, I thought it relied too much on viewing the system through the microphonic potential. Von Békésy's "Experiments in Hearing" had a much wider scope than just the treatment of the auditory periphery, and it was a collection of research papers, not a monograph with continuity. Thus I set out to fill what I perceived as a void. Now, some years later, the same void still exists even though there is more tutorial material available as chapters in various compendia.

This book attempts to provide a detailed and relatively complete account of the biophysics and physiology of the peripheral auditory system. It is aimed at a relatively heterogeneous audience, since workers in many fields have an interest in various aspects of the functioning of the hearing organ. I am hopeful that the work will be useful to biophysicists and bioengineers as well as to physiologists, otolaryngologists, and speech and hearing scientists. Because of the desire to provide a comprehensive account of the operation of the auditory system, the inclusion of considerable mathematical detail was deemed necessary. The heterogeneity of the envisioned readership, however, dictated that certain mathematical steps and procedures be explained. My rationale for choosing what knowledge to assume and what to explain is as follows. More and more young practitioners of the life sciences are acquainted

xi

with differential calculus and have some knowledge of differential equations. However, probably relatively few would be familiar with, for example, the use of Laplace transforms in systems analysis. Thus the latter technique is used more sparingly and on an elementary level. A considerable amount of mathematics is included in Chapters III and IV, but I believe that even these segments of the book will prove to be readable by the nonmathematically oriented reader.

To make the book self-contained, the first chapter provides some background in the anatomy of the peripheral auditory system and the second describes the most common experimental techniques. I conceive of the "auditory periphery" as extending to, but not including, the cochlear nerve. Consequently, neural phenomena are treated in the book only to the extent that they highlight cochlear events. This is arbitrary and clearly reflects my orientation and approach. The referenced material is necessarily selective, and I apologize to all colleagues whose pertinent work was overlooked, particularly to those—most likely to be in this category—whose work is not in English.

There are many individuals who directly or indirectly contributed to the realization of this book. Dr. Raymond Carhart, Director of the Auditory Research Laboratory at Northwestern University, provided the appropriate milieu and freedom during the past ten years to make my laboratory flourish and allow me to grow professionally. He has also given his friendship and much valuable advice. George W. Allen, M. D., first introduced me to the use of animal preparations and physiological techniques. Much credit is due to my students and collaborators: P. Allaire, M. Billone, B. Chesnutt, J. R. Boston, J. Durrant, I. Hung, C. O. Linnell, L. Pinto, R. G. Robbins, Z. G. Schoeny, R. H. Sweetman, C-y. Wang, and D. W. Worthington. W. Ballad provided valuable help in preparing photographic material for the book. Dr. C. Laszlo gave me wise suggestions for Chapters II and III. Very special thanks are due to my associate, Mary Ann Cheatham, for her good work and invaluable help in the preparation of this book. Mrs. Laura Reiter and her typists, Mrs. B. Duffin and Mrs. N. Seitz, did an outstanding job in preparing the manuscript. I thank the various publishers for their permission to reproduce copyrighted material and the many authors who helped me by providing photographs and drawings for illustrations.

The National Institute of Neurological Diseases and Stroke is thanked for the continuing support of my laboratory and my research efforts. Appreciation is expressed to the Research Committee of Northwestern University for defraying the costs of preparing this manuscript.

Finally, my wife Cirla has provided an atmosphere of love, patience, and understanding without which this work could not have been undertaken, much less completed.

PETER DALLOS

CHAPTER 1

Introduction

This introduction provides a framework for the detailed discussions that follow in subsequent chapters. Here, a presentation of the functional organization of the auditory system is followed by a rather sketchy description of the gross and neuroanatomy of the hearing organ.

I. Functional Organization of the Auditory System

In Fig. 1.1 a block diagram of the system is presented. The individual boxes represent the logical structural divisions within the overall system. The subdivisions above the actual block diagram indicate the function of any group of blocks, while those below pertain to the predominant mode of operation within a given block or group of blocks.

The first block represents the outer ear, whose external visible portion is the auricle or pinna and whose "inside the head" portion is the earcanal or external auditory meatus. The auricle in man has very little acoustic effect. In some animals, however, it is enlarged and quite movable and thus serves a useful role in the localization of sound in space. The earcanal, a long narrow tube, funnels the incoming sound to the eardrum, which is its inner boundary. The main function of the canal is to protect the delicate middle ear from noxious outside agents. The canal also introduces its own acoustic resonance into the transmission process; thus it exerts an effect on

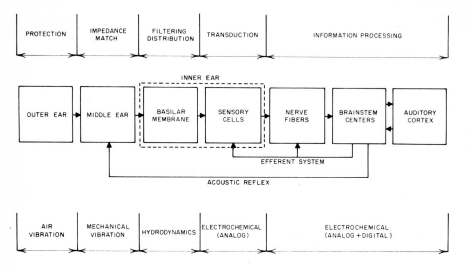

Fig. 1.1. Block diagram of the auditory system. In the center the anatomical subdivisions are shown, with the arrows indicating the direction of information flow. At the top the function of the various segments is indicated, while at the bottom the dominant mode of operation is described.

the actual information flow in the auditory organ. Within the earcanal sound is conducted by the vibration of air molecules. This fluctuating air pressure sets the eardrum into vibration and thus activates the mechanical lever, pressure transformer of the middle ear: the ossicular chain. The airborne sound is then translated into the vibrations of the bones of the middle ear.

The function of the middle ear is to translate airborne vibrations into pressure waves in the fluid that fills the inner ear (cochlea) and to match impedances between this fluid and air. The middle ear fulfills this role by boosting sound pressure through a combined force–pressure amplification process. The middle ear is endowed with muscles that can contract reflexively and thus subserve one of the feedback mechanisms that operate in the auditory system: the middle ear muscle reflex. The vibrations of the innermost bone of the ossicular chain are delivered to the fluid that fills the inner ear cavity. There the pressure wave sets the membranous portions of the inner ear into vibration and causes local deformations within the complex cellular structure that forms an important portion of this membrane complex. The sensory cells of the hearing organ are situated within the cell matrix attached to the membranous structure, and these cells are deformed in the above process. The deformation of these cells is the final mechanical event in the chain that starts with airborne vibrations and continues with mechanical movements within the middle ear, followed by hydrodynamic and fine mechanical events in the inner ear.

The sensory cells are transducers that convert mechanical deformation to electrical and chemical processes, the latter of which serves as the communicating link to the auditory nerve. The fibers of the nerve carry all information pertaining to the auditory environment in the form of nerve spikes whose temporal pattern (density) codes this information. The function of the inner ear is to perform appropriate filtering of the incoming acoustic signal coupled with the distribution of acoustic energy to differing groups of sensory cells, depending largely on the spectral content of the signal. The sensory cells are the critical transducers in the auditory chain. Feedback signals are transmitted to the inner ear by the well-developed efferent auditory system. All variables up to the initiation of spikes in the auditory nerve are in analog form; in other words, they are smoothly graded functions of the parameters of the incoming sound.

The information carried in the auditory nerve passes up, through various brainstem centers, to the auditory cortex. There is a great deal of cross connection between the two sides (left and right) beyond the first way station in the brainstem, and there is also a great deal of centrifugal information flow from the cortex down to the various brainstem nuclei via the efferent auditory system and the reticular formation. We can consider the entire neural network beyond the cochlea to serve the function of auditory information processing. One more feedback system should be mentioned for the sake of completeness. This is the sympathetic innervation of the auditory nerve fibers and of the blood vessels that serve the inner ear.

The aim of the chapters to follow is to provide the details of operation of the various subcomponents of the system that form the "auditory periphery." These include the middle ear and the inner ear up to and including the initiation of impulses in the auditory nerve but excluding the delineation of the code whereby these impulses carry information. Similarly excluded are the properties of functioning of the subcortical and cortical auditory centers. We shall include a treatment of the peripheral portions of the various feedback mechanisms.

II. Anatomy of the Auditory System

A. GROSS ANATOMY*

The overall anatomical structure of the ear can be followed with great clarity in Fig. 1.2, which is a reproduction of Brödel's well-known illustration of the cross section of the human ear.

* Zemlin (1968), Wever and Lawrence (1954), Polyak (1946).

1. The External Ear

The auricle is the externally visible, flaplike portion of the ear that is attached to the sides of the head. It is largely cartilaginous and has many convoluted folds that lead to the opening of the external meatus. This is an irregularly shaped canal, and in the human being is about 3 cm long with a diameter of approximately 7 mm. The size and shape vary greatly among species. In the cat, for example, it consists of a narrow peripheral portion about 1.5 cm long and a wider central portion approximately 0.5 cm in length.

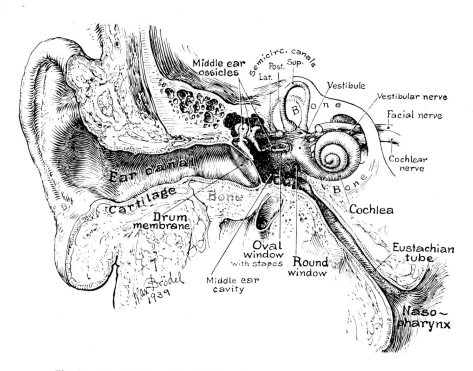

Fig. 1.2. Reproduction of M. Brödel's classical drawing of the cross section of the human ear. (From Brödel, 1946.)

These two segments of the canal are almost perpendicular to one another. A peripheral segment of the canal has cartilaginous walls, while the medial segment has bony walls. The relative lengths of these two portions vary among species. In human beings the two segments are about equal in length, while in the cat there is virtually no bony segment. The inner wall of the meatus is lined with skin bearing numerous hairs and wax-producing glands.

These serve a protective function and keep intrusion of foreign matter to a minimum.

2. The Middle Ear

The middle ear is an air-filled volume situated in a cavity which in higher mammals is surrounded by the temporal bone of the skull but which in most laboratory animals is surrounded by a thin bony compartment, the auditory bulla, attached to the skull. The middle ear cavity extends from the eardrum on its lateral border to the bony cochlear wall on its medial extreme. It communicates with the cochlea through two openings in the bony wall, the oval and round windows, and it also communicates with the nasopharynx via the eustachian tube. In humans the middle ear volume is customarily divided into two portions: the superior attic and the inferior tympanic cavities. The former communicates via the tympanic antrum with the mastoid air cells; thus the effective volume of the middle ear is considerably in excess of the volume of the tympanic cavity proper. The entire cavity, including the antrum and the mastoid air cells, is covered with a smooth mucous membrane lining. In animals that possess auditory bullae, the middle ear space is divided by a partition (bony septum) into two volumes. One of these is analogous to the tympanic cavity and houses the ossicular chain, while the other communicates with the round window. The relative size of the cavities and the size of the opening between these volumes are highly species variable. In some rodents (e.g., chinchilla, kangaroo rat) the bulla is hypertrophied and it contains several communicating air-filled compartments that greatly increase the effective volume of the middle ear cavity.

The lateral border of the middle ear, the eardrum or tympanic membrane, is a cone-shaped structure held in place by its own thickened, fibrous border, the annulus, which is inserted into a groove in the bony wall of the earcanal. The membrane itself is made up of three layers. The outermost layer is continuous with the lining of the earcanal, while the innermost layer is continuous with the lining of the middle ear. The structure that gives the membrane its characteristic cone shape and its structural stability is the central fibrous layer. This layer is composed of two groups of fibers, one radially oriented and one concentrically arranged. A long process (manubrium) of the most peripheral ossicle, the malleus, is firmly attached to the tympanic membrane, covering the full radius at 12 o'clock. Thus movements of the tympanic membrane are transmitted into movements of the malleus. The other two bones of the ossicular chain, the incus and the stapes, transmit the malleolar vibrations to the oval window of the cochlea, to which a portion of the stapes is flexibly affixed. The three bones form a functional unit; the joints between the adjacent bones are relatively firm. In most rodents the malleus and the incus are actually fused and thus there is only one joint in these species.

In humans the ossicular chain is suspended in the middle ear cavity by five ligaments. Three of these attach to the malleus, one to the incus, and one, the so-called annular ligament, holds the stapes in the oval window.

The ossicles are complex in shape. The human malleus has a large head, a neck, and three processes: the manubrium, the anterior process, and the lateral process. The manubrium is attached to the eardrum, the head is supported by the superior ligament, the anterior ligament attaches to the anterior process, and the tendon of the tensor tympani muscle is inserted opposite to the lateral process on the manubrium. On the head of the malleus there is an articular facet that joins the matching facet of the incus and forms the relatively rigid malleoincudal joint. The incus itself consists of a body and two processes that emerge from it at approximately right angles. The short process is anchored by the posterior ligament in the epitympanic recess (attic). The long process of the incus is parallel to the manubrium of the malleus; its inferior end is called the lenticular process, which forms the articulation with the stapes in the incudostapedial joint. The stapes is the smallest bone in the body; it consists of a head, a neck, two crura, and the footplate. The anterior crus and the posterior crus connect the footplate to the neck of the stapes. The footplate fits into the oval window; it is held in place by the annular ligament. The tendon of the stapedius muscle is inserted at the neck of the stapes. The articulation between incus and stapes is similar to a ball and socket joint. The entire ossicular chain is covered with a mucous lining, the same sort that covers the walls of the middle ear cavity. Figure 1.3a is a schematic drawing of the human ossicular chain as seen from the inside. It is notable that the entire system is suspended so that it can rotate about an axis formed by the short process of the incus and the anterior process of the malleus. Figure 1.3b, a drawing of the guinea pig ossicular chain, is given for comparison. The similarity between the two systems is quite striking even though in the guinea pig the two outer ossicles are fused to form a single unit. As the chain performs a rotary movement about its major axis a lever action takes place because of the unequal lengths of the manubrium (input arm of the lever) and the long process of the incus (output arm). This is a reducing lever, which means that the force exerted on the stapes is greater than the force communicated to the manubrium by the eardrum.

We have already described the attachments of the two middle ear muscles to the ossicular chain. These muscles are the effectors of the middle ear muscle reflex, which forms one of the important auditory feedback mechanisms. Both muscles are striated, pennate types (generating great tension with minimal displacement) having extremely rich innervation. The tensor tympani muscle runs in a bony canal parallel to the eustachian tube and only its tendon emerges into the middle ear cavity. The stapedius is in a bony canal in the posterior wall of the tympanic cavity, again only its tendon

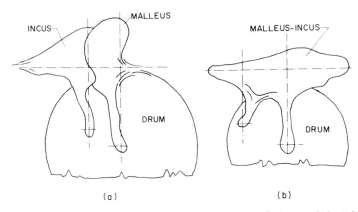

Fig. 1.3. Schematic diagram of the ossicular lever system in the human being (a) and in the guinea pig (b).

protruding from the canal. The stapedius, when contracted, pulls the head of the stapes in a posterior direction, almost at a right angle to the plane of rotation of the chain. The tensor pulls on the manubrium of the malleus in an anterior–medial direction, again roughly perpendicularly to the direction of the ossicular chain rotation. Thus the two muscles exert their force in opposing directions; they are anatomical antagonists even though functionally they are synergists. Contraction of the two muscles produces a stiffening effect on the chain.

3. The Inner Ear

The inner ear is enclosed in a system of cavities within the temporal bone (or within the thickened wall of the bulla). These interconnecting cavities form the bony labyrinth within which the organs of equilibrium and hearing are in intimate contact. Inside the bony labyrinth, and closely conforming to its shape, is the membranous labyrinth that contains the actual sense organs. Since our interest is in the hearing organ, the description of the bony and membranous vestibular system that follows is at best sketchy, while major attention is given to the osseous and membranous cochlea.

The bony labyrinth has three major subdivisions: the bony cochlea, the bony vestibule, and the bony semicircular canals. The outline of these can be discerned in Fig. 1.2. It should be emphasized that what one sees are the boundaries of a series of canals and cavities that are encased in bone. The openings to the osseous labyrinth are the oval and round windows, the cochlear aqueduct, the vestibular aqueduct, and the openings to the brain cavity through which the nerve and vascular supply of the labyrinth enter. The two aqueducts facilitate fluid exchange and regulation between the two labyrinthine fluids (perilymph and endolymph) and the cerebrospinal fluid space and the endolymphatic sac, respectively. For our purposes the most important portion of the bony labyrinth is the coiled bony cochlea. This snail-shaped structure can contain from two to five complete turns in mammals, while it is relatively straight in lower animal forms. The bony cochlea is coiled around its bony central core, the modiolus. From the modiolus a thin bony shelf protrudes into the cochlear cavity. This osseous spiral lamina incompletely divides the cochlear spiral into two compartments. The lower compartment (scala tympani) communicates with the tympanic cavity via the round window, while the upper compartment (scala vestibuli) opens through the oval window and is also contiguous with the vestibule. The larger-diameter portion of the cochlea that faces medially is called the base, while the top of the spiral is named the apex. In certain rodents (such as guinea pig and chinchilla) the bony cochlea is not a mere cavity within the temporal bone, but it actually consists of a bony shell that juts into the middle ear cavity, providing easy surgical access to the various turns. The entire inner surface of the bony labyrinth is lined with an epithelial membrane (periosteum) that is probably responsible for the secretion of the fluid that fills the bony labyrinth, the perilymph.

The vestibular portion of the membranous labyrinth is subdivided into

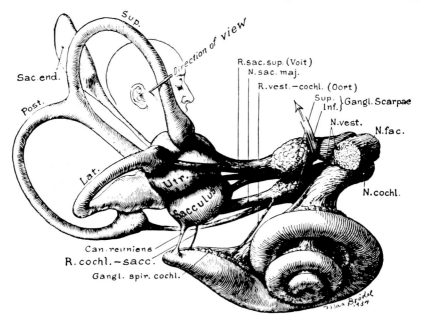

Fig. 1.4. Brödel's detailed drawing of the membranous labyrinth and its innervation. (From Hardy, 1934, p. 412.)

the semicircular canals, the utricle, and the saccule. The latter communicates with the membranous cochlea through a slender canal, the ductus reuniens. The entire system is shown in Fig. 1.4. The utricle and saccule are within the bony vestibule. The membranous labyrinth is filled with a fluid, the endolymph. The system communicates with the endolymphatic sac (located under the dural lining of the posterior cranial fossa) via the endolymphatic duct that courses within the vestibular aqueduct. It should be clearly understood that on the outside of the membranous labyrinth, between its walls and the bony labyrinth, there is a fluid-filled space containing perilymph. The inside of the membranous labyrinth is filled with another fluid, the endolymph.

The membranous cochlea, or cochlear duct, is formed by two membranes and is attached to the outer wall of the bony cochlea. One of the membranes, the basilar membrane, forms the floor of the cochlear duct. It is attached to the osseous spiral lamina on the modiolar side and to the spiral ligament (an enlargement of the periosteum) at its outer edge. The duct is completed on its vestibular side by Reissner's membrane. This membrane is also attached to the spiral ligament at its outer edge and to the thickened periosteum (spiral limbus) that covers the vestibular side of the osseous spiral lamina. The cochlear duct terminates prior to the termination of the cochlear canal at the apex, and thus it provides for communication between scalae vestibuli and tympani through an opening, the helicotrema. At any other point within the cochlea the two outer scalae, vestibuli and tympani, are completely separated from one another by the osseous spiral lamina and the membranous cochlea, which forms the third scala, the scala media. The cross-sectional areas of the cochlear scalae, the width of the basilar membrane and that of the osseous spiral lamina all change along the length of the cochlea. The cross-sectional areas become gradually smaller from base to apex and so does the width of the osseous spiral lamina. In conjunction with these changes the basilar membrane becomes wider at the apex; the variation in its width can be as great as 1:10. The cochlear duct is lined with a cell-rich vascular layer of tissue on its outer wall. This layer, known as the stria vascularis, plays an important role in the maintenance of the ionic balance of the endolymph. The ionic composition of the cochlear fluids is presented in Table 1.1. We should immediately note the differences between endolymph and perilymph. The former is similar to intracellular fluid in composition; that is, it has a high potassium concentration and a low sodium concentration. The perilymph in contrast is like interstitial fluid, having high sodium and low potassium content.

Within the cochlear duct and in intimate contact with the basilar membrane is the organ of Corti complex of cells. This structure is the actual sensory receptor of the auditory organ. Before we examine it in detail (Section II,

TABLE 1.1

CHEMICAL COMPOSITION OF COCHLEAR FLUIDS AND SPINAL FLUID[a]

Fluid	Potassium (mM)	Sodium (mM)	Chloride (mM)
Perilymph	7	140	120
Endolymph	154	1	110
Spinal fluid	4.2	152	122.4

[a] From Davis, 1958, p. 372, and Johnstone, 1970, p. 171.

B,1), however, we should get acquainted with the blood supply to the cochlea.

4. The Blood Supply of the Cochlea

The arterial supply of the inner ear is obtained from the cochlear artery, a branch of the labyrinthine artery. Another branch of the labyrinthine artery (the posterior vestibular artery) supplies part of the vestibular system. The labyrinthine artery derives from the anterior inferior cerebellar artery, which in turn is a branch of the basilar artery. The labyrinthine artery enters the inner ear through the internal auditory meatus together with the nerve supply of the cochlea. Small branches of the cochlear artery are directed toward the outer cochlear wall, where through radiating arterioles they provide the supply for the capillary network of the stria vascularis. Other branches supply the spiral vessels that run longitudinally under the basilar membrane. The venous blood is removed primarily through the internal auditory vein that passes through the internal auditory meatus and empties into the inferior petrosal sinus.

Oxidative metabolism is extremely high in the cochlea; it is subserved by the very extensive capillary network of the stria vascularis. The actual sense organ, the organ of Corti, receives its nutrition via the cochlear fluids and also, probably more importantly, from the spiral vessel that runs under the basilar membrane.

B. FINE ANATOMY

1. The Organ of Corti*

The organ is a complex cellular structure that sits on top of the basilar membrane and runs the entire length of the cochlear duct. It consists of a framework of supporting cells, within which the sensory cells are imbedded,

* Spoendlin (1966), Polyak (1946).

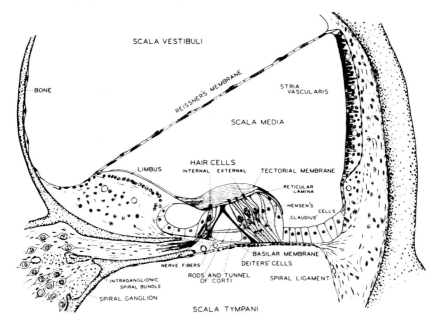

Fig. 1.5. Drawing of the cross section of one turn of the cochlea. Prepared from a midmodiolar section of a cat's cochlea. The drawing depicts the second turn. (From Davis and associates, 1953, p. 1182.)

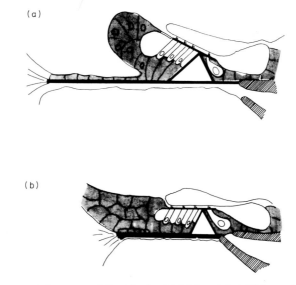

Fig. 1.6. Sketch of the organ of Corti in the third (a) and first (b) turn of the cochlea. (Adapted from Spoendlin, 1970, p. 4.)

and the terminal plexus of the auditory nerve fibres that innervate the sensory cells. The detailed drawing in Fig. 1.5 depicts the organ of Corti as it is situated within the cochlear cross section, while the two sketches in Fig. 1.6 illustrate how the dominant features of the organ change along the length of the cochlea. Figure 1.6a shows the appearance of the organ of Corti toward the apical end of the cochlear canal, while Fig. 1.6b depicts it in the basal region. In Fig. 1.7 a scanning electron microgram of the organ is

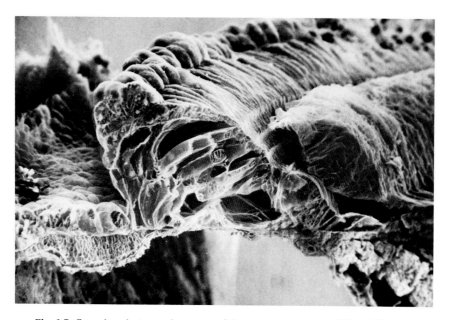

Fig. 1.7. Scanning electron microgram of the guinea pig organ of Corti. The organ is seen through a fracture in the preparation. The relationships among outer hair cells, supporting cells, the tunnel of Corti, and the basilar membrane are very clearly seen. The tectorial membrane is somewhat receded. (From Bredberg *et al.*, 1970, p. 861.)

presented to provide some appreciation of the spatial relationships. It is apparent that the detailed cross-sectional drawing of Fig. 1.5 shows the organ of Corti as it appears in the more basal region, while the scanning electron microgram was taken from a higher turn of the guinea pig cochlea. It should be mentioned for the sake of clarity that the latter picture was obtained from a specimen that had a natural fracture across the organ of Corti. Thus one can view both the cross-sectional area and a longitudinal extent of the organ. The following discussion of the various features of Corti's organ can proceed most profitably by utilizing Figs. 1.5, 1.6, and 1.7.

The lower boundary of the organ is the basilar membrane. On this membrane there is a relatively rigid framework formed by specialized cells that provide the structural support for the organ of Corti. The most conspicuous of these special cells are the inner and outer pillar cells, which form the triangular main support of the structure. Other primary supporting elements are the outer phalangeal cells of Deiters and the inner phalangeal cells. These cells, whose base rests on the basilar membrane, envelop the bottom portions of the sensory cells and thus hold them in place. These same cells extend rigid phalangeal processes that reach up to the apex of the sensory cells. There they flatten out and, together with the apical extensions of the pillar cells, form the reticular lamina, which is a flat plate that fills the spaces between the uppermost portions of the sensory cells. In other words, the reticular membrane provides the support for the top ends of the sensory cells and at the same time provides isolation between the inner spaces of the organ of Corti and the endolymphatic space. It is notable from the structural viewpoint that the phalangeal processes course upward with an oblique angle; the point at which they reach the reticular membrane is about two or three sensory cells more apicalward than the origin of their cell bodies. The entire supporting cell matrix strongly resembles the structure of a strutted bridge; it is clearly developed to provide considerable stability. A particularly clear view of the relationship among hair cells, supporting cells, and the reticular lamina is provided in the scanning electron microgram of Fig. 1.8.

The actual sensory cells are arranged on the two sides of the pillar cells. On the modiolus side there is a single row of inner hair cells, while on the other side there are three or four rows of outer hair cells. The inner hair cells are completely surrounded by the border cells of Held and the inner phalangeal cells that we have already mentioned. The outer hair cells are completely free of surrounding cells. Only their apex is supported in the reticular membrane and their base in the cup-shaped process of the Deiters' cells. Away from the outer hair cells toward the spiral ligament the organ of Corti is completed by the tall cells of Hensen, followed by the cells of Claudius, which hug the basilar membrane in a narrow layer. Spaced between the Claudius' cells and the basilar membrane are sparsely spaced so-called Boettcher's cells.

The basilar membrane itself is largely noncellular. It is composed mainly of fine (50 Å thick) radial fibers that are covered with an approximately 200 Å thick basement membrane on the organ of Corti side. On the tympanic side of the basilar membrane there is an irregular layer of cells, the number of which increases toward the apex of the cochlea. The spiral blood vessel that runs under the basilar membrane is imbedded in this layer of cells.

Between the supporting and sensory cellular structure of the organ of Corti is a network of extensive fluid-filled tunnels and spaces. The most prominent of these is the triangular space between the pillars of Corti,

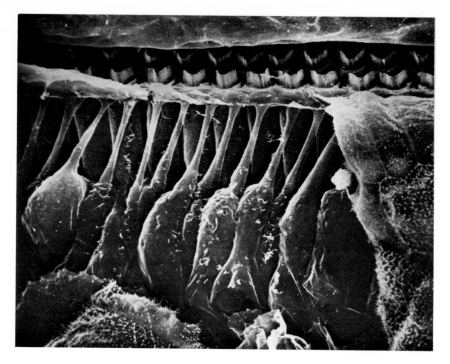

Fig. 1.8. Scanning electron microgram of a segment of the organ of Corti showing Deiters' cells and their phalangeal processes (foreground) and a row of outer hair cells (behind Deiters' cells). The reticular lamina and the stereocilia are also clearly seen, as is the tectorial membrane (top of picture). (Courtesy of G. Bredberg; from Bredberg *et al.*, 1972.)

which is termed the tunnel of Corti. The space between the outer pillar cells and the outer hair cells is the space of Nuel, while the opening between the outer hair cells and the cells of Hensen is called the outer tunnel. All these spaces are filled with a fluid that was named cortilymph by Engström. This fluid has the ionic composition of perilymph even though its protein content might be different.

Above the organ of Corti and in close proximity with it is an important structure that we have not yet mentioned: the tectorial membrane. On the modiolus side this membrane is attached to the top of the spiral limbus and is probably also attached to the cells of Hensen at its other extreme. The tectorial membrane itself is completely noncellular. It is composed of 93% protein substance (Iurato, 1962b); it is not collagenous but made up of fine filaments (approximately 96 Å diameter) that run transversely. The entire structure has the consistency and properties of a gel. Not possessing any sort of cell membrane, the tectorial membrane is not likely to present an electrical or ionic barrier but to subserve mechanical functions only.

The dominant group of sensory cells in the organ of Corti is comprised of the outer hair cells. These are slender cylindrically shaped cells with a diameter of about 5 μ and a length that varies from 20 μ in the base to 50 μ in the apical end. As we have said before the cells are anchored only at their apex and at their base, while the entire extent of the cell body is surrounded by the fluid within the organ of Corti. In Fig. 1.9a an electron micrograph of an outer hair cell is shown. The entire cell is surrounded by a typical unit membrane, and the lower one-third of the cell body is almost completely occupied by the cell nucleus. The apical pole of the cell is almost completely covered with a thick, rigid structure, the cuticular plate. Out of this plate protrude from 100 to 200 stiff hairs or stereocilia arranged in an orderly matrix. As Fig. 1.10 shows the hairs describe a W pattern formed of three rows of cilia. The W is oriented in the same direction on all outer hair cells, the top of the W facing the modiolus. Between the bottom extremities of the W is the only cuticle-free region of the hair cell. In this opening of the cuticular plate a basal body is present during embryonic development, but at least in some species this body disappears after birth. The cilia are stiff structures. Their length is graduated in that those in the innermost row are the shortest, and those in the outer row are the longest. The average length is about 2 μ in the basal region and it increases to approximately 6 μ in the apex. The diameter of the cilium is about 0.15 μ. The tops of the longest cilia extend into shallow indentations in the bottom surface of the tectorial membrane. Thus mechanical contact between the tectorial membrane and the hairs is firmly established. Within the cell body, at the apical end near the cuticular opening and all along the periphery of the cylindrical shaft, there is a significant concentration of mitochondria, which suggests that in these regions there is high metabolic activity. In the infranuclear area there is again a great concentration of mitochondria along with specialized presynaptic structures, indicating that this area functions as a presynaptic region.

The inner hair cells as shown in Fig. 1.9b are usually described as flask shaped; they are completely surrounded by supporting cells. From their apical cuticular plate about 60 stereocilia emerge. These are arranged in three very slightly curved rows, whose long axis is perpendicular to the cochlear radius. An asymmetrically placed cuticular opening with a basal body is also present in the inner hair cells. The cilia are much coarser (diameter 0.35 μ) than those belonging to the outer hair cells. Their length increases from base to apex and varies considerably from row to row, being the greatest in the outermost row. There is no evidence that even the longest cilia make contact with the tectorial membrane. As opposed to the outer hair cells, where the receptor cell–neural junctions are confined to the very bottom part of the cell,

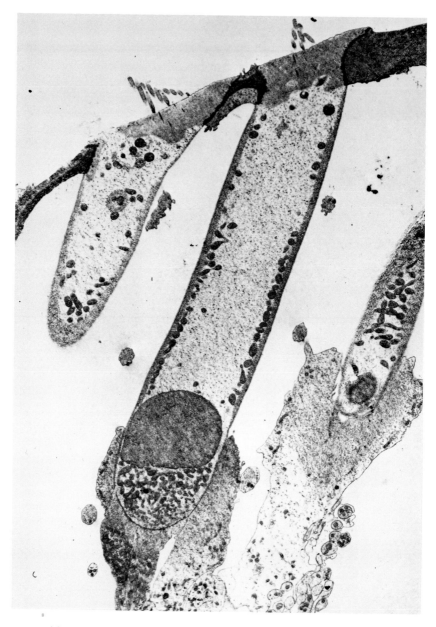

Fig. 1.9a. Electron microgram of three outer hair cells of the chinchilla. Only the center cell is shown in full cross section. Note the support of the cells at their apex by the surrounding reticular lamina and at their base by Deiters' cups. Some nerve endings are visible at the base of the hair cells. Note the large number of mitochondria just inside the cell membrane and the accumulation of vesicles and presynaptic structures below the cell nucleus. (From Smith, 1968, p. 424.)

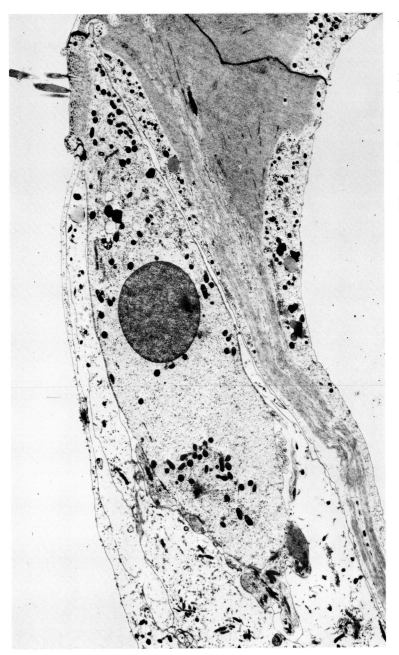

Fig. 1.9b. Electron microgram of the inner hair cell of the chinchilla. Note that the cell is completely surrounded by supporting cells, that the nucleus is much more centrally located than in the outer hair cell, and that mitochondria are not so conspicuously concentrated just inside the cell boundaries. Nerve endings are seen around the basal one-third of the cell. (Courtesy of C. Smith; adapted from Smith and Takasaka, 1971, p. 160.)

these junctions are widely scattered along the surface of the inner hair cell and they extend as high as two-thirds of the total height. It is important to emphasize here the many significant differences between the two hair cell groups, for we shall return to their discussion in Chapter 5. The scanning electron microgram of Fig. 1.10 provides an overall view of the top of the

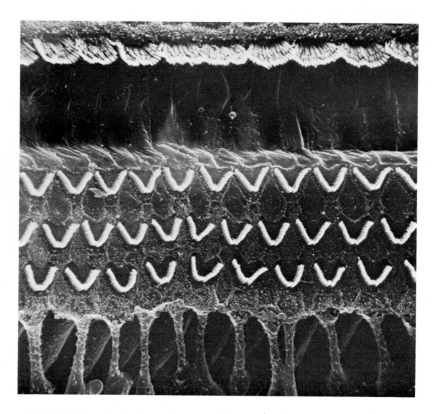

Fig. 1.10. Scanning electron microgram of the organ of Corti as viewed from the scala media (tectorial membrane is removed). This picture clearly indicates the spatial arrangement of the stereocilia of the single row of inner hair cells (top) and of the three rows of outer hair cells (center). The processes of the Deiters' cells forming the support of the reticular lamina are seen at the bottom of the picture. (Courtesy of G. Bredberg; from Bredberg *et al.*, 1972.)

organ of Corti with the tectorial membrane removed. This picture illustrates the spatial arrangement of stereocilia on both inner and outer hair cells. The differences between the two groups that we have discussed are clearly seen here, as are other spatial features that we have mentioned.

2. The Innervation of the Organ of Corti*

a. The Afferent Innervation. Ascending neural communication between each cochlea and the homolateral cochlear nucleus (the first auditory brainstem center) is accomplished with the approximately 30,000 fibers that form the afferent portion of the acoustic or 8th cranial nerve. These auditory neurons are of the bipolar variety. Their cell bodies form the spiral ganglion that is located in a bony canal (Rosenthal's canal) at the junction of the modiolus and the osseous spiral lamina. The dendritic portion of the neurons is within the organ of Corti, while the telodendria are in the cochlear nucleus. From the spiral ganglion the fibers travel peripherally within fine channels between the bony layers of the osseous spiral lamina, and they enter the organ of Corti at the junction of the lamina and the basilar membrane through openings in the lamina, which are designated as the habenula perforata. The fibers are myelinated central to the habenula, but they are bare (not even possessing Schwann cells) within the organ of Corti, even though they might be invaginated in between and in the folds of the supporting cells. The diameter of the myelinated fibers is approximately 3–5 μ; they are severely constricted in the habenular openings to about 0.25–0.7 μ, and vary between 0.2 and 1.5 μ within the organ of Corti.

Approximately 30 fibers enter the organ of Corti through each habenular opening. The majority of these fibers go directly to the nearest inner hair cell; each of these is innervated by about 20 fibers. These dendrites with their nerve endings are distributed fairly evenly over a large segment of the surface of the inner hair cell. A small number of the incoming fibers approach the inner pillar cells and pass through between adjacent cells. Only one or two fibers cross between any pair of pillar cells, and thus the total number of fibers that innervate the outer hair cells is quite small, approximately 1/10 of the total afferent population. After passing between pillar cells the afferent dendrites are buried in enfoldings of the pillar cells in the bottom of the tunnel of Corti. Within the tunnel floor the fibers course radially and toward the base. The fibers pass between the outer pillar cells and then make a distinct right-angle turn toward the base. They extend a considerable distance in their spiral course and form the so-called outer spiral bundle. These bundles are formed by about 20 fibers, each in single vertical extent between the rows of Deiters' cells. The schematic diagram of Fig. 1.11 depicts the fiber arrangement and clearly shows the very extensive, tortuous course of these outer spiral fibers. The maximal length of a given afferent dendrite innervating the outer hair cells is hard to measure, but it might be as great as 1 mm. As the fibers run their spiral course they gradually approach the base of the outer hair cells. Any spiral fiber gives off several collaterals that innervate

* Spoendlin (1966, 1970).

effector cells around the basilar, inferior anterior cerebellar, and labyrinthine arteries. The network does not extend further peripherally than the modiolar branches of the cochlear artery. This system of neurons is clearly connected with the general homeostatic function of the sympathetic nervous system. The other group of sympathetic or adrenergic fibers forms a very extensive network within the osseous spiral lamina and terminates just centrally from the habenula perforata. Since the actual terminations of these fibers have not yet been demonstrated, we do not know if they form synaptic contacts with the afferent or efferent nerve fibers. The function of this extensive adrenergic plexus in the region of the habenula perforata is not known.

CHAPTER 2

Experimental Techniques

I. The Quantities to be Measured

In this chapter the most commonly used measuring tools and techniques are discussed. The importance of knowing the underlying principles, ranges of applicability, virtues and limitations of a given method cannot be over-emphasized. Today more than ever before the proliferation of complex instruments enables the experimenter to ferret out more useful information from his raw data and to obtain hitherto unmeasurable data. On the other hand the ever more sophisticated methods and instruments can provide fascinatingly "well-behaved" artifacts. The only way to separate out the meaningful data is to know the power and the limitations of the method used in gathering the information in question.

The starting-point in our inquiry must of necessity be the discussion of the quantity to be measured. We shall be concerned with a number of such quantities: electrical potentials, mechanical motion, impedance, and sound pressure. Aside from the obvious distinction among these major categories we must pay particular attention to such issues as, for example in case of electrical recording, the nature of the potential to be measured. This will clearly determine which probe or electrode will be most appropriate for any particular measurement. It is equally important to choose an appropriate position for the location of the electrode, or if this is not possible one should at least be familiar with the meaning of the quantities recorded from any particular location. No matter how well the electrode and its position are chosen, the processing of the signals picked up by this electrode still has a radical influence on the experimental results. Special techniques can enhance the value of raw data, but they can also lead to erroneous interpretation if not used with discretion.

In order to cover such areas adequately, this chapter first presents the salient facts about the quantities that can be recorded from the peripheral auditory system. This discussion is followed by an introduction to electrical measuring techniques. Subsequent topics include the methods commonly used to measure motion; impedance measurement, both acoustic and electrical; and finally the elements of sound pressure measurements.

A. POTENTIALS TO BE RECORDED

Chapter 5 is a detailed account of the present status of knowledge of cochlear potentials. Because of this, only the salient features of the various potentials are discussed here, and only to the extent that these features influence the experimental method used to measure a given electrical phenomenon. The various potentials that we shall treat here are the cochlear microphonic (CM), the summating potential (SP), the resting potentials (EP, OCP), the generator potential (GP), the whole-nerve action potential (AP), and finally the single-unit response. Of these potentials the CM has been known since 1929 and has been studied to a tremendous extent, while the GP has not been isolated as yet with certainty. The other potentials fit between these extremes as far as our knowledge of their properties is concerned.

1. The Cochlear Microphonic (CM)

At moderate levels of the acoustic stimulus the CM potential duplicates to a great extent the displacement-time pattern of the cochlear partition. Since for any type of stimulus the partition exhibits an oscillatory motion pattern about its resting position, the CM itself possesses an ac (alternating current) waveform. This simply means that this potential changes its polarity between positive and negative signs with a time pattern that largely depends on the stimulus waveform. Figure 2.1 demonstrates the CM in response to an acoustic click and a tone burst. The waveforms of the sound stimulus are also shown in this figure. It is quite striking that the CM provides a fair representation of the driving signal.

This ac potential, the CM, is generally proportional in magnitude to the intensity of the stimulus. The proportionality holds for low and moderate levels, but at high intensities the CM generators saturate and the CM magni-

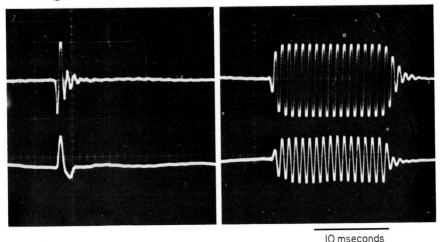

10 mseconds

Fig. 2.1. Cochlear microphonic responses to an acoustic click and tone burst. The upper traces show the CM, while the lower traces depict the waveforms of the sound monitored at the eardrum. The CM is recorded with differential electrodes in the first turn of the guinea pig cochlea.

tude ceases to increase with growing stimulus strength. The lower intensity limit at which CM is measurable depends solely on the experimental techniques used. In other words, there is no reason to assume that a real threshold (aside from that set by system noise) exists for CM. The upper limit of CM is dependent on species, frequency, and electrode location. In mammals, at low frequencies, and recorded from the endolymph, the CM can reach about 2–10 mV, but in lower animals the CM is generally smaller. The maximal CM decreases with increasing frequency. While the CM potentials can be picked up *anywhere* from the vicinity of the cochlea (popular "targets" have been the round window, the bony cochlea, and the cochlear fluids), they are the biggest if the recording electrode is located in the scala media. Recording from the other cochlear scalae reduces the CM by about a factor of 2–10, and further decreases are evident with additional distance between the electrode and the generating site.

When stimulated with pure tones, the cochlea responds with sinusoidal CM voltage. The frequency of the CM is of course the same as that of the stimulus. The question naturally arises as to the frequency limits within which one can record CM. The answer is complex, since the CM-producing ability of the cochlea is intimately tied to its ability to respond with mechanical motion to a stimulus. This ability is highly species dependent. Most laboratory animals respond from a few hertz to 20,000–40,000 Hz. Some animals, primarily those that utilize echolocation as an important source of information, respond far into the ultrasonic range. In general there is a best-frequency region for any species, and their ability to respond with a CM for either lesser or greater frequencies rapidly diminishes outside this range.

2. The Summating Potential (SP)

While this potential was identified quite some time ago, we still do not have adequate and conclusive evidence about many of its properties. To a large extent this is due to the fact that the SP is made up of a number of components and the limited measurement techniques that were employed in studying this phenomenon could not reveal all its complexities. At this point it is sufficient to note that the SP is a dc (direct-current) potential that somewhat mimics the envelope of the eliciting stimulus. Figure 2.2 depicts SP

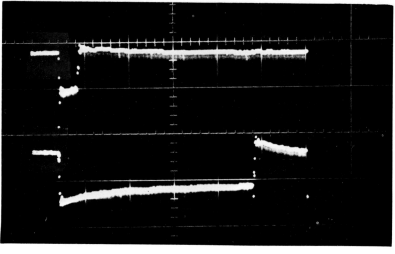

40 mseconds

Fig. 2.2. Summating potential responses to short and long tone bursts. Differential-electrode recording from the first turn of the guinea pig cochlea. The CM is removed from these traces by averaging several non-phase-locked responses.

responses to a short and a long tone pip. We see that the SP persists as long as the stimulation lasts. This potential, just like the CM, can be measured from any location in the vicinity of the cochlea but, again like the CM, its magnitude is greatest in the scala media. Experimental evidence indicates that the magnitude and the polarity of the SP depend on the complex interaction of intensity, frequency, and electrode location. It is significant that the time course of the SP is different in scala media and in the perilymphatic scalae. Depending on the combination of recording site and stimulus parameters, the SP can have the same or opposing polarity in the two perilymphatic scalae. With increasing stimulus strength the SP function does not show a tendency toward saturation, and within the physiologically significant intensity range it can reach a magnitude of several millivolts.

3. Single-Fiber Responses in the 8th Nerve

The afferent portion of the auditory nerve responds to sound stimulation by increased firing rate, synchronization of activity, or both. These changes in firing pattern are in reference to a resting discharge that is evident even without measurable sound stimulation. All afferent fibers demonstrate a spontaneous discharge. The rate of this activity can be as slow as a few spikes per minute and as fast as 100 spikes per second.

All primary auditory fibers respond to tone stimuli with some degree of frequency selectivity. For any given unit there is a best, or characteristic frequency at which the fiber responds to a least stimulus intensity. At higher levels an ever-widening band of frequencies can elicit responses. In response to low-frequency pure tones, the neural spikes occur in synchrony with the stimulus waveform. Above approximately 5000 Hz such time lacking is no longer observed.

Recording of single-unit neural responses is readily accomplished with microelectrodes thrust into the auditory nerve trunk. These electrodes pick up the extracellular electric field that is generated by the spikes traveling along the myelinated axons of the auditory nerve. Typical spike trains in response to tone bursts are shown in Fig. 2.3. The spike *magnitude varies*

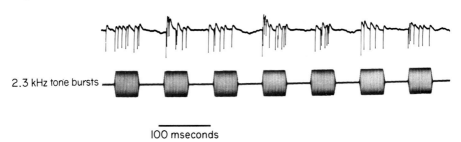

2.3 kHz tone bursts

100 mseconds

Fig. 2.3. Sample spike trains from a single auditory nerve fiber in response to repetitive tone bursts. (From Kiang, 1965, p. 15.)

greatly with the distance of the electrode tip from the fiber and with the characteristics of the electrode itself. The spike height can thus change from approximately 100 μV to several millivolts.

4. The Whole-Nerve Action Potential (AP)

Electrodes located in the vicinity of the cochlea can also pick up summated neural responses. These neural components (AP) result from the synchronous firing of a large number of fibers. Such synchronous activity is usually seen at the onset of tone bursts or in response to clicks, for it requires well-localized events in time to synchronize adequate populations of neurons. The AP is manifested as a series of predominantly negative brief potential peaks. Such an AP response is shown in Fig. 2.4. Since auditory nerve fibers

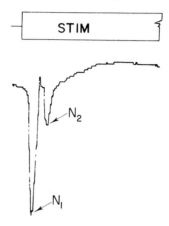

Fig. 2.4. Whole-nerve action potential response at the onset of a tone burst of 8000 Hz. Average potential of the two perilymphatic scalae [AVE = (SV + ST)/2]. The CM is removed from the trace by averaging several non-phase-locked responses. Note the N_1 and N_2 components of the response.

are fairly uniform in diameter, the magnitude of the AP is related to the number of fibers discharging simultaneously. This is because uniform fiber diameter results in uniform conduction velocity, and thus from any given region all firings arrive at the recording electrode at the same time and thus summate.

It should be mentioned that, in addition to AP responses at the onset of tone pips or due to clicks, such responses can be seen riding on each individual cycle of the CM with pure tone stimuli at relatively low frequencies.

5. The Generator Potential (GP)

It has become increasingly evident that, in sense organs, graded electrical activity precedes the initiation of nerve impulses. It appears to be sound practice to discriminate between two types of graded activity (Davis, 1961a) The "generator potential" is, by definition, the electrical activity that triggers the neural impulses in the initial segment of an axon. In contrast, the "receptor potential" (RP) is generated in a specialized receptor cell in response to external energy. In the auditory system the CM and the SP have been described as either GP or RP. It is useful to consider them as RP and to assume that a separate GP ought to exist. This GP has not yet been experimentally identified with certainty. Its probable location is in the initial, nonmyelinated segment of the auditory nerve.

6. The Endocochlear Potential (EP)

Thus far we have discussed stimulus-related electrical events in the peripheral auditory system. Aside from these potentials, one can measure a dc polarization of the endolymph of the scala media with respect to the rest of the body. This potential (EP) is approximately $+80$ mV. It is unique in that the scala media is the only place in the body where a fluid-filled region has such high positive polarization. This potential apparently originates in a layer of vascular tissue covering the wall of the scala media (stria vascularis).

7. The Organ of Corti Potential (OCP)

When a recording electrode passes through the organ of Corti it registers a negative potential of the order of -70 mV. This potential can be a manifestation of the resting polarization of the cells in Corti's organ or, as has been suggested by some, it might be a dc polarization of the fluid space within the organ.

B. Motion Patterns

Since the auditory periphery is a mechanohydraulic as well as an electrical system, information about it is sought not only from electrical measurements, but also from investigations of various motion patterns within the system. Some of the most fundamental knowledge about the operation of the auditory system has in fact been garnered by other than electrical measurements. For example, von Békésy's now-classic studies on the motion patterns of the basilar membrane were conducted with optical measuring techniques.

The basic problems to be investigated concern the amplitude and pattern of vibrations of the various middle ear structures, the eardrum and the ossicles; the vibratory pattern of the basilar membrane; and finally the mode of displacement of the various subcomponents of the organ of Corti. Clearly, as one proceeds more and more centrally the problems of accurate measurement are compounded. Because the middle ear is a relatively gross and easily accessible structure, present-day measuring techniques appear to be adequate to provide a complete description of its vibratory properties. The necessary measurements involve the delineation of the absolute and relative motion of the ossicles and the pattern of vibration of the tympanic membrane. The former tasks can be now accomplished over almost the entire dynamic range of the middle ear with such methods as laser interferometry or the Mössbauer technique. The former, because of its wider dynamic range, is probably more suitable for these measurements. The actual vibratory pattern of the eardrum can be studied both qualitatively and quantitatively with acoustic holography.

Aside from direct observation of the vibrations of the basilar membrane the Mössbauer method has been used quite successfully to obtain accurate data on its displacement. This endeavor, of course, is a very severe technical challenge. The movements are very small (10^{-10}–10^{-3} cm), the place of measurement is difficult to approach, the measurements should be made in a fluid medium, and other problems abound. Not the least of these is the restricted dynamic range of the Mössbauer method itself.

Only some very rudimentary qualitative observations have been made to date on the fine motion patterns of the organ of Corti. Small size, small movements, and inaccessibility are some of the reasons why no major progress is likely to occur with present methodology.

II. Measurement of Electrical Potentials

A. ELECTRODES

Electrodes serve as connecting links between biological tissue and measuring instruments. Their function is to pick up electrical activity and to deliver it, with as little distortion as possible, to the first stage of instrumentation. This first "head stage" or preamplifier is intimately tied to the electrode in its properties. It is the electrode–head-stage combination that determines the range of applicability of the measuring system.

Depending on the size of the electrode tip one can distinguish gross and microelectrodes. There is no clear-cut demarcation between the two types; they are separated by the criterion that microelectrodes are supposed to be capable of recording electrical activity from single neural units, while gross electrodes in general pick up responses from large populations of units. Both types of electrode have been used extensively in auditory research. Gross electrodes are used primarily in recording cochlear potentials, although microelectrodes are being used for this purpose more and more. The primary use of microelectrodes is in the recording of single-unit activity from the auditory nerve and from higher centers.

1. Gross Electrodes

Large electrodes used for measuring cochlear potentials are divided into two categories depending on their placement during recording. One class of electrodes is used to pick up potentials from the round-window membrane (RW); another type of electrode directly contacts the cochlear fluids. The latter, intracochlear (IC) electrode is inserted into the cochlea through fine holes drilled in the bony cochlear wall. Round-window and intracochlear electrodes alike have certain peculiarities, limitations, and advantages. Most of the limitations stem from the common property of all large electrodes that they pick up the summated or averaged responses of a very large number of biological generators. In many studies of the functioning of the cochlea, investigators seek to discern the response of a narrow segment of inner ear active tissue to certain acoustic stimuli. Experiments that immediately come to mind are those designed to determine the distribution of electrical events along the length of the inner ear and those that seek to describe the effects of certain damaging agents, or electrical or mechanical modifications of the peripheral auditory system, on the electrical responses from the cochlea. In order that valid conclusions can be gleaned from experimental data obtained with gross electrodes, the investigator must know the properties of his most important instrument, the electrode. In the following sections some characteristics of customary gross recording techniques are discussed in some detail in order to alert the reader to some limitations and pitfalls.

a. Single Active Electrode Recording. This discussion is equally applicable to the popular round-window recording technique and to the not infrequently used single intracochlear electrode method. The conclusions also apply to the older method of placing electrodes in contact with the cochlear bone. The latter technique suffers from all problems of the single-electrode method with the added disadvantage of generally reduced potential pickup.

The physical form of the gross cochlear electrode is usually quite simple. Round-window (RW) electrodes are made either of saline-soaked wicks or of metal. The latter type has been more popular. The simplest metal RW electrode is made of enamel-insulated silver wire of approximately 100-μ diameter. The enamel is first scraped back about 1 mm from the tip, and then the bare end is flattened into a foil. The foil part is then bent so that it forms an angle of approximately 120° with the shaft, and the electrode is ready for placement.

A sturdier RW electrode can be made, again from enameled silver wire, by forming a silver ball at the end of the electrode by repeatedly plunging the wire into the flame of a Bunsen burner. Very nice balls can be formed by this method, but it is rather difficult to prevent the burning of the enamel off from the wire over several millimeters from the ball. Another method of creating a ball electrode without damaging the insulation is to dip the wire into mercury and then pass approximately 1 A current through the junction for a few seconds.

Intracochlear electrodes are usually made of either tungsten or stainless steel wire. A wire diameter of approximately 20 μ has been found to be quite satisfactory. The most common method is to dip short pieces of wire into some glue or wax so that this substance will form beads on the wire. The wire is then cut so that a bead is present a short distance from the tip. The bead is used to stop the electrode against the bony cochlear wall and to resist the outflow of perilymph. The wire is usually twisted around colored silk thread to facilitate identification and handling.

In our laboratory we prefer to use a somewhat more rigid intracochlear electrode. This electrode consists of a 24-μ tungsten wire, which is sealed into a glass capillary tube. First an ordinary glass pipette is made with an electrode puller, and then the tip is broken so that it has an inner diameter of approximately 30–50 μ. A precut piece of wire is then threaded into the pipette. The wire is sealed into the glass by dipping the electrode tip into the flame of a Bunsen burner for a few seconds. In Fig. 2.5 a photograph of such

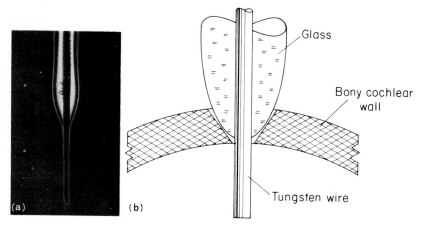

Fig. 2.5. (a) Photograph of glass-insulated tungsten electrode used to record from the perilymphatic scalae. (b) Schematic cross section of guinea pig cochlear bone with glass-coated wire electrode in place. The glass itself is effective in stopping fluid escape.

an electrode is shown along with a schematic diagram of the electrode in place in the cochlea. As can be seen, the glass envelope itself is used to seal the hole drilled into the cochlear bone.

The main difficulty facing the user of a simple gross electrode is the classification of the components that constitute the picked-up electrical signal, and the identification of the site of origin of these components. Let us begin with the first problem. It is well known that if pure tones are used as stimuli then, up to 4–5 kHz, synchronized neural firings occur at every cycle of eliciting sound. This volleying of the auditory nerve is manifested by negative potential peaks seemingly mixed with the CM. These AP peaks occur on every cycle, and they can be quite difficult to distinguish from bona fide CM. To dramatize the ambiguity of the single-electrode pickup, Fig. 2.6 shows

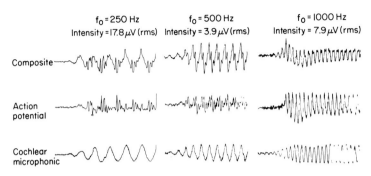

Fig. 2.6. Electrical potentials recorded from the cat round window in response to tone pips of three frequencies. Top traces show the raw data, the middle traces show the whole-nerve action potential after rejection of the CM, and the lower traces show the CM alone.

round-window-recorded responses to tone pips with stimulus frequencies of 250, 500, and 1000 Hz. The upper traces show the response as recorded. The lower two traces depict the CM and the AP components after these were separated by a combined masking–computer technique. At low frequencies (250 Hz) it is seemingly easy to visually separate the AP from the CM in the composite response trace. The AP here is predominantly of higher frequency than the fundamental CM response, even though a considerable amount of the AP voltage does appear at the fundamental frequency. The higher-frequency components form a Fourier series, and the individual voltage values can be measured with a selective voltmeter (wave analyzer). This method, however, does not separate the CM and AP components that appear at the fundamental frequency. Moreover, the method can be used only at low sound levels, for nonlinear distortion of the CM is also manifested by the appearance of harmonic components that are indistinguishable (as far as the wave analyzer is able to measure them) from components of the AP. At higher frequencies (see especially the traces for 1000 Hz) most of the energy contained in the AP appears at the fundamental frequency. Clearly, there is no way to visually break down the 1000-Hz composite trace and to so determine the AP and CM portions. Similarly a wave analyzer would be of no use here. It is striking to note how serious this problem of AP–CM mixing can be around 1000 Hz. Observe that the composite signal is smaller than either the AP or CM alone. This is due to the peculiar phase relationship between CM and AP in this frequency and intensity region. The two voltages are almost in phase opposition, and thus when added they partially cancel one another. The phase of the AP as referred to the CM is both frequency and intensity dependent. Clearly, measurement of the composite signal from a single electrode cannot reveal the true size of either the CM or the AP.

This conclusion is valid whether the electrical potential is measured with a wide-band (vacuum tube voltmeter) or narrow-band (wave analyzer) instrument. These uncertainties of measurement make the drawing of certain conclusions somewhat hazardous. The experimenter must be aware that changes in recorded potentials during the course of an experiment might be due to alterations of AP or CM or both.

Another problem that always arises with single cochlear recording is the question of the origin of the electrical signals picked up by the electrode. To explain, microphonic potentials are generated over various size patches along the basilar membrane. Depending on the stimulus frequency and intensity the size of the active region changes as does the location of maximal activity. Consider a round-window electrode located close to a segment of the basilar membrane which is maximally sensitive to high frequencies but which also responds to low frequencies. The question naturally arises, during the course of low-frequency stimulation does the RW electrode respond to the proximally generated small CM, to the distally generated large CM, or to both? Some authorities (Wever, 1949; Lawrence et al., 1959) feel that round-window-recorded potentials represent the integration of the outputs of generators that are widely distributed over the length of the basilar membrane and thus that it is not possible on the basis of this composite potential to draw conclusions about the pattern of electrical activity of the cochlea. Other authorities (Tasaki and Fernández, 1952; Simmons and Beatty, 1962; Davis, 1957), however, feel that RW electrodes measure CM generated within a region 1–2 mm, at most, from the electrode site. If this were the case then single cochlear electrodes would be adequate to accurately describe highly localized cochlear events—a very attractive proposition. We shall pick up this line of thought and draw some conclusions after the differential-electrode recording method is discussed.

   b. Differential-Electrode Recording. Differential-electrode recording simply means that one uses two active electrodes, one in scala tympani and one in scala vestibuli of a particular turn of the cochlea, the outputs of which are either added or subtracted to provide the desired electrical information. As we shall discuss below, the potential difference between the two electrodes is measured when the local cochlear microphonic (CM) is to be emphasized, while the sum of the two electrode potentials is studied when action potentials (AP) are of interest. Tasaki and Fernández (1952) and Tasaki et al. (1952) developed the techniques of differential recording, and the latter authors gave the theoretical considerations on which the method is based. It has become increasingly clear that this system of recording cochlear potentials provides the best means of studying localized electrical events and thus of delineating amplitude and phase distribution patterns.

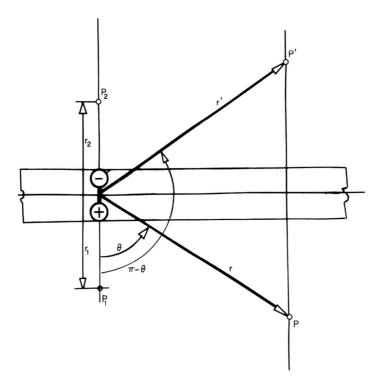

Fig. 2.7. Schematic representation of a dipole source. (From Dallos, 1969a, p. 1000.)

In order to clarify the theory of differential recording, let us consider a much simplified scheme. Assume that an elementary source of CM can be represented in a given instant as a dipole. With this assumption, a simple calculation can be made of the magnitude of the electric field at any point in the vicinity of the dipole. The appropriate geometry is shown in Fig. 2.7. The dipole is symbolized by the two opposite charges close to one another, arranged perpendicularly to the cochlear partition, which is denoted by shading. The distance from any point P to the center of the dipole is denoted by r, while the angle subtended between the axis of the dipole and the line connecting the dipole to the point P is denoted by θ. The magnitude of the potential at point P due to the dipole can be expressed as

$$E = (K \cos \theta)/r^2 \tag{2.1}$$

where K is a constant dependent on the strength of the dipole. An electrode whose tip is situated in point P_1 would record $E_1 = K/r_1^2$, since the angle θ is zero. An electrode at point P_2 would record $E_2 = -K/r_2^2$, since here the angle is 180°. Note that, if $r_1 = r_2$, then $E_1 = -E_2$. Similarly, all points that are symmetrical to the $\theta = 90°$ line (i.e., the cochlear partition) see the same potential magnitude but with opposite sign. This can be seen by comparing the potential at points P and P', Since $r = r'$, $E = (K \cos \theta)/r^2$, while $E' = [K \cos(\pi - \theta)]/r^2$. But since $\cos(\pi - \theta) = -\cos \theta$, it follows that $E = -E'$. It is thus clear that electrodes situated symmetrically on two sides of the source would pick up potentials of the same magnitude and of opposite polarity. If the potentials recorded by two symmetrically placed electrodes are amplified by a differential amplifier, we obtain

$$E_{out} = A(E - E') = A \cdot 2E \qquad (2.2)$$

where A is the amplification factor. Note then that a pair of electrodes in conjunction with a differential amplifier provides signals that are due to all generators situated in a plane equidistant from the two electrodes.

If an electrode is far away from a particular dipole source, then two effects take place. First, since the potential is inversely proportional to the square of the distance, the contribution of distant dipoles decreases rapidly with increasing separation. Second, since the increase in r takes place with θ gradually approaching 90°, the diminution of the potential is even more rapid. Consequently, if r is large the potential pickup due to a distant dipole is very small. If the cochlear partition is flat, then, even though very small, the potentials in the two electrodes (on opposite sides of the cochlear partition) are of opposing signs. consequently, they are additively amplified by the differential amplifier to which the electrodes are connected. When the cochlear partition is curved, however, both electrodes subtend approximately the same angle from the dipole, and thus the small contribution of the remote source tends to cancel in the differential amplification. These arguments point out that remotely generated CM is not canceled out as an inherent property of the differential-electrode method; instead, it is the angle effect that, coupled with the differential-electrode technique, is responsible for whatever cancellation might be seen for distant CM generators. In the first turn of the cochlea, the curvature is relatively mild; thus for sources located there, the angle effect is not pronounced. Electrodes situated in the higher cochlear turns are more likely to be influenced by the sharper curvature of the cochlea, and thus one would expect them to be more responsive to narrower cochlear segments than the basal-turn electrodes.

A very important remote source that is seen at the same angle by both electrodes of any pair is the one that generates the AP. Thus action potentials appear at equal magnitudes and with the same sign in both electrodes of a pair. If the potentials are amplified with a differential amplifier, the AP can be canceled from the total response. Conversely, if the potentials from the two electrodes are added, the AP is emphasized while the CM can be canceled. This ability of separating CM from AP was probably the main motivation for the development of the differential-electrode technique and has remained the main incentive in using the method. In fact, the major interest is usually the rejection of CM in favor of AP (Teas *et al.*, 1962; Fernández, 1955).

It ought to be pointed out that the theoretical structure presented above should be considered only as a first approximation. All considerations have tacitly assumed that the dipole source is situated in a homogeneous electric medium. Considering the complex structure of the membranous labyrynth, this assumption clearly does not represent reality. The inhomogeneity of the medium is primarily manifested in that the two recording electrodes see any source through complex, and not necessarily equal, impedances. Thus an apparent imbalance between the recording electrodes could occur at certain frequencies. The imbalances would be manifested by incomplete cancellation of remote activity and asymmetrical pickup of local activity.

A single electrode of great importance is the round-window electrode. In Fig. 2.8, three isopotential curves are shown for one experimental animal. A round-window, a single intracochlear, and a differential recording plot are shown in this figure. Of course, the two latter curves were obtained from electrodes in the basal turn. As was pointed out by Tasaki (1957), the fre-

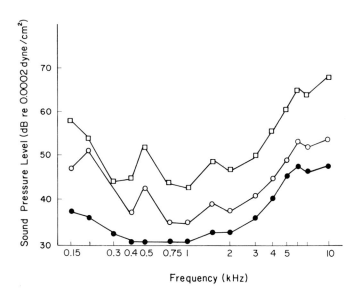

Fig. 2.8. Isopotential curves obtained from one guinea pig with single (○) and differential (●) basal-turn electrodes as well as with a round-window (□) electrode. (Adapted from Dallos, 1969a, p. 1003.)

quency dependence of the round-window electrode is very much the same as that of the basal-turn intracochlear electrodes. More specifically, as Fig. 2.8 demonstrates, the correspondence is particularly good between single intracochlear and round-window recording. Both of these techniques respond to a mixture of local CM, remote CM, and AP, and both show considerable fluctuation in sensitivity from one frequency to another. The fluctuations in sensitivity are largely eliminated by the differential recording technique. One very important difference between the single intracochlear and round-window electrodes is in the overall sensitivity of the two. Our experience is that the round-window electrode is approximately 10 dB less sensitive than the intracochlear wire at all frequencies.

The superiority of the differential-electrode technique over measurements with single intracochlear electrodes can be demonstrated by studying some third-turn CM responses of the guinea pig. In Fig. 2.9 we can distinguish

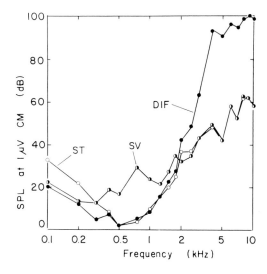

Fig. 2.9. Isopotential curves obtained from one guinea pig with third-turn electrodes. Single scala tympani and vestibuli electrodes, as well as their differential combination, were used.

two general frequency regions. In this animal, we see—especially at the midfrequencies but, in general, also at low frequencies—wide departures between the single-electrode outputs, indicating the intermixing of local and remote responses. The remote response is a mixture of AP and CM generated in distant cochlear regions. Above 2000 Hz, the two single-electrode traces are quite close to one another, indicating that both electrodes pick up approximately the same amount of electricity. It is significant that the differential-electrode trace diverges widely from the two single-electrode curves. The reason for this discrepancy between single and differential third-turn recording is simple. At frequencies above approximately 1000 Hz, an ever-increasing proportion of the response that is picked up by either electrode is remotely generated CM. The fraction of the remote response that is seen by both electrodes at the same relative phase is rejected in the differential amplification process. Whatever fraction is not in the same phase (and also all local response) continues to be amplified. One can estimate the relative contributions to the potential recorded by a single electrode in the third turn of local and remote out-of-phase responses on the one hand, and remote in-phase responses on the other hand. At 3000 Hz, for example, the differential-electrode response is 20 dB smaller than either of the single-electrode responses. If we assume that the activity reflected in the differential recording is of local origin, then clearly about 90 % of the potential picked up by a single electrode does not appear to originate in the immediate vicinity of that electrode. This fraction increases to approximately 99 % at 10,000 Hz. It should be pointed out that the rate of high-frequency cutoff with the differential-electrode recording is of the order of 100 dB/decade. The corresponding rate with single electrodes is approximately 45 dB/decade. The single-electrode technique is clearly much less selective, and probably much less reflective of the true vibratory pattern of the cochlear partition in its vicinity, than the differential-electrode method.

c. Performance Criteria. We should now consider methods for evaluating the adequacy of a pair of differential electrodes after these electrodes have been placed. The need for some objective criterion is very real; this becomes clear when one considers the difficulties attendant on placing pairs of electrodes in, especially, the higher cochlear turns. Interestingly, this problem has not received much attention in the literature. Tasaki *et al.* (1952) give the theory of use of differential electrodes but do not discuss how a given placement might be evaluated. Tonndorf (1958b) briefly states that "faulty electrode positioning was assumed whenever the responses from two electrodes of a pair (single electrode versus neck) were unequal or were not in exact phase opposition." Teas *et al.* (1962) rely on accumulated experience for adjusting the balancing circuit that follows their differential electrodes to optimize their recording. They use a standard 7000-Hz tone pip, and, since the AP and CM in response to this pip are quite different, they do not have great difficulty in balancing out either undesired potential. Presumably this method is used with their basal-turn electrodes. There is no indication of the method used in checking, or balancing, electrodes located in higher turns.

We have found no easy way to solve the problem of checking differential-electrode performance. The method suggested by Tonndorf appears to be attractive, but closer examination reveals that it is inadequate by itself. It is true that ideally positioned differential electrodes should individually pick up the same magnitude and, in opposite phase, the CM, which is generated in the region of their tips. However, AP and possibly remote CM contribute to the electric potential seen by the two electrodes about equally and with about the same phase. Consequently, even though the electrodes might be perfectly placed, the resultant voltages registered by them are by no means equal in magnitude nor 180° apart in phase. Thus this method does not provide an adequate general criterion. However, if the adequacy of first-turn electrodes is to be evaluated, then this method is appropriate, provided that a high-frequency test tone is used. This is because at high frequencies there is no synchronized AP, nor is there significant remote CM. We usually plot complete sets of isopotential curves from all electrodes placed. Characteristic plots of this nature are shown in Figs. 2.9 and 2.10. To evaluate

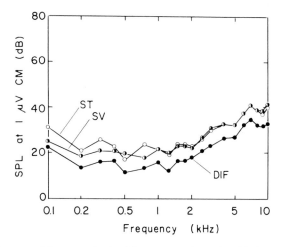

Fig. 2.10. Isopotential curves obtained from one guinea pig with first-turn electrodes. Single scala tympani and vestibuli electrodes, as well as their differential combination, were used.

the basal-turn placement, we use a modified form of the Tonndorf criterion. For a placement to be accepted as good, the two single-electrode plots, above 3000 Hz, should superimpose within 2 dB and should be separated from the differential electrode plot by 6 dB. Of course, this is equivalent to saying that the two electrodes should pick up local CM in opposite phase and with the same magnitude.

To evaluate the placement of third-turn electrodes, we again look at their high-frequency behavior. Here again, the single electrodes should record approximately equal magnitudes of CM above 3000 Hz, but now the differential-electrode curve should depart widely from the individual curves. Separation between these should be of the order of 30 dB or more at 10,000 Hz. Simply comparing the differential-electrode isopotential curves from the first and third turns can also give a fair estimate of the adequacy of the entire preparation (but comparison with single-electrode plots is necessary to determine which placement is faulty in case the total picture is judged inadequate). If one has good electrode positioning, then in the range 500–700 Hz the third-turn electrodes should be about 10–15 dB more sensitive, while at 10,000 Hz the first-turn electrode pair should be superior by at least 40 dB, but preferably 50 dB. The crossover of the two curves is around 1500 Hz. The difference in sensitivity of the third-turn electrode between its best frequency and 10,000 Hz should exceed 60 dB, but 80 dB is preferable. As we have seen, the first-turn response curve is relatively flat. Criteria for the evaluation of second- and fourth-turn electrodes have not been worked out in similar detail, but the same general principles of course apply. It should be mentioned that in our experience it is almost impossible to obtain adequate differential recording from the fourth turn due to the difficulty of placing electrodes in the scala tympani.

The last items that we should consider here in connection with the differential-electrode technique are the effects of electrode imbalance and circuit asymmetries on the obtained potentials and, in addition, the interpretation of the meaning of potentials when imbalances and asymmetries between the recording electrodes exist. First, it is necessary to define our terms and indicate what is meant by electrode imbalance and circuit asymmetry. The first concept simply reflects the adequacy of electrode placement, in that it is assumed that two similar electrodes placed across the cochlear partition in a perfectly symmetrical manner are balanced. Circuit asymmetry means that the electrical paths from sources within the cochlea to the two recording

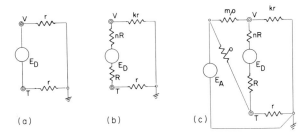

Fig. 2.11. Three electrical equivalent circuits of the cochlear cross section to aid in the discussion of the effects of circuit asymmetries on electrical recording. See text for details. (Modified from Dallos *et al.*, 1972, p. 12.)

electrodes are unequal. The following discussion will clarify and quantify these concepts.

In Fig. 2.11a the simplest possible circuit representation of the differential-electrode scheme is shown. Here we merely assume that there is a single voltage source (E_D) within the organ of Corti, that this source is symmetrical with respect to ground, and that measurements are made in scala vestibuli (V) and in scala tympani (T). One-half of the source voltage drops in this case on the vestibuli-to-ground resistor, and one-half drops on the tympani-to-ground resistor. Thus the voltages measured are $E_V = E_D/2$ and $E_T = -E_D/2$. If the difference and sum of the vestibuli and tympani voltages are formed, we obtain

$$\text{DIF} = E_V - E_T = E_D \quad \text{and} \quad \text{AVE} = \tfrac{1}{2}(E_V + E_T) = 0 \qquad (2.3)$$

Note that here we define the differential component as simply the voltage difference between the two electrodes, while the sum component is taken as the average of the two voltages. This definition conforms to the actual measurements that are performed when either AP or CM are minimized in the usual differential-electrode recording situation. We note that in this vastly oversimplified representation of the cochlear circuit the differential component represents the organ of Corti source (E_D), while the average component is zero. If the resistance paths from the electrodes to the source are unequal, which is analogous with what we called an electrode imbalance, or if the vestibuli-to-ground and tympani-to-ground resistance paths are unequal, then we have a more realistic view of the cochlear circuit. In order to study the effect of such asymmetries on differential-electrode recording, let us expand the circuit diagram of Fig. 2.11a in the form shown in Fig. 2.11b. Here we still have only one source of potentials, E_D, assumed to be within the cochlear partition between the electrodes. The scala vestibuli and tympani recording points, however, have asymmetrical resistance paths to the source and to the common reference. The asymmetry is expressed by the multipliers k and n. In this case the following relationships hold:

$$\text{DIF} = E_V - E_T = \frac{(1+k)rE_D}{(1+k)r + (1+n)R}$$

$$\text{AVE} = (E_V + E_T)/2 = \frac{\tfrac{1}{2}(k-1)rE_D}{(1+k)r + (1+n)R} \qquad (2.4)$$

It is quite clear that unless $k = 1$ both the AVE and DIF components are influenced by the source. When $k = 1$ the AVE component vanishes. The greater k becomes, the more the AVE component approaches the magnitude of the DIF component. It is interesting that the asymmetry of the resistance path between the source and the nodes does not influence the DIF and AVE components in a selective manner.

A more general, although still quite simplified, picture of the recording situation of interest can be studied with the aid of the circuit diagram shown in Fig. 2.11c. This diagram is a refinement of Fig. 2.11b. In it we assume the presence of two sources. One (E_D) is a source within the organ of Corti between the electrode tips, and the other (E_A) is a remote, possibly extra-partition source. The two nodes, V and T, represent the points of measurement in scala vestibuli and tympani. It is simply assumed that the resistance paths from the nodes to the sources and to the reference point are unequal. The resistance differences are symbolized by the multipliers k, m, and n. In the desired optimal case the voltage difference between nodes V and T (DIF $= E_V - E_T$) would reflect E_D only, while the sum of these voltages [AVE $= (E_V + E_T)/2$] would reflect E_A only. It is a relatively straightforward matter to show that such conditions arise only if $k = m = n = 1$. Whenever there are asymmetries in the resistance paths, both E_D and E_A contribute to both the DIF and AVE measurements. The analysis of this circuit is straightforward. The solutions for DIF and AVE voltages are given as follows:

$$\text{DIF} = \frac{rE_D}{D} \left[k(m+1)r\rho + (k+1)m\rho^2 \right] + \frac{rE_A}{D} \left[(n+1)(k-m)\rho R \right]$$

$$\text{AVE} = \frac{rE_D}{2D} \left[(k-1)m\rho^2 + k(m-1)r\rho \right]$$

$$+ \frac{rE_A}{2D} \left[k(n+1)(r+\rho)R + k(m+1)r\rho \right] \quad (2.5)$$

where

$$D = r[(m+1)kr\rho + (k+1)m\rho^2] + R(n+1)[kr + (r+\rho)m\rho] \quad (2.6)$$

There are a few obvious relationships between DIF, AVE, E_D, and E_A that one can see by inspecting these formulas. In the case when $k = m$ the DIF potential does not depend on E_A, but is completely determined by E_D. When $R = 0$, the DIF potential is of course identical to E_D. In order for the AVE potential to be independent of E_D, it is necessary that both k and m be equal to unity. Since we would like to construe the DIF component as being primarily reflective of the source E_D, and conversely the AVE component as representative of E_A, it would be desirable to know how good such representations are. Error coefficients can be expressed in the following manner:

$$e_{\text{DIF}} = \frac{E_D - \text{DIF}}{E_D} = 1 - \frac{\text{DIF}}{E_D} \quad \text{and} \quad e_{\text{AVE}} = \frac{E_A - \text{AVE}}{E_A} = 1 - \frac{\text{AVE}}{E_A} \quad (2.7)$$

One can substitute the expressions for DIF and AVE that were obtained above, and after that formulas for the error coefficients are obtained in the following form:

$$e_{DIF} = A + B\,\frac{E_A}{E_D} \quad \text{and} \quad e_{AVE} = F\,\frac{E_D}{E_A} + G \qquad (2.8)$$

In these formulas A, B, F, and G are all functions of r, R, ρ, and k, m, n. Notice that in the case when, for example, $E_A = 0$ the error in the DIF component is constant and it is determined by the asymmetry of the circuit. If however, E_A is not zero then in addition to the constant error we have an error component that increases with E_A/E_D. This means that the error in the DIF component increases without bound when E_A becomes much larger than E_D. The converse is of course also true; the error in the AVE measurement becomes larger and larger as the output of the E_D source exceeds that of the E_A source. These relationships can be expressed by saying that the most accurate measurement of the DIF component can be obtained in situations when E_A is small compared with E_D. In the recording situation when E_D is small in comparison with E_A, the DIF component is likely to severely misrepresent the former source. The converse is true for the relation between AVE and E_A. It should be mentioned that the influences of extrapartition sources on the DIF, and of local sources within the partition on the AVE component that result from the various asymmetries of the circuit, are not particularly troublesome when the only purpose of the differential-electrode recording is to separate CM from onset AP. These two electrical signals are so different in their waveforms that contamination of one by the other can usually be recognized with relative ease. Problems could arise from the circuit asymmetries if one wished to separate local and remote CM components or SP components that arise from differing sources. In these cases the waveforms are not different and they do not help in distinguishing a legitimate response from a contaminant. In these situations it is important to make judicious use of the estimated error in order to assess the validity of the recording.

2. Microelectrodes

While probably the preponderance of electrical data obtained from the cochlea were collected with gross electrodes, certain tasks call for the use of finer recording tools. Such applications are the measurement of intracochlear dc potentials, the search for generator potentials, and any attempt to record potentials from the scala media. Let us first discuss some of the requirements placed on electrodes that have to perform the above-listed tasks. Direct-current potentials in the cochlea are usually measured by introducing fine electrodes through the round-window membrane and advancing them to the desired region. Clearly the electrode must be of small diameter so that damage to and interference with the motion of the round window be kept at a minimum. Since these electrodes are usually thrust through the basilar membrane also, the matter of size is even more critical. As we shall discuss in detail, in order to measure dc potentials the experimenter must use fluid-filled micropipettes. Metal electrodes do not give reliable dc recording. Thus the most common form of microelectrode used for intracochlear recording is a glass pipette drawn to a fine tip and filled with an appropriate electrolyte into which the actual electrode wire (usually Ag–AgCl) is introduced. This type of electrode is also used whenever potentials are to be recorded from the scala media. There the approach is to drill through the cochlear bone without damaging the stria vascularis and then to introduce the microelectrode through the stria. The electrode size is quite critical, for the vascular stria is extremely sensitive, and the smaller the diameter of the object forced through it the less damage it is likely to sustain.

Finally, any attempt to discern the enigmatic generator processes in the cochlea, i.e., recordings from hair cells, dendrites, or the axon initial segments, necessitates the use of hyperfine electrodes. Recording of these generator events might require the use of both fluid and metal microelectrodes, the former to record from cell bodies and the latter to record from axonal processes.

There are two classes of microelectrodes: fluid-filled pipettes and metal electrodes. Both types possess advantages as well as limitations. No electrode is usable in all situations; that is, *there is no universal electrode.* In very simple terms the metal microelectrode can be considered as a highpass filter. As such it is completely useless for the measurement of dc potentials and membrane processes, but it is quite excellent when one is interested in propagated signals or in extracellular events in general. In contrast the fluid-filled probe is essentially a low-pass filter. Thus it is best suited to measuring dc or slow potentials, but it is inferior in picking up rapid extracellular voltages (Gesteland *et al.*, 1959). We shall now discuss the features of both types of electrode in some detail.

*a. Metal Microelectrodes.** Body tissues from which electrical activity is recorded should be considered to form electrolytes in which ions of various concentration are present. The operation of the electrode depends on the properties of the metal–electrolyte (electrode–body fluid) junction. Theoretical treatment of the electrochemistry of even the simplest metal–electrolyte interface is quite difficult. When organic molecules are present in the solution around the electrode, such theoretical treatment becomes extremely involved

* These discussions follow Frank and Becker (1964).

if not impossible with present-day techniques. For our purposes a very simple consideration of some common metal–electrolyte junctions will suffice.

When an electrode is used to pick up potentials from a fluid medium, electrical charges are transported from the metal to the electrolyte or vice versa. At the interface an electrochemical reaction takes place which is manifested by the liberation of certain chemicals and the depletion of others in the junction region. Because of this chemical change a potential difference builds up across the metal–electrolyte interface. Such a potential difference opposes the free flow of charges between electrode and electrolyte and thus effectively increases the electrode resistance. The process of this potential buildup is called electrode polarization. In a completely polarized (or nonreversible) electrode the separation of charges creates an electrical double layer around the electrode which acts as a capacitor in blocking the passage of ions. Such an electrode cannot pass dc current, but just as a capacitor it is capable of conducting ac current.

In contrast with the polarized electrode is the reversible type, which allows ions to move freely from and into the solution surrounding it. Such a nonpolarizable metal electrode is capable of sustaining dc current. However, as the size of the electrode tip decreases the degree of reversibility also decreases, directly dependent on current density and frequency.

Practical electrodes are always a mixture of ideal reversible and nonreversible types. Consequently *no metal electrode with very fine tip diameter is capable of reliably measuring dc potentials.* Metal electrodes, however, are extremely useful for picking up rapid potential changes. This is because the electrode resistance decreases with increasing frequency. The rate of resistance decrease with frequency depends on both the electrode material and the chemical composition of the fluid.

b. Fluid Microelectrodes. The major problems of recording with metal microelectrodes stem from the minute contact area of the metal–liquid junction. The primary consequence of the small area is large current density at the junction during recording. This can be overcome by artificially increasing the area between metal and fluid by using a glass pipette filled with electrolyte to serve as a bridge between biological tissue and metal electrode. The fine tip of the pipette is inserted into the tissue from which the recording is to be made and the electrode wire is inserted into the large end of the pipette where it makes contact with the electrolyte over a large surface area. Glass pipettes are made by pulling out heated glass tubes, first gently, but after the glass softens, rapidly. At the end of the pull, the glass necks down to a fine diameter tip and separates. Tip diameters of between 0.2 and 1.0 μ can be pulled consistently with commercially available micropipette pullers. After the pulling, the pipette is filled with a suitable electrolyte, usually KCl solution. The advantage of using KCl is that the mobilities of the K^+ ions with outward current and of the Cl^- ions with inward current are very similar, which has the desirable consequence that the liquid junction potential is quite small, of the order of 4 mV between the 3 M KCl electrode and axoplasm (Cole and Moore, 1960).

The contact between the fluid bridge in the pipette and the electronic recording apparatus is usually made by immersing an Ag–AgCl wire in the electrolyte. Since the silver–silver chloride electrode is not in contact with biological fluid and since, due to the large contact area, the current density is very small, this electrode is reversible. Thus the fluid-filled pipette with the Ag–AgCl electrode is dc stable and consequently it is usable for the measurement of membrane potentials and other dc phenomena.

Fluid-filled pipettes possess a complex electrical impedance. This impedance can be expressed as the parallel combination of a large resistance and small capacitance. The resistance is concentrated at the tip and depending on the tip diameter can vary from a few megohms to several hundred megohms. The shunt capacitance is the resultant of distributed capacitance along the fluid-immersed shank of the electrode. If one is recording highly localized electrical events from regions near the electrode tip, then the shunt capacitance can be combined with the capacitance of the connecting wire to ground. Under these conditions the equivalent circuit shown in Fig. 2.12a represents

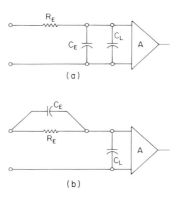

Fig. 2.12. (a) Equivalent circuit of a fluid microelectrode. (b) Equivalent circuit of a fluid microelectrode deep in tissue.

the recording situation. Here R_E is the electrode resistance, C_E is the electrode capacitance, C_L is the lead capacitance, and A is the amplifier. It is clear that the $C = C_E + C_L$ capacitance has the effect of shunting high-frequency components to ground. With a modest electrode resistance of 10 MΩ and a shunt capacitance of 10 pF, signal components above 1600 Hz are severely deteriorated. Methods for counteracting the shunt capacitance will be discussed in the next section.

If the potentials recorded with the pipette are not concentrated at the tip, but present in the fluid surrounding the pipette, then the capacitance C_E is effectively across the resistance R_E and the equivalent circuit in Fig. 2.12b applies. The result of the distributed capacitance C_E is an apparent improvement in high-frequency response, for rapid changes in potential that are present in the fluid can be transmitted through C_E, while similar changes that are concentrated at the tip are attenuated by R_E. This type of recording situation would apply, for example, if an experimenter were attempting to record from the organ of Corti. High-frequency CM potentials would be transmitted through C_E to the recording electronics even though they might not have been present at the electrode tip. Thus the investigator could draw incorrect conclusions about the electrical activity in the region where the pipette tip is situated, especially at high frequencies. For example, if $R_E = 75$ MΩ and $C_E = 10$ pF then the shunt reactance of the distributed capacitance would drop to a value that is one-tenth of the tip resistance at a frequency as low as 2100 Hz.

B. MEASURING INSTRUMENTS

1. *Preamplifiers*

The success of measuring electrical events from living tissue depends not only on the appropriate choice of recording electrode but equally well on the proper processing of the electrical information gathered by the electrode. The most important link between electrode and the recording apparatus is the preamplifier. Most electronic instruments used in data evaluation or storage cannot operate satisfactorily if the signal input is excessively small. Most cochlear potentials are in the microvolt range and they must be boosted before processing. To provide the initial boost in voltage level the pickup electrode is connected to a preamplifier. When gross electrodes are used, the properties of the preamplifier are not too critical. For CM recording, any low-level ac amplifier providing a gain of about 60 dB and having a moderately low noise figure (less than 10–15 μV rms referred to the input) will suffice. It is considered imperative that the experimenter use a differential amplifier whether he picks up his signals with single or with differential electrodes. As is well known a differential amplifier accepts two signal inputs (e_1 and e_2) and amplifies the difference of these voltages,

$$e_{\text{out}} = A(e_1 - e_2) \tag{2.9}$$

If both e_1 and e_2 contain a common component, that is, if

$$e_1 = e_n + e_1' \qquad e_2 = e_n + e_2' \qquad (2.10)$$

then

$$e_{out} = A(e_1' - e_2') \qquad (2.11)$$

Now if differential-electrode technique is used then the outputs of the two electrodes are led to the two inputs of the differential amplifier. In this case the common component is AP and remote CM, plus whatever interference the electrodes pick up from the environment. All these extraneous signals are rejected by the differential preamplifier, and only the proximal CM component is amplified.

If single-electrode technique is utilized in recording cochlear potentials, the differential amplifier is still a must. In this case the electrode is connected to one of the amplifier inputs, while the other input is connected to some indifferent tissue of the animal. Whatever electrical interference the active electrode might pick up the other indifferent electrode is just as likely to be exposed to. Thus this interference is rejected by the differential amplifier and the signal-to-noise ratio of the recording process is greatly enhanced.

The desired frequency response of the preamplifier depends a great deal on which animal species are studied. In recording CM from the most common laboratory animals used in hearing research, guinea pig and cat, a range from 0.1 Hz to 40 kHz is quite sufficient. Most often the lower frequency limit is artificially truncated to obtain stable base lines for recording and to reduce 60-Hz interference. The above recommended lower limit (0.1 Hz) is useful when one wishes to record SP as well as CM in response to tone pips. If the low-frequency cutoff point is higher, then the shape of the SP response becomes unduly distorted due to the high-pass filtering action of the amplifier.

The requirements placed on the preamplifier (or head stage) are more severe if microelectrodes are used for recording electrical events. Under these circumstances the main function of the head-stage is not amplification but instead the matching of the electrode to the rest of the instrumentation. This matching has different aspects depending on whether fluid electrodes or metal electrodes are used.

When fluid-filled pipettes are used the experimenter is confronted with two major difficulties. First, fine micropipettes can have tip resistances in excess of 100 MΩ. Clearly whatever amplifier follows the electrode, it must possess an input impedance that is much greater than the electrode impedance. If this condition were not fulfilled, the amplifier would load down the source (the electrode) and a completely false voltage recording would obtain. Thus the first criterion for a good preamplifier to be used with fluid electrodes is that it must have extremely high input impedance. Commercially available units have input resistances of the order of 10^{11}–10^{12} Ω These amplifiers are usually built with input stages containing either an electrometer tube or a field-effect transistor. Both of these devices are distinguished by their high input resistance.

The second difficulty is that with such high input resistance, the stray capacitance (C_L) existing between the electrode lead and ground forms an extremely effective low-pass filter. Any high-frequency component that might be picked up by the electrode is lost if somehow the stray capacitance is not counteracted. The method most commonly used to cancel the stray capacitance utilizes positive feedback around the amplifier (Amatniak, 1958). Through the positive feedback process an effectively "negative capacitance" appears across the amplifier input. If carefully adjusted this negative capacitance equals the stray capacitance and thus cancels it. While negative capacitance input amplifiers have greatly improved frequency characteristics, the method is inherently noisy. As a consequence very small signals cannot as a rule be recorded successfully with a fluid electrode and its complement the negative capacitance amplifier.

Finally, going hand in hand with the requirement of high input impedance, the amplifier used in conjunction with fluid electrodes must have extremely low input current. This is required because any steady current flowing through the liquid electrode junction would create a junction potential that would yield false readings of dc potentials. In addition, it is undesirable to allow dc current to flow into the biological tissue because of its potentially damaging or polarizing effects on cells.

The requirements placed on a head stage that is to be used with metal microelectrodes are quite different. The most distinguishing feature of the metal microelectrode is its low noise figure, and it is important that the head stage does not impair this feature. Thus the most important requirement is that the preamplifier be a low-noise device. This is accomplished by using cathode or source followers having high transconductance. The input is connected to the electrode through a coupling capacitor to prevent any dc current from flowing through the electrode and thus polarizing it.

2. Signal Analyzers

Modern electronics has provided the physiological investigator with a fantastic array of instruments. Imaginative use of these tools can open up hitherto unavailable avenues of processing bioelectric information. Most conventionally used instruments such as the oscilloscope, oscillograph, vacuum tube voltmeter (VTVM), and electronic wave analyzer are so well known that there is no need for describing their theory of operation here. I would like to confine this section to a few remarks on techniques that have become standard in physiological acoustics, their advantages, and pitfalls.

One of the most fundamental and most often performed measurements is the determination of CM pseudothreshold or isopotential curves. These curves represent the sound pressure levels (SPL) required to produce a given CM level at various frequencies. There are real advantages in setting the criterion level low since, especially at low frequencies, distortion of the CM can occur even at relatively low sound levels, and it is not desirable to measure isopotential curves in the nonlinear region of the CM input–output function. The lowest usable criterion CM level is determined largely by the instrument that is used to measure it. If conventional low-level preamplifiers are used to boost CM, then it is likely that the output noise level of these amplifiers is not better than 10–20 mV peak-to-peak signal if the amplifier gain is 1000 fold. Wide frequency band VTVM's and oscilloscopes respond to all frequency components present in the signal. Thus if an oscilloscope is used, it is unlikely that the criterion level can be set any lower than $10\mu V$ peak-to-peak. With a VTVM the corresponding limit is poorer, for the eye can recognize the presence of sinusoidal pattern in an oscilloscope trace, but the signal-to-noise ratio has to be quite good if a positive identification of the signal is to be made on the basis of a meter deflection. It is unlikely that the criterion level can be set any lower than $10\mu V$ rms if the measuring instrument is a VTVM. Isopotential curves at much lower levels can be obtained with narrow-band wave analyzers. Since these instruments are activated by voltages in only a limited frequency band, their limit of operation is set by the noise components in that band. It is a relatively easy task to measure CM voltages down to approximately 0.1–$0.5 \mu V$ rms (with 1000-fold preamplification) with wave analyzers.

If feasible, a wave analyzer should always be used for the measurement of CM input–output functions. The advantages of the wave analyzer over the VTVM or the oscilloscope are twofold in this application. First, because of the reduced noise interference, the dynamic range of the wave analyzer is greater; hence the input–output function can be measured over a wider range of intensities. Second, since the wave analyzer is tuned to the fundamental microphonic frequency, at high levels where nonlinear distortion introduces harmonic components into the CM, the measurement is not contaminated by the harmonics but is confined to the fundamental. The VTVM would in this case measure the total electrical activity, fundamental and harmonics combined.

Another instrument, less widely known, which can provide the same advantages as the wave analyzer is the phase-sensitive demodulator, or lock-in amplifier. This instrument can also perform some tasks that would overtax the wave analyzer's capabilities. The phase-sensitive demodulator is essentially a voltmeter which is, however, sensitive to the relative phase of the signal that it measures. The reading of the phase-sensitive demodulator

is marginal even though the number of samples averaged was quadrupled. One can clearly find an optimum for adequate improvement of signal with minimum number of averaging cycles.

The mechanics of operation is quite straightforward. Signals are presented repetitively, and with every presentation the computer is instructed to store in its memory the voltage values that correspond to the response. As we see in Fig. 2.13 the first such stored response is the instantaneous value of both true response and noise. After the addition of another response the signal doubles in size but the noise is randomly modified. After several presentations the signal has grown in proportion to the number of samples averaged, but the noise tends to cancel. Actually all operations are performed at discrete points in time following the initiation of the averaging. The total duration of the averaging operation is divided into many equal intervals, each interval being monitored by one specific memory location. Thus the information contained in any given memory location of the computer describes the sum of a series of voltage readings taken always at the same instant after the delivery of the stimulus or, more precisely, after the "triggering" of the computing cycle. The information in any memory location is stored in digital form, that is, as a number and not as an actual voltage level. The process of converting voltages to corresponding numbers is called analog-to-digital (A–D) conversion. During averaging the computer progresses from one memory location to another and adds the current voltage reading to the content of the memory. At the end of the averaging process the content of the memory is "read out," i.e., made available in some form, but again serially: one memory location after the other.

The definition one obtains depends directly on the number of data points (memory locations) that a particular machine uses to delineate the signal in the time dimension. More locations allow for the display of more fine detail in the signal. Of course, more points mean a greater memory and increased cost. The frequency response of the averager depends on the rate at which the machine is capable of sweeping from one memory location to the next. Assume that in order to perform all necessary computations the machine must dwell at each memory location for at least 100 μseconds. Since theoretically a sine wave can be described by two values per one period, the highest frequency that could be processed by our hypothetical averager would be 5000 Hz. In practice one wants to have at least 10 samples per period; thus this machine would produce fair-quality averaging if the highest-frequency components in the signal did not exceed 1000 Hz.

Some practical applications of averagers in the study of cochlear potentials are the recording of responses (CM, SP, and AP) to very low level stimuli. Figure 2.14 shows the oscilloscope trace of a round-window-recorded potential. Clearly no distinct feature is detectable above the basic noise

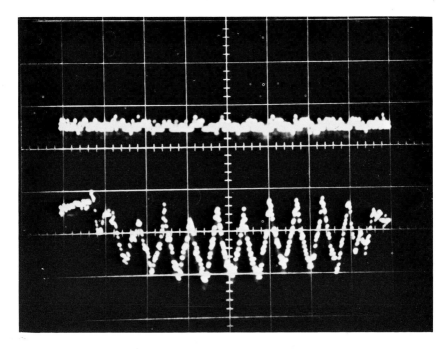

Fig. 2.14. Appearance on the oscilloscope screen of a small (1 μV) CM response (upper trace) and the same response averaged over 256 samples. The ability of the averaging process to recover very small signals from noise is clearly demonstrated here.

level. In the same figure the CM and SP responses are also shown after they are "pulled out" of the base-line activity after the averaging of 256 samples. Note that the CM level in this case is 1 μV, completely undetectable with an oscilloscope.

Summating potentials and AP responses at the onset of a tone pip are very easy to average, and one can also obtain these potentials without the CM if so desired. Here the trick is to make sure that the tone stimulus and the pip envelope are not phase locked. This simply means that the consecutive tone pips do not begin at the same phase of the tone. If the initiation of the computing process is locked to the beginning of the pip then the CM response, not being phase locked with the timing of the computer, averages out, leaving those potentials (SP, and AP at the onset) that are related to the envelope of the stimulus. If only the AP is desired, then the same procedure is used but the signal is first high-pass filtered before it is led to the computer. The filtering blocks the low-frequency SP, and the lack of phase locking eliminates the CM. Very clear traces of the onset AP can be obtained with this method. Figure 2.15 shows examples of the situation when the *same* response is avera-

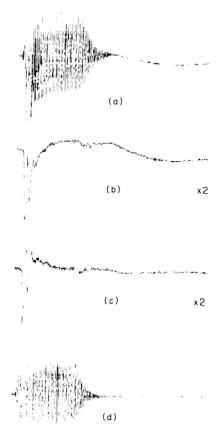

Fig. 2.15. The same biological response to sound, a mixture of CM, SP, and AP, processed three different ways. (a) Computer is phase locked to sinusoidal stimulus; all three response components are preserved. (b) Computer is phase locked to the onset of the sinusoidal burst but not to the carrier frequency itself; AP and SP are preserved, but CM is eliminated. (c) Same processing as in (b), but before computation the signal is high-pass filtered; only the onset AP is preserved. (d) Sound stimulus.

ged three different ways. In (a) the averager is phase locked to the stimulus sine wave; the averaged response contains CM, AP, and SP. In (b) the averager is not synchronized with the stimulus sine wave, only with the onset of the pip. Here the response contains only the onset AP and SP. In (c) the signal is high-pass filtered before averaging and the result is onset AP alone.

Averagers can also be used to eliminate the synchronized whole-nerve AP that rides on every cycle of low-frequency CM responses. The method here is to introduce masking noise into the sound signal, which, if appropriately chosen, is capable of degrading the AP. Since the added masking noise is random, it averages out and quite pure CM response remains. A little additional computation allows one to eliminate the CM in turn and leave only the synchronized low-frequency AP. First, one stores in the computer memory n samples of the response which is obtained without any masking noise. This is the sum of AP and CM. Next, one inverts the phase of the electrical signal led to the computer and on top of the already stored data adds n samples of the signal but with adequate masking. These n samples are pure CM, but they are in phase opposition and thus subtract from the content of the memory. That which remains after processing the $2n$ samples is AP alone. The set of traces shown in Fig. 2.6 was obtained with this method.

III. Recording of Mechanical Motion

From the standpoint of deciphering the mode of operation of the peripheral auditory system, mechanical motion measurements are on a par in importance with measurements of electrical phenomena. The hearing organ is a mechanoreceptor and it possesses a complex mechanohydraulic accessory structure (basilar membrane—organ of Corti) which performs a great deal of signal analysis. Knowledge of the intricate motion patterns of and within the accessory structure is highly desirable, for only armed with such knowledge can we hope to describe the first stages of transduction of information in the auditory sense modality.

Motion patterns of interest are those of the middle ear structures, the cochlear partition as a whole, and various structures within the cochlear partition. The more detailed the information that is desired, the harder the experimental task becomes. Investigation of ossicular motion with present-day techniques is no longer considered a very difficult task. The study of basilar membrane motion is more feasible than it was a decade ago, but it is still extremely challenging. The investigation of the ultimate mechanical motion of the cochlea, hair cell deformation, and ciliary movement is beyond the scope of existing experimental skills. Clearly there is a definite parallel between mechanical and electrical measurements. As we progress from gross movements or potentials to micromovements or generator potentials, the experimental difficulties skyrocket. New techniques are needed and are being developed, especially in mechanical recording. Here the alert experimenter can borrow from other disciplines, such as physics, to supplement his armamentarium. Interestingly, progress in mechanical motion measurement is presently quite rapid. The first noteworthy efforts to duplicate von Békésy's 1949 results on basilar membrane vibratory patterns were not made until 1967. It is certain that further studies will emerge with the adoption of techniques developed by other disciplines.

A. Optical Methods

1. Stroboscopy

One of the simplest, and thus far most productive, methods of measuring small vibratory motion characteristics is the direct observation of the moving structure under a high-power microscope. Actual measurements are made feasible by using stroboscopic illumination (von Békésy, 1953; Guinan and Peake, 1967). The technique is as follows. The experimenter selects a small but prominent feature on the structure to be studied or, and this is a better method, creates one by placing small highly reflective specks of material (silver particles, for example) on the vibrating object. These features are viewed through a microscope and their motion, which faithfully follows that of the object, can be measured.

The heart of the measuring scheme is the stroboscope, a device that provides sharp light flashes at preselected rates. The stroboscope is synchronized with the signal that is used to set the object under study in vibration. One version of the general instrumentation scheme is shown in Fig. 2.16.

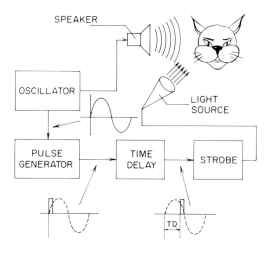

Fig. 2.16. Block diagram of stroboscopic measurement of movement.

The audiooscillator provides the acoustic stimulus and also drives a pulse generator. The output of the pulse generator is fed through a variable time delay unit, which in turn provides the stroboscope triggering signal. The strobe light is triggered once per cycle. As the duration of the light flash is extremely short, the vibrating object is illuminated for a very brief time only, once every cycle. The point in time at which this illumination occurs is controlled by the time delay imposed on the triggering pulse. If one views the vibrating structure, one sees a bright point corresponding to the reference particle, which is illuminated always at the same time instant and hence appears stationary. If the instant of illumination is changed with the aid of the time delay unit then the bright spot moves to any preselected point on the excursion path. Clearly there are two points that correspond to maximal excursion; the distance between them is equal to the peak-to-peak amplitude of the motion of the object. If the microscope is equipped with a calibrated scale, the vibratory amplitude can be measured.

With an ordinary operating microscope (magnification ×40) the motion of the ossicles can just be detected when the sound pressure is over 130 dB and the frequency is less than 5000 Hz. If the total microscope magnification is about 140-fold, and very small (2–3 μ) silver particles are used, then the accuracy of measurements can be as good as a fraction of a micron. With this magnification the apparent vibratory amplitude of the basilar membrane is about 1 mm if the low-frequency sound stimulus is at 140 dB SPL. Since this is about the upper physiological limit, measurements should be made below this intensity. At the "safe" intensity of 120 dB, the apparent size of stapes movement is 0.8 mm, while that of basilar membrane movement is 0.1 mm. These figures apply to stimulating frequencies below 1000 Hz. Clearly the measurement of visual distances as small as these is extremely tiring and time-consuming. Guinan and Peake (1967) reported that to obtain stapes displacement and phase functions over the audio range took them up to 36 hours of experimental time.

Aside from measuring motions of various middle ear elements and the gross movements of the cochlear partition, von Békésy (1953) also made qualitative observations on the fine motion pattern of several structures of the organ of Corti. Such observations constitute the limit of utility of the optical method.

Two special variants of the optical method should also be mentioned. Both of these methods are "optical" in the sense that they utilize light beams reflected from the moving object for measuring displacement. Neither method, however, requires the human eye as the detector of motion. This would appear as a distinct advantage, but it should be noted that man's sensory capabilities in "pulling out" meaningful patterns from background interference are often superior to the best of our electronic instrumentation.

2. *"Photonic Sensor"*

One of these methods (Jako *et al.*, 1967) utilizes two very fine fiber optics bundles, one to shine light on the vibrating structure, the other to pick up the reflected light. As the object moves toward and away from the probe bundle the amount of light flux changes, and these changes in light can be detected with a photocell or photomultiplier. The inverted-V-shaped operating characteristics of the bifurcated fiber bundle indicate that there are two operating regions, one with high gain, the other with relatively low gain. Because of the extreme proximity between object and probe which is required to operate on the high-gain slope, the feasibility of such operation is not good, particularly in moist preparations. Working on the low-sensitivity slope and using a photomultiplier pickup combined with phase-sensitive demodulation techniques, I could detect round-window movements at 60 dB SPL at low frequencies.

3. Laser Interferometry

Interferometric techniques, utilizing both light and sound, are among the oldest methods in physicists' armamentaria for the accurate measurement of length, vibratory amplitude, or some physical properties of gases and liquids. The essence of the method is that two wavefronts, a reference wave and an object wave, are made to interact or interfere with one another. Depending on the phase difference between the two waves, a variable wave amplitude is produced at the plane of measurement, and this resulting amplitude reflects the relative position or movement of the sources of the interfering waves. The scheme of operation of an optical interferometer can be understood with the aid of Fig. 2.17. From the light source a focused

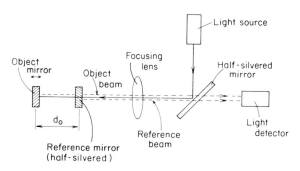

Fig. 2.17. Scheme of laser interferometry.

light beam passes through the reference mirror on to the object mirror. A portion of the beam is reflected from the reference mirror to the light detector, as is the beam from the object mirror. The two light beams interact at the detector surface, and depending on their relative phase they can either reinforce or cancel one another. If the object mirror is attached to a vibrating structure, the successive reinforcements and cancellations are in harmony with the structure's vibratory pattern. The path difference between the reference beam and the object beam is twice the distance between the two mirrors; this distance is denoted as θ. Then θ can be expressed as a multiple of the wavelength of the light (λ) or as an angle,

$$\theta = 2d_0 = 4\pi d_0/\lambda \quad \text{(radians)} \tag{2.13}$$

Since the resultant amplitude at the face of the detector is the vectorial sum of the two incoming waves, that is,

$$A^2 = A_1^2 + A_2^2 + 2A_1A_2 \cos \theta \tag{2.14}$$

the intensity of the resultant at the face of the detector can be written in terms of the intensities of the incoming waves as

$$I = I_1 + I_2 + 2(I_1 I_2)^{1/2} \cos \theta \tag{2.15}$$

Note that the detector output will contain a constant and a variable term; thus it can be written as

$$I = A + B \cos \theta \tag{2.16}$$

Assume now that the object mirror vibrates and that its amplitude function is $F(t)$. Then $\theta = (4\pi/\lambda)[d_0 + F(t)]$, and $I = A + B \cos[4\pi d_0/\lambda + 4\pi F(t)/\lambda]$. This expression can be rewritten as follows:

$$I = A + B[\cos 4\pi d_0/\lambda \cos 4\pi F(t)/\lambda - \sin 4\pi d_0/\lambda \sin 4\pi F(t)/\lambda] \tag{2.17}$$

If the resting distance d_0 is originally adjusted so that $d_0 = (2n+1)\lambda/8$, with $n = 1, 2, 3$, then the last expression is greatly simplified and appears as

$$I = A + B \sin 4\pi F(t)/\lambda \tag{2.18}$$

For very small displacements the above expression is further simplified and it yields

$$I = A + B[4\pi F(t)/\lambda] \tag{2.19}$$

Clearly the output of the interferometer is equal to a constant plus a term that is proportional to the displacement of the object mirror. It is also clear that the actual time function of the displacement, $F(t)$, is present in the detector output in an undistorted form. When the displacement of the object is sinusoidal then the detector output is expressed as a Bessel series of the amplitude of the object. In this most important case, at low vibratory amplitudes the detector output is linearly related to the displacement magnitude of the object. As amplitude increases an output peak is reached, beyond which there is a whole series of valleys and secondary peaks. It is obvious that measurements must be confined to the initial linear segment of the function. The positions of the various maxima and minima are directly determined by the wavelength of the light that is used in the interferometer. For any wavelength the extent of the linear region can be readily calculated. For a helium–neon laser that has been used by Khanna *et al.* (1968b) the wavelength is 6.328×10^{-5} cm, the first maximum corresponds to a peak vibratory amplitude of 0.92×10^{-5} cm, and the linear range extends to approximately 10^{-6} cm amplitude. The method is insensitive to the frequency of the vibration of the object.

The utilization of coherent laser light in the interferometer permits its operation at a sensitivity that is considerably superior to that of devices using incoherent light. A laser interferometer operated together with narrowband filters has such favorable signal-to-noise properties that vibratory amplitudes of the order of 3×10^{-10} cm can be detected with it. Consequently the device possesses a dynamic range of approximately 90 dB.

Khanna *et al.* (1968b) could routinely measure tympanic membrane vibrations in living cats of the order of 10^{-5} cm amplitude. The repeatability of the measurements was approximately 1 dB in amplitude and 5° in phase. Apparently this is a very sensitive and promising method for measuring the vibratory patterns of middle ear and inner ear structures. Severe problems still exist in utilizing the method to its fullest potential, however. These problems are primarily connected with the extreme sensitivity of the device; extraneous vibrations, movement connected with respiration, etc., can play havoc with quantitative studies. Another problem concerns the preparation of adequate mirrors that are to be placed on the vibrating object. The mirrors have to be flat, of good optical quality, and yet light enough not to interfere with the object's motion. Khanna *et al.* utilize mica split into small strips. Their mirrors are about 0.1 mm^2 in area and weigh less than 1 μg. Thus far successful measurements have been confined to the delineation of the vibratory pattern of various middle ear structures (Tonndorf and Khanna, 1968b).

B. CAPACITIVE PROBES

If a small metal plate is brought in the proximity of a vibrating object, the two can be construed as forming a capacitor whose capacitance changes with the varying distance between them. It is a fairly straightforward task to design electronic circuits that can detect capacitance changes. The most common method (von Békésy, 1941) utilizes the object–probe capacitance in the resonance circuit of a high-frequency oscillator. As the capacitance changes the oscillator frequency changes with it. The frequency-modulated signal can be demodulated with any appropriate discriminator circuit and thus a voltage proportional to the capacitance is obtained. The sensitivity of this probe is of the order of 10^{-6} cm (100 Å). In a similar scheme (Fischler *et al.*, 1964) the vibrating object and the probe form the coupling capacitance between a high-frequency oscillator and amplifier. As the capacitance changes the amplifier input voltage becomes modulated in amplitude. If the system parameters are appropriately chosen then the depth of modulation is linearly related to the vibratory amplitude. The output of the high-frequency amplifier is demodulated, filtered, and recorded. Such a capacitive system is sensitive down to vibratory amplitudes of 30 Å (Rubinstein *et al.*, 1966). Combining the capacitive probe and averaging techniques allowed measurements of vibratory motions of some middle ear structures with a sensitivity of approximately 2 Å (Fischler *et al.*, 1967).

C. THE MÖSSBAUER TECHNIQUE

The Mössbauer technique is ideally suitable for the measurement of velocity. If one is interested in displacement measurement this method is still useful because, during sinusoidal motion, displacement and velocity are very simply related. Velocity is the first derivative of displacement; if the latter is

$$x = x_0 \sin \omega t \qquad (2.20)$$

then the velocity $v = x_0 \omega \cos \omega t$. Thus $|v| = x_0 \omega$ and, conversely, $x_0 = |v|/\omega$. Clearly then, if we can measure velocity, and the frequency $(\omega = 2\pi f)$ is known, it is an easy matter to obtain the amplitude of the motion.

If the nucleus of an atom is excited, it is set in vibration and in consequence it radiates energy in the form of gamma rays. With the emission of these rays the nucleus loses energy and thus the amplitude of vibration decays. The duration of such nuclear vibration is characterized by the "half-life," the time it takes for the radiation energy to decrease by one-half. During radiation the frequency of vibrations is perfectly stable, and thus the vibrating nucleus can be used like a miniature pendulum: the heart of a clock. If in the vicinity of the vibrating nucleus there is a second nucleus, it will begin to vibrate with the same frequency as the first. This is the same phenomenon on an atomic scale as the familiar sympathetic resonance in acoustics. The phenomenon is known as nuclear resonance, and it has been familiar to physicists for quite some time. While the phenomenon is well known, its measurement is beset with one particular difficulty. In order for nuclear resonance (absorption of gamma rays by the nucleus) to take place both the emitting and the absorbing nucleus must have the same oscillation rate within extremely narrow tolerance. Same oscillation rate means that both nuclei should possess the same energy. If during emission and absorption there were no loss of energy then the absorbed photon would set the absorbing nucleus in vibration at the same rate at which the emitting nucleus vibrated. However, during emission the nucleus itself "recoils" (like a gun firing a bullet) and part of the available energy is taken up by the recoil and is not carried away by the gamma ray. Similarly, during absorption the receiving nucleus also recoils, and again part of the energy of the gamma ray is used up in this recoil. As a consequence the energy of the emitter nucleus is quite different from that of the absorber nucleus, which in turn means that their natural frequencies are quite different. This being the case no resonance can be established. Mössbauer circumvented the loss of energy by the clever trick of anchoring the participating nuclei within crystal lattices, thus preventing recoil. This way, the gamma ray carries the total vibratory energy of the emitter and delivers it undiminished to the absorber, thus setting the latter in vibration.

In practice one usually uses the isotope cobalt-57 as the emitter. This isotope has a half-life of 280 days. During its active life the radioactive cobalt decays into iron-57, which is an excited iron isotope. The nuclei of the iron atoms vibrate at a frequency of 3×10^{18} Hz. In resonance measurement a beam of gamma rays emitted by the unstable iron-57 nuclei is aimed at a hunk of stable ^{57}Fe. These nuclei absorb the gamma rays so that, if one places a so-called scintillation counter behind this absorber during resonance, there is a pronounced dip in the counting rate, indicating the absorption of gamma rays.

What makes this technique so powerful, and incidentally of any use to us, is the fact that in order for resonance to take place, as we have already said, the frequencies of the emitting and absorbing nuclei must be practically identical. Now if the emitter moves toward or away from the absorber, a slight but all-important change takes place in the frequency of the gamma rays. This phenomenon, the Doppler effect, is well known in acoustics; it simply means that the apparent frequency of a receding source of sound decreases, while that of an approaching source increases. The Doppler effect, of course, is also observable in optics, where again if the source moves then the light rays emitted by it change their frequency depending on the direction of motion.

Because of the extreme sharpness of nuclear resonance (i.e., the necessity for very limited frequency differences between emitting and absorbing nuclei), incredibly small relative velocities between source and absorber can create enough of a frequency shift to destroy resonance. Thus the velocity of even slow (compared to nuclear speeds) motions can be measured by noting changes in absorption between conditions of rest and motion.

Two laboratories have thus far utilized the Mössbauer technique in auditory research. Johnstone and Boyle (1967) placed a tiny emitter (0.3 μg) of ^{57}Co on the basilar membrane of the basal turn of a guinea pig cochlea; the absorber was a small foil of ^{57}Fe. They used two counters, one to measure absorption rate in quiet and one to measure the rate during sound application. The difference in count rate was calibrated in terms of velocity by simulating the experimental conditions using known vibration velocities. Johnstone and Boyle determined mechanical tuning curves for the basilar membrane with this method for a wide range of frequencies. While the method is extremely promising, it should be kept in mind that its primary limitation is the necessary duration of any measurement. In order to insure sufficient accuracy in counting rate, counting should continue for several minutes for any one data point. Thus it takes several hours to obtain a single tuning curve.

Rhode (1971) measured basilar membrane motion in the cochlea of squirrel monkeys with this technique over a relatively wide frequency range.

IV. Impedance Measurement Techniques

A. ACOUSTIC IMPEDANCE

While not a direct measure of displacement or movement, acoustic impedance can provide extremely valuable information about the properties of vibrating structures, especially the middle ear (Møller, 1965; Mundie, 1963; Zwislocki, 1957). Several acoustic impedance bridges have been constructed (Metz, 1946; Møller, 1960; Zwislocki, 1961; Pinto and Dallos, 1968), most of which could be adapted for work with physiological preparations.

In essence, impedance bridges make use of Ohm's law for acoustical circuits,

$$P = ZU \qquad (2.21)$$

where P is pressure, Z is acoustic impedance, and U is volume velocity of sound. If one has a constant volume velocity source then the measured sound pressure is directly proportional to the acoustic impedance of the medium or enclosure in which the pressure is developed. In practice, the difficulty with such a measuring scheme lies in the construction of an adequate volume velocity source in combination with a pressure transducer that does not load down the impedance to be measured.

Figure 2.18 is a block diagram representing an apparatus used to measure both absolute impedance of the eardrum and changes in impedance about the resting value. Since impedance is a vector quantity, it is necessary that both the real and imaginary parts be measured in both the static and dynamic conditions. In this scheme static impedance is measured by electronically balancing the bridge; dynamic changes are observed by recording the imbalance of the bridge caused by the alteration of the measured impedance. The volume velocity source of the bridge (a sound source in series with a high-resistance coupling tube) is powered by a sinusoidal voltage; thus it generates a pure tone. A high-impedance microphone measures the sound pressure in front of the eardrum. This sound pressure is directly dependent

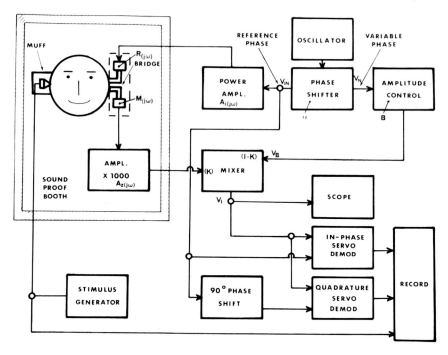

Fig. 2.18. Scheme for the measurement of static and dynamic components of the acoustic resistance and reactance of the ear. (From Pinto and Dallos, 1968, p. 14.)

on the input impedance of the drum membrane, which is of course a function of the state of the middle ear. The sound measured by the microphone is the resultant of the field generated by the source and the field reflected by the eardrum. The latter sound field is determined by the laws pertaining to acoustic reflection at the boundary between two dissimilar media (in this case air and the drum membrane). It is well known [see Eqs. (3.8)–(3.14) for derivation] that the properties of the reflected wave are determined by the ratio of impedances of the two media on either side of the boundary. The more dissimilar these impedances are as sound travels from air to the second medium, the more energy is reflected at the boundary. Thus higher eardrum impedance corresponds to increased sound pressure in front of the drum and vice versa.

The output of the microphone is amplified and mixed with an electrical signal, which is derived from the same oscillator that powers the sound source. This electrical signal can be controlled in amplitude and phase before the mixing takes place. If the system is properly calibrated this electrical signal can be made to represent an electrical analog of the input impedance of the eardrum. In other words, the settings of the amplitude controller and phase shifter can be directly converted to magnitude and phase information pertaining to the measured impedance. Such conversion can be made when the bridge is balanced, i.e., when the magnitude of the analog signal is identical to the microphone output and when these two voltages are in phase opposition. Under such balance condition the null detector instrument reads zero voltage at the mixer output.

Changes from the static impedance can be measured as a function of time, for it can be shown (Pinto and Dallos, 1968) that, after the bridge is balanced, the departure of the mixer output from zero is proportional to the change of impedance since its balance value–vector components (in-phase and quadrature) can be obtained by feeding the mixer output to two phase-sensitive demodulators. The reference signals to these demodulators are obtained from the audio oscillator, which drives the sound source. If the oscillator signal is used directly as the reference, the output of the phase-sensitive demodulator provides the in-phase signal. If the oscillator output is first given a 90° phase shift, the demodulator gives the quadrature component. Both of these components are written out on a paper chart recorder.

An important consideration in this type of measurement, already alluded to, is the matter of insuring that the impedance bridge does not "load down" the impedance to be measured. Assume that P_o is the pressure output of a low-impedance sound source, R_s is the series resistance of its coupling tube, P_M is the sound pressure measured by the microphone whose coupling tube has a resistance of R_P, while the unknown impedance is Z. The value of P_M can be obtained as

$$P_M = Z \frac{P_o R_L}{R_s(R_L + Z)} \quad \text{where} \quad R_L = \frac{R_s R_P}{R_s + R_P} \quad (2.22)$$

Ideal measurement can be obtained if $R_L \to \infty$. Then

$$P_M \text{ (ideal)} \to P_o Z / R_s \quad (2.23)$$

The fractional error due to less than ideal measuring conditions is expressed as

$$e = \frac{P_M \text{ (ideal)} - P_M}{P_M \text{ (ideal)}} = \frac{Z}{R_L + Z} \quad (2.24)$$

The error e approaches zero as the shunting resistance R_L approaches infinity. However, the losses associated with high values of R_L set a practical limit on the reduction of e. The practical value of $R_L = 20 |Z|$ gives a fractional error in measuring Z of about 5% in magnitude and 3° in phase.

B. Electrical Impedance

The measurement of the impedance characteristics of various biological structures is an extremely important tool of contemporary physiological research. This method of investigation has been applied to the study of cochlear function (von Békésy, 1952; Misrahy *et al.*, 1958a; Johnstone *et al.*, 1966; Matsouka *et al.*, 1956) but probably not to the extent that its real potential has been fulfilled. Impedance measurements can be utilized to detect dimensional or conductivity changes of a biological structure. In either case, two electrodes are attached to the structure in such a manner that the biological event that the experimenter desires to detect should take place between the electrodes. The event changes the current density pattern between the electrodes, and the change is detected as an impedance variation from the resting value. Aside from the measurement of impedance changes in order to infer to causal biological events, the measurement of absolute electrical impedance of certain structures can also be of great value. In cochlear research the latter has received most attention: Investigators have been curious to determine the various resistance paths that form the electrical cochlear network.

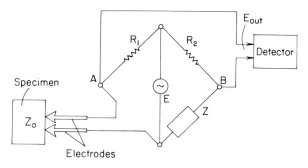

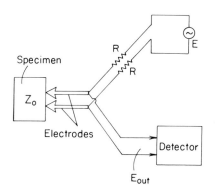

Fig. 2.19. Two types of electrical impedance measurement.

The most common circuits for the measurement of impedance are shown in Fig. 2.19 (Geddes and Baker, 1968). The first circuit is a bridge in which two measuring electrodes are applied to the specimen, which forms one arm of the bridge. Two other arms are fixed (R_1, R_2) while the fourth arm is adjustable (Z). An oscillator supplies the measuring signal (E) and a detector indicates whether the bridge is balanced. It is well known that in the circuit configuration shown in the figure, the bridge is in a so-called balanced condition (there is no potential difference between nodes A and B) when $R_1 Z = R_2 Z_0$. Consequently if the variable impedance is calibrated, the unknown impedance (Z_0) can be obtained by adjusting Z until the detector indicates a null and then reading the value of Z. After the bridge is nulled and the static impedance is obtained, the bridge becomes unbalanced and thus an output voltage is obtained whenever, due to some biological event, Z_0 is altered. Any change in the generally complex Z_0 produces an output voltage, and consequently if it is of interest to determine what fraction of the changes is due to resistive and what fraction to reactive (capacitive) changes in the specimen's impedance, then a phase-sensitive demodulator must be used to resolve the two components.

The second commonly utilized circuit is quite simple. It consists of the source oscillator that delivers the measuring signal to the electrodes through high series resistances (R). The voltage drop across the electrodes is measured with a suitable detector. This voltage drop is equal to $E_{out} = EZ_0/(2R + Z_0)$. A prerequisite for the proper operation of this scheme is that the series resistance R should be much greater than $|Z_0|$. In this case, assuming that $Z_0 = R_0 + jX_0$, we can write

$$\frac{E_{out}}{E} = \frac{Z_0}{2R + Z_0} = \frac{R_0 + jX_0}{2R + R_0 + jX_0}$$

$$= \frac{2R(R_0 + jX_0) + (R_0^2 + X_0^2)}{4R^2 + 4RR_0 + R_0^2 + X_0^2} \simeq \frac{R_0 + jX_0}{2R} + \frac{R_0^2 + X_0^2}{4R^2} \simeq \frac{Z_0}{2R} \quad (2.25)$$

We note that the output voltage is proportional to the impedance to be measured; if this impedance is composed of a static part (Z_0') and a changing part (ΔZ_0) then the output voltage is the sum of a dc component ($Z_0'/2R$) and a changing component ($\Delta Z_0/2R$). The latter can be resolved with the aid of a phase-sensitive demodulator into resistive and reactive portions.

If only resistive changes of the specimen are of interest, the source voltage can be a dc signal; whenever the total impedance or its change is sought, an ac source is the practical choice. Whatever the source, it is imperative to choose the measuring voltage so that its mere presence will not alter the condition of the biological specimen. In other words, one wishes to avoid the use of measuring signals that can produce stimulation or electrolytic effects. In practice this necessitates the use of low current densities and high-frequency signals.

V. Measurement of Sound Pressure

The accurate specification of stimulus quality and strength has always been one of the most difficult, and often most neglected, tasks of the physiological experimenter. Students of the auditory system are fortunate, however, in that they at least have the availability of well-established methods and usually the instrumentation for measuring stimulus parameters. Scientists studying the olfactory system, taste, or simple mechanoreceptors, for example, are not that fortunate. It is regrettable that, in spite of the availability of techniques, stimulus specification in auditory research has often been grossly neglected. It should be emphasized that quite frequently even the most beautiful and significant physiological measurement can prove useless if all that is reported about the stimuli is that they were "loud" or "soft," "low frequency" or "high pitched." In a review on cochlear potentials, Wever (1966) pleads for the adequate specification of the sound stimuli in experiments on auditory physiology. This section is written mainly to underscore his plea. The items that we wish to consider are (a) experiments with open and closed systems, (b) calibration of sound pressure at the eardrum, and (c) some specific problems that arise in studies of aural distortion.

A. CLOSED VERSUS OPEN SYSTEMS

The majority of acute experiments on the auditory system are done with a so-called closed sound system. This means that the sound source is coupled to the ear so that the eardrum, meatus, coupling device, and sound source form a closed cavity. There are as many arrangements as experimenters, but two types of system have emerged as most common. In the first, a high-power acoustic driver is connected to the external meatus with a rubber or plastic hose that terminates in a speculum. The speculum itself can be inserted into either the bony or the cartilaginous meatus, and the pinna can be removed or left intact. These details depend on how much surgery the experimenter wants to do and how exacting his requirements are. In rodents probably the best strategy is to resect the cartilaginous meatus at its insertion and couple the speculum directly to the bony meatus. In cats the bony meatus is so short that this approach does not work; in this animal the meatus is resected about 0.5 cm from its insertion and the speculum is secured in the stump. A somewhat sloppier, but often adequate, coupling can be achieved by introducing the speculum into the intact external meatus. In a truly closed system one would wish to achieve good acoustic seal between the cavity and the surrounding air. This is much easier to do if the speculum is in contact with the bony meatus than when it is just inserted into the intact ear.

The length of the connecting hose is not critical when only low-frequency measurements are made. It should be kept in mind, however, that standing waves will appear in a long tube, and the longer the tube the lower the frequency at which these might become troublesome. It should also be mentioned that the use of long coupling tubes precludes the delivery of sharp, well-defined acoustic transients. Whenever such transients are required the experimenter should place the sound source in the immediate vicinity of the eardrum. The greatest advantage of using acoustic drivers is of course their considerable power handling ability and thus the possibility of generating intense acoustic fields. One additional consideration that might enter into the choice of the length of the connecting tube arises when, in addition to air-conducted tones, bone-conducted stimuli are also utilized in an experiment. It is well known that a closed ear effect operates at low frequencies during the delivery of bone stimulation that is manifested in enhancement of the response at low frequencies (Tonndorf, 1966). The effect can be eliminated if the volume of air enclosing the eardrum is sufficiently large.

Another commonly used method of delivering sound in a closed system is to couple the sound source directly to the meatus, usually with the aid of a rigid speculum assembly. This scheme is most useful when the sound source itself is small; otherwise the assembly becomes unwieldy. Most commonly such a small sound source is a reverse-driven condenser microphone. Whenever very sharp transients, or pure tones considerably above 10 kHz in frequency, are desired, the condenser microphone becomes the most suitable sound source. Its only disadvantages are cost and limited power handling capacity. The basic operation of the condenser microphone as a sound source is also inherently nonlinear. A compensating circuit has been described (Molnar *et al.*, 1968) that can be utilized to linearize the driving system and thus to extend its utility.

No matter what the sound source or the method of coupling to the ear, closed acoustic systems afford much greater ease of calibration than the so-called free-field sound systems. In addition, more acoustic power can be provided by a given source in a closed system than in an open system. Open systems are of course much easier to instrument than closed systems; one needs only to hang a loudspeaker in the vicinity of the animal's head. If this is done in a reverberant environment then of course echoes will arise, making transient measurements rather tenuous. Free-field measurements have their greatest use in behavioral studies. In such cases the animal is placed in an anechoic environment and is usually semirestrained. Clearly, the technical difficulties in using a closed sound system in such a situation would be formidable. Accurate calibration of the sound field at the eardrum of an unrestrained animal is of course an almost impossible task. The usual method is to establish the sound pressure at the entrance of the earcanal and then use appropriate transformations to correct for the effect of the meatus (Wiener *et al.*, 1966). We shall discuss some of these corrections in Chapter 3. When establishing the sound pressure at the entrance of the meatus, one must, for accurate results, take into account the baffle effects of head and body of the animal. In other words, it is not appropriate to measure the sound field in the absence of the animal at the point where the meatus usually is in space and to assume that the measured value will be the same when the animal is in place. Especially at higher frequencies, the differences due to body and head baffle effects can be significant.

B. CALIBRATION OF SOUND PRESSURE*

There are three common methods for establishing sound pressure values during experiments. The first is to measure the sound pressure at the eardrum during each experiment. The second is to measure the sound pressure at the eardrum of a large number of animals of a given species and to use the mean of these measurements in lieu of any further calibration during the experiment. The third method is to measure the sound pressure in a small cavity, the coupler, and use these figures to specify an approximate sound pressure at the animal's eardrum. Let us compare these methods.

The difference in SPL between the conditions when measurements are made at the guinea pig's eardrum and when they are made in a 2-cm^3 coupler, with identical voltages across the speaker at all frequencies and in all conditions, reveals that depending on frequency the two measures can be quite discrepant. At low frequencies, more pressure develops in the coupler than in the earcanal, but the discrepancies are not too great and are relatively constant. In contrast, at higher frequencies the pressure is greater in the earcanal, and the difference is substantial indeed, exceeding 30 dB. These results are quite consistent, and they indicate that the experimenter can severely underestimate the stimulus sound pressure if he relies solely on coupler calibration of his sound system. This contention is also stressed by Laszlo (1968). The reasons for the observed discrepancies are relatively simple. For simplicity, we have used a standard coupler that certainly was not designed to serve as an artificial ear for guinea pigs. Undoubtedly, appropriate couplers could be designed and constructed that would have impedance characteristics similar to that of guinea pig ears (or those of any other experimental animal). If such couplers were available, calibration of experimental apparatus with their aid would yield fairly acceptable results. However it is probably fair to say that in the absence of adequate artificial ears the

---

* Based on Dallos *et al.* (1969b).

experimenter is well advised to use actual animal ears for calibration purposes in place of couplers.

The optimal procedure is to monitor the sound field at the animal's eardrum during every experiment. Only this method can provide the experimenter with adequate accuracy in measurements when exact specification of sound levels is of critical importance. A method that is second best, but usable in less demanding circumstances, is to obtain the average response characteristic of the apparatus on the basis of measurements of sound pressure at the eardrum of a fairly large number of experimental animals. If the experimental apparatus, the preparation of the animals (i.e., bulla open or closed, etc.), and the approximate size of the experimental animals are unchanged in subsequent measurements, then the average sound pressure at any frequency is a fairly accurate indication of the actual pressure level. Our experience is that sound pressures generated by a given apparatus generally do not vary more than about 15 dB from animal to animal. If such a margin of error is tolerable, the experimenter might forego sound calibration during every experiment. Figure 2.20 illustrates the variability of sound

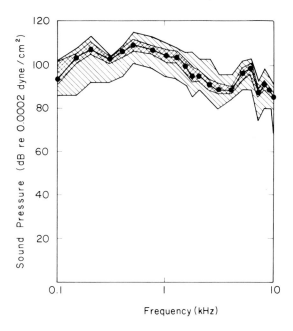

Fig. 2.20. Median, interquartile range, and full range of maximum sound pressure levels produced by a particular experimental setup at the eardrum of guinea pigs. The sound source, the voltage across it, and all experimental procedures are identical in all cases ($N = 40$).

pressure levels at the eardrum in a closed system. The median, interquartile range, and full range of such values across frequency are shown as obtained with a particular experimental setup on a large number of guinea pigs ($N = 40$). The third, and regrettably quite commonly used, method is calibration in a coupler. As we have pointed out above, unless the coupler is specifically designed to mimic the acoustic characteristics of the experimental animal's ear, this method can yield very substantial errors in sound pressure estimation.

It is recommended that probe tube measurement techniques be used as routinely as possible in experiments on auditory physiology. Of course, these measurements are only as good as the calibration of the probe tube itself. The measurement of probe tube characteristics is a relatively straightforward task for frequencies below approximately 8000 Hz. Above that, it becomes more and more difficult to accurately calibrate a probe tube microphone, and probably the results are not reliable enough to justify the efforts.

In analyzing the behavior of a probe tube it should be realized that this device is essentially an acoustic transmission line in which multiple resonances occur but whose overall characteristics are otherwise like that of a low-pass filter. From the theory of transmission lines one can obtain expressions that describe the impedance and transmission properties of the probe tube. The input impedance of the transmission line, Z, can be computed from

$$Z = Z_0 \frac{Z_M + Z_0 \tanh \gamma l}{Z_0 + Z_M \tanh \gamma l} \tag{2.26}$$

In this expression Z_0 is the characteristic impedance of the transmission line, Z_M is the terminating impedance, in our case the acoustic impedance of the microphone, γ is the so-called propagation constant of the line, and l is the length of the line. We can obtain the characteristic impedance by assuming that the acoustic medium enclosed in the tube has a distributed acoustic inertance M per unit length, a distributed acoustic compliance C per unit length, and a distributed acoustic resistance R per unit length, and by also assuming that losses through the walls of the tube are negligible. Then $Z_0 = [(R + j\omega M)/j\omega C]^{1/2}$. Expressions for M, C, and R are as follows:

$$M = \frac{\rho_0}{S} \qquad C = \frac{S}{\rho_0 c^2} \qquad R = \frac{R_0}{S} \tag{2.27}$$

where S is the cross-sectional area of the tube, and R_0 is the viscous resistance of air. Combining the above expressions yields

$$Z_0 = \frac{\rho_0 c}{S} \left(1 - j \frac{R_0}{\rho_0 \omega}\right)^{1/2} \tag{2.28}$$

When R_0 can be neglected, i.e., if the tube is not exceedingly narrow, then the above expression reduces to a real number: $Z_0 = \rho_0 c / S$.

The propagation constant γ is by definition $\gamma = [(R + j\omega M)j\omega C]^{1/2}$. After substituting the appropriate expressions we obtain

$$\gamma = \left(j\omega \frac{R_0}{\rho_0 c^2} - \frac{\omega^2}{c^2} \right)^{1/2} \tag{2.29}$$

It is customary to express γ as a complex number, $\gamma = \alpha + j\beta$, where α is the propagation constant (expressed in nepers per unit length) and β is the phase constant (expressed in radians per unit length). With these designations the mathematical description of the wave traveling in the tube is

$$p = P_1 \exp(-\gamma x) + P_2 \exp(\gamma x) \tag{2.30}$$

One can solve for α and β.

$$\beta^2 = \frac{\omega^2}{2c^2} \pm \frac{\omega^2}{2c^2} \left[1 + \left(\frac{R_0}{\rho_0 \omega} \right)^2 \right]^{1/2} \tag{2.31}$$

and

$$\alpha = \frac{R_0}{2\rho_0 c^2} \frac{1}{\beta} \tag{2.32}$$

If the resistance can be neglected then the attenuation and phase constants assume much simpler forms. Thus $\beta = \omega/c$ (this is of course the wave number, usually designated as k), while $\alpha = 0$. In this case the traveling wave has the particularly simple description

$$p = P_1' \cos kx + P_2' j \sin kx \tag{2.33}$$

A general expression for the pressure transformation in the probe tube can be obtained in the following form:

$$\frac{p_M}{p_{in}} = \frac{1}{\cosh \gamma l + (Z_0/Z_M) \sinh \gamma l} \tag{2.34}$$

In this expression p_M is the pressure at the microphone diaphragm, p_{in} is the pressure to be measured, and l is the length of the tube. This pressure transformation, or probe tube loss as it is generally called, is of course frequency dependent. In principle the probe tube loss could be calculated from this expression; unfortunately, however, this is not an easy task. First, the computation itself is rather tedious and, second, there is some degree of difficulty in accurately specifying Z_M, Z_0, and γ. Probably the most troublesome item is the specification of Z_M. This impedance includes the acoustic impedance of the microphone diaphragm, the small coupling cavity between the diaphragm and the entrance of the probe tube, and whatever leakage resistance might exist due to imperfect seal between the microphone and the tube. None of these factors can be easily computed. Because of these uncertainties, one rarely attempts the exact calculation of probe tube losses; instead these are determined experimentally. Some general conclusions can be drawn from the theory, however, and can help in determining the approximate characteristics of a probe tube.

At very low frequencies the probe tube loss is completely negligible, but above a cutoff or corner frequency the loss gradually accumulates. The rate of accumulation can be approximated with good accuracy as 6 dB/octave. The actual probe tube loss versus frequency function is not a smooth curve. Around the line approximating the 6 dB/octave loss characteristic the function fluctuates due to resonances.

If one assumes that the microphone presents a virtual short circuit to the probe tube, one can predict the approximate frequencies at which resonances in the tube are likely to occur. The argument is as follows. If the resistance is neglected and $Z_M = 0$ is assumed, then the expression for the impedance [Eq. (2.26)] takes the form

$$Z = Z_0 \tanh \gamma l = j Z_0 \tan kl = j \frac{\rho_0 c}{S} \tan \frac{\omega}{c} l \qquad (2.35)$$

Since the open end of tube represents $Z = 0$, we can write

$$\tan \frac{\omega l}{c} = 0 \quad \text{or} \quad \frac{\omega l}{c} = n\pi \qquad (2.36)$$

where n is any integer. Consequently the resonant frequencies of the tube can be written as

$$f_r = nc/2 \qquad (2.37)$$

whereas the resonant wavelengths are

$$\lambda_r = 2l/n \qquad (2.38)$$

The probe tube used most often in our laboratory has a length of 9.0 cm. Consequently we can expect it to have its first few resonances at 1920, 3840, 5760, and 7680 Hz. The expected 0 dB/octave and -6 dB/octave slopes are shown as dashed lines in Fig. 2.21 and the expected resonance frequencies are indicated by arrows. The experimentally obtained calibration curve of this probe tube is also shown in the figure. It is clear that the general character of the frequency-dependent probe tube loss can be deduced from simple theoretical considerations but that the actual curve is quite complex. The resonant peaks can be reduced by packing the tube with damping material.

A few words should be said about the method of calibrating probe tubes.

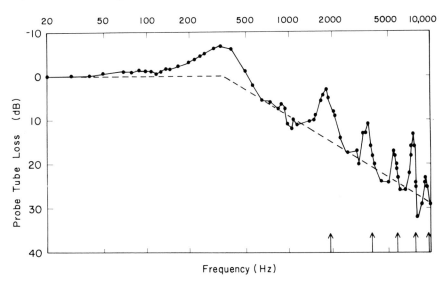

Fig. 2.21. Comparison of computed and measured losses of a particular probe tube. The arrows indicate the computed resonance frequencies.

Such calibrations can be done either with the aid of suitable rigid-walled couplers or in a free field (Benson, 1953). Since the coupler calibration is simpler, only this will be described. The preferred procedure is to have a coupler that is symmetrical about a plane which is perpendicular to the diaphragm of the sound source and which passes through the center of the sound source. The cavity is open on two sides, the openings being parallel with the aforementioned hypothetical plane. In these openings one can insert a microphone or a dummy plug whose dimensions (facing the cavity) are identical to those of the microphone. In Fig. 2.22 an exploded view of the measuring setup is shown. Two measurements are required. First, with a solid dummy plug closing the coupler, the sound field is measured across the frequency range with microphone M_1. Then the solid dummy plug is replaced with one that has a hole in its center through which the probe tube is introduced so that its end is flush with the inner surface of the dummy plug. The probe tube is connected to another microphone, M_2. The relationship between the characteristics of M_1 and M_2 is assumed to be known, probably on the basis of prior reciprocity calibration. With the probe tube in place the measurements are repeated with both M_1 and M_2. Ideally the introduction of the probe tube should not disturb the field in the cavity; this can be ascertained by comparing the two sets of measurements with M_1. In practice the differences between the two sets of measurements should be within 1 dB, provided the bore of the probe tube is small enough, of the order

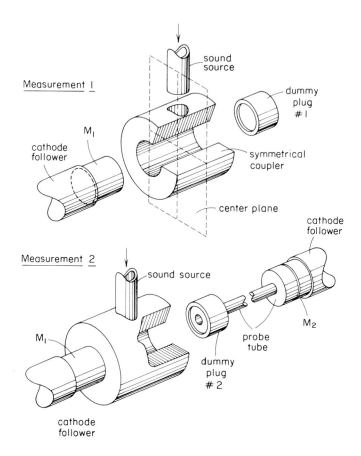

Fig. 2.22. Scheme of calibrating a probe tube in a symmetrical coupler. See text for details.

of 0.05 cm (Benson, 1953). If the sensitivity of M_1 is the same as that of M_2, and the probe does not change the field in the cavity, then the probe tube loss is simply the difference between the measurements with M_1 and M_2. This of course presupposes a perfectly symmetrical cavity. The latter can be checked by repeating the measurements with the cavity turned around. Whatever asymmetries exist, either in the cavity or between M_1 and M_2, can be taken into account as correction factors on the basis of these measurements.

C. Special Problems in Distortion Calibration*

At intense sound levels *all* acoustic systems behave nonlinearly and thus

* Based on Dallos *et al.* (1969b).

produce harmonic and intermodulation distortion. The experimenter's task is to determine the amount of distortion present in a given situation and to judge whether, depending on his experiment, that amount is tolerable. In treating distortion, our main contention is again the desirability, indeed the necessity, of measuring the sound stimulus at the eardrum during actual experiments. First, we wish to establish that, depending on the exact nature of coupler measurements, one can easily under- or overestimate the amount of distortion that might actually be present in the sound field at the eardrum of the experimental animal. We have made extensive comparison measurements of intermodulation and harmonic distortion generated in various couplers and at the guinea pig eardrum (Dallos *et al.*, 1969b). We found that, for example, the 500-Hz difference tone is vastly overestimated when measured in a standard 2-cm^3 coupler for most of the frequency range. This can happen in spite of the fact that in this coupler less sound pressure develops at a constant speaker voltage than in the real ear.

In general, specifying equipment distortion on the basis of coupler measurements is an unreliable enterprise at best. The question naturally arises as to whether it is possible to specify a level of distortion that can be considered tolerable. It appears that a general answer to this question is not available and that acceptable distortion in the sound field depends on the purpose and technique of any particular experiment. This contention can be explained with the aid of Fig. 2.23, in which cochlear microphonic input–output functions are shown for two distortion components and for pure tones of the same frequency. All were recorded from the third turn of a guinea pig cochlea, with the differential electrode technique and with the auditory bulla open. The right panel of Fig. 2.23 shows the third-harmonic component (2280 Hz) in the microphonic potential in response to a 760-Hz fundamental. The input–output function for a pure tone of 2280 Hz is also given. In addition, the 2280-Hz sound component recorded in front of the animal's eardrum is also given as the function of the intensity of the fundamental. It is seen that, at the most intense fundamental level (100 dB SPL), the third-harmonic component in the sound has a strength of 56 dB SPL. Thus this particular distortion component is 44 dB down from the fundamental or, stating it differently, it is approximately at the 0.5% level. With the aid of this sound pressure (of distortion) versus sound pressure (of fundamental) function and the microphonic versus sound pressure function for the pure tone at the frequency of the third harmonic, one can easily construct a microphonic versus SPL function for the anticipated distortion. This function is also shown. It is quite clear that in this case the distortion anticipated in the microphonic, as the result of distortion in the sound, is significantly less than the actually observed third-harmonic content of the microphonic potential. The anticipated distortion is at least 20 dB down from the observed distortion; thus the

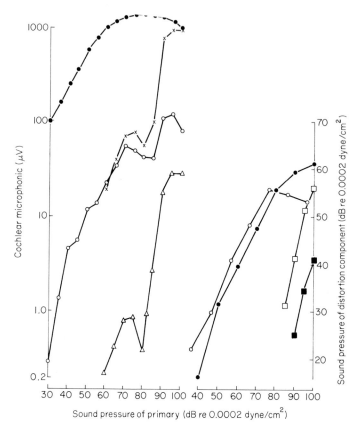

Fig. 2.23. Right panel: Cochlear microphonic versus sound pressure functions for a third-harmonic component of 2280 Hz (fundamental frequency: 760 Hz), ●; for a 2280-Hz pure tone, ○; and for an estimated 2280-Hz third harmonic, ■. The latter function is obtained with the aid of the sound pressure function shown for the 2280-Hz distortion component, □. Bulla open. Left panel: Cochlear microphonic versus sound pressure functions for a 500-Hz pure tone, ●; for a 500-Hz difference tone (plotted at the eliciting primaries), ○; and for an estimated 500-Hz difference tone, X. The latter function is obtained with the aid of the sound pressure functions shown for the 500-Hz distortion component, △. Bulla open. Left-hand ordinate, rms magnitude of cochlear microphonic potential (microvolts); right-hand ordinate, SPL of distortion components (decibels re 0.0002 dyne/cm²); abscissa, SPL of pure tones and fundamental components. (From Dallos *et al.*, 1969b, p. 359.)

latter is not contaminated by distortion originating in the experimental apparatus to any significant degree. Thus, in this specific case, a distortion component in the sound that is 44 dB down from the strength of the fundamental turns out to be totally inconsequential.

In the left panel of Fig. 2.23, a similar set of functions is shown. Here we are interested in a first difference tone (500 Hz) elicited by 260- and 760-Hz primaries. The function for the difference tone is shown along with the input–output function for a 500-Hz pure tone. The 500-Hz distortion component as measured in the sound is also plotted. Note that at maximum intensity of the primaries (100 db SPL), the strength of the difference tone in the sound is 59 dB SPL. This component is then 41 dB down from the primaries, or it appears at the approximate level of 1 %. As before, by using the sound pressure function of the distortion component and the input–output function for the 500-Hz pure tone, one can construct a microphonic function for the 500-Hz component that is directly due to the distortion in the sound. Clearly, this function mimics the shape of the actually observed plot, and it is equal to it or greater in magnitude. One is forced to draw the conclusion that most, and probably all, of the measured 500-Hz microphonic component is simply a direct consequence of the distortion in the experimental apparatus.

Let us now contrast the two situations discussed above. In both cases the actual amount of distortion in the sound field is quite similar, 44 versus 41 dB down from the level of the fundamentals. Yet this distortion could be completely neglected in one case, while in the other case it was altogether the dominant factor. Of course, the difference between the two situations can be explained easily by noting the relative sensitivity of the third-turn electrodes to the two frequencies at which distortion is measured. Five hundred hertz is the most sensitive frequency for the third-turn preparation, while at 2280 Hz the sensitivity is down by about 46 dB (for this specific animal). Thus the distortion is actually accentuated at 500 Hz by the extreme sensitivity of the third-turn microphonic to this frequency, while the effect of the distortion at 2280 Hz is effectively diminished by the reduced sensitivity of the preparation to this frequency. Our general conclusion is that the absolute specification of distortion level can be extremely misleading and should be avoided, unless, of course, one can insure a phenomenally low level of equipment distortion of the order of approximately −70 to −80 dB. Since commonly available equipment cannot, in general, produce high-level sound signals of such purity, we feel that the investigator whose main interest is the study of distortion originating in the auditory system (as opposed to the experimental apparatus) is well advised to obtain estimated microphonic distortion functions of the type shown in Fig. 2.23 in order to allay any doubt about the legitimacy of his measurements.

A word should be said about the estimated microphonic for the 500-Hz distortion component in Fig. 2.23. At high intensities, the estimated 500-Hz microphonic is considerably greater than the actually measured potential at that frequency. We believe that the explanation for this discrepancy is relatively simple and that it is to be sought in the well-known interference phenomenon (Wever *et al.*, 1940d). Note that we have computed the anticipated 500-Hz function from the response function for a 500-Hz pure tone. During the measurement of the actual 500-Hz distortion function, the two primary tones at frequencies of 260 and 760 Hz were also present. These high-intensity tones in the same frequency region as the 500-Hz component generate considerable decrease in the magnitude of the response to the 500-Hz component in the sound, in comparison to the situation when the 500-Hz tone is presented alone. Thus, owing to interference, we overestimate the distortion above approximately 70 db SPL. Of course, this process keeps us on the safe side. It is better to overestimate the contamination from equipment distortion than to underestimate it. More accurate estimation can be obtained by working from microphonic functions that are measured by presenting the stimulus tone in the presence of a secondary tone. The secondary tone should be chosen to mimic the strength and approximate frequency of tones that create interference during the actual experimental conditions, namely, the primary tones.

CHAPTER 3

The Middle Ear

I. The Concept of a Transfer Function

The analysis of linear systems can most fruitfully proceed with the aid of the transfer function concept. In the simplest case the system has one excitation (or input) and one response (or output) function. In general the input and output are both functions of time. The transfer function relates the system output to the input in an indirect manner. To explain, the transfer function does not directly provide a relationship between the input and output time functions; instead it relates their respective Laplace transforms. For those readers to whom Laplace transformation is unfamiliar* it will be sufficient to note that Laplace transformation substitutes a function whose independent variable is generalized frequency for a given function whose independent variable is time. This pairing of functions is accomplished via the following mathematical vehicle:

$$L[f(t)] = F(s) = \int_0^\infty f(t)e^{-st}\, dt \qquad (3.1)$$

This simply means that one multiplies the time function $f(t)$ in question by the factor e^{-st} and then the product is integrated for all times between zero and infinity. The resulting function of the generalized frequency s is the

* For a lucid treatment see, for example, Goldman (1949).

Laplace transform $F(s)$. The frequency s is a complex number, $s = \sigma + j\omega$. One can view this entire operation as a convenience measure, performed in order to convert a time function into a form that is more amenable to simple arithmetic operations than the original function. To clarify the meaning of the type of operation that we call a "transformation" let us consider one of the simplest and most familiar transformations which is often used to simplify knotty arithmetic problems. This is the logarithmic transformation, which is used to simplify difficult numerical computations such as obtaining exponentials. One can diagram the transformation process that is embodied by the taking of logarithms, for example in the case of multiplication, as shown in Fig. 3.1a. Thus to perform the multiplication, we first transform

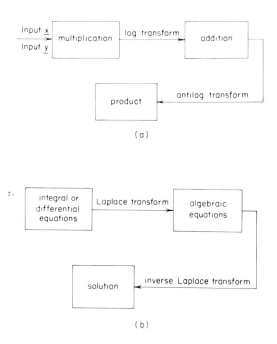

Fig. 3.1. (a) Schematic representation of the log and antilog transformations. (b) Schematic representation of the Laplace and inverse Laplace transformations.

the numbers to be multiplied by taking their logarithms, and at the same time we also transform the multiplication operation into addition. To obtain the numerical result we must perform an inverse transformation on the logarithmic sum; this is of course the obtaining of the antilog. To sum up, by making a transformation we are able to reduce the degree of difficulty of the numerical operation to be performed. The use of this transformation approach can be appreciated by the reader if he considers performing the operation $327^{2.45}$. The direct computation in this case is hardly feasible, but the logarithmic transformation reduces this problem to simple multiplication.

The Laplace transformation is a similar convenience measure which reduces the solution of differential and integral equations to the solution of algebraic equations. In order to compare this process with the logarithmic transformation, one can depict the Laplace transformation in diagram form, as shown in Fig. 3.1b.

Operationally what happens is that differential equations that are most commonly set up in terms of the independent variable, time, are transformed into algebraic equations expressed in terms of a generalized frequency as the independent variable. The transformation is obtained by performing Laplace transformations on the various time functions. The algebraic equations can usually be solved quite readily, and the resultant function can be transformed back into the time domain by inverse Laplace transformation. The analogy with the simple log operation is quite clear. Thus the Laplace transformation is a means of simplifying the operations on *functions*, just as, for example, the logarithmic transformation is a means of simplifying opera-tions on *numbers*. This can be seen by considering that if one were to obtain the output of a system that corresponded to a given input in terms of the familiar time variable, then one would have to solve a set of probably complicated differential equations. If, however, the transform of the input function were available along with the transfer function of the system, then the transform of the output could be obtained by multiplying the transform of the input and the transfer function. Symbolically,

$$G(s) = F(s)Q(s) \qquad (3.2)$$

where $G(s)$ and $F(s)$ are the transforms of the output and the input, respect-ively, and $Q(s)$ is the transfer function. Actually one could define the system transfer function with the aid of the above relationship as the ratio of the Laplace transform of the output and input time functions.

$$Q(s) = G(s)/F(s) \qquad (3.3)$$

As we have seen, the mathematical manipulation which is called Laplace transformation involves a change in variable from time t to a generalized frequency s. The corresponding functions $f(t) \longleftrightarrow F(s)$ are called trans-form pairs. They are compiled in tables, just as logarithms are given in approp-riate tables. Thus the process of integration does not have to be performed every time anew. Understanding the basic principles of the transformation process and the perusal of tables permits one to use this method.

To understand the meaning and significance of the real and imaginary parts of the complex frequency s, let us consider a somewhat simplified situation. If the output of a system $Q(s)$ is $g(t)$, then the transform $G(s)$ can be written in most practical situations as the following series:

$$G(s) = \frac{A_1}{s - s_1} + \frac{A_2}{s - s_2} + \cdots + \frac{A_i}{s - s_i} + \cdots \tag{3.4}$$

The inverse transformation of this series can be written as

$$g(t) = A_1 e^{s_1 t} + A_2 e^{s_2 t} + \cdots + A_i e^{s_i t} + \cdots \tag{3.5}$$

Let us examine the ith term in this series. The s_i terms are in general complex numbers, i.e., $s_i = \sigma_i + j\omega_i$. Thus

$$A_i e^{s_i t} = A_i e^{(\sigma_i + j\omega_i)t} = A_i e^{\sigma_i t} e^{j\omega_i t} \tag{3.6}$$

$$= A_i e^{\sigma_i t} (\cos \omega_i t + j \sin \omega_i t)$$

Notice that this time solution is a sinusoid whose amplitude changes as $A_i e^{\sigma_i t}$. Now, depending on σ_i, this function can decay ($\sigma_i < 0$), stay constant ($\sigma_i = 0$), or grow indefinitely ($\sigma_i > 0$). The last situation does not have much physical significance in passive systems; thus we are interested in the first two cases. The general situation is when $\sigma_i < 0$. This corresponds to a sinusoid that decreases in time, depicting a *transient* component of the solution. The magnitude of σ_i determines the speed with which a given transient dies out. The $\sigma_i = 0$ situation portrays a sinusoidal solution whose amplitude does not change in time. This is a so-called *steady-state* solution. Of course, if $\omega_i = 0$ then we are dealing with a nonoscillatory component in the total solution. This component can be decaying (transient) if $\sigma_i < 0$, or it can be a dc component (steady state) when $\sigma_i = 0$. We can thus appreciate the meaning of the real and imaginary parts in the generalized frequency s. The real part governs the transient properties of the response, while the imaginary part dictates the oscillatory properties. If only steady-state solutions are of interest, then instead of expressing the transfer functions in terms of s, the $\sigma = 0$ substitution allows us to express them in terms of $j\omega$. These functions are then usually referred to as frequency response functions.

Let us assume that the input sine wave is expressed as $f(t) = F \sin \omega t = F \sin 2\pi f t$, while the output sine wave is $g(t) = G \sin(\omega t + \theta) = G \sin(2\pi f t + \theta)$. Here F and G are the amplitudes of input and output, respectively, while θ is the phase difference between them. Then if we change the frequency ω, in general both G and θ change. These changes are expressed by the transfer function, or frequency response function, for

$$\frac{G}{F}(\omega) = |Q(j\omega)| \quad \text{and} \quad \theta(\omega) = \angle Q(j\omega) \tag{3.7}$$

or, in words, the ratio of the output and input amplitudes as the function of frequency is equal to the absolute value of the transfer function, while the phase difference as the function of frequency is equal to the phase of the transfer function. Of course, this discussion immediately suggests the simplest method of determining the steady-state transfer function (or frequency response function). We need a test stimulus, a sinusoid with known amplitude and variable frequency. This test stimulus is impressed on the system and the amplitude of the resultant output is measured along with the phase difference between input and output for a number of frequencies. The ratio of output and input amplitudes provides the magnitude response function for the range of frequencies that is of interest, while the phase difference between input and output provides the phase response function. For simplicity it is customary to keep the input amplitude constant at all frequencies during measurement. In order to completely describe a system one needs to have both the magnitude and phase functions. Only in simple cases, for so-called minimum phase* systems, are the magnitude and phase functions uniquely related, so that if one obtains either of them the other function can be determined by computation.

A few words ought to be said about the determination of the system transfer function for the general case when both transient and steady-state behavior are of interest. The method is again to use a test function and to measure the response. The best test function is the so-called impulse function, which as the name implies is an extremely brief, strong disturbance of the system. The impulse function is ideal, for its Laplace transform happens to be equal to unity; thus $F(s) = 1$ and consequently $Q(s) = G(s)/1 = G(s)$. This implies that the system response to an impulsive disturbance, the so-called impulse response function, is nothing but the time function whose Laplace transform is equal to the transfer function of the system under investigation. Clearly this is probably the most economical way of obtaining the system transfer function, if one considers that there is need for only a single measurement; namely, one has to plot the response of the system to an impulsive input. Then the Laplace transform of the obtained function must be taken to yield the transfer function. Of course, the usual problem is the last step, for if the impulse response of the system is complicated then obtaining its Laplace transform is not a simple matter. Nevertheless, one should appreciate the beauty and simplicity of obtaining the system transfer function on the basis of a single measurement. This can be contrasted with the necessary task of measuring output magnitude and phase for a wide

---

* Assuming that the transfer function of a system can be written in the form $Q(s) = f(s)/g(s)$, and if $f(s) = 0$ has no solutions $s_i = \sigma_i + j\omega_i$ with $\sigma_i > 0$, then $Q(s)$ is said to describe a minimum phase system. The most common nonminimum phase systems incorporate time delays.

array of sinusoidal inputs when one wishes to determine the steady-state frequency response functions.

It is important to emphasize that, if a system is linear and time invariant, its properties are completely determined by its transfer function. In contrast, for a so-called nonlinear system the transfer function concept and Laplace transformation methods are not particularly useful. In this case a frequency response function might describe the system's operation for a particular set of parameters—but *not* in general. In contrast, the knowledge of the transfer function implies the complete knowledge of a linear system.

It should be recognized that the transfer function is no more than a mathematical model of the behavior of a linear system. Another type of model that can be and has been used to study the operation of the middle ear is the network model. For a lumped-parameter, minimum phase system one can always obtain a network model whose transfer function is the same as that of the system. Such a network model is not unique; many networks can be constructed to yield identical transfer functions. In general, an indefinite number of network models can be constructed for any particular transfer function. Such a network is strictly analogous to the physical system that it purports to model only if the elements and the configuration are so chosen that there is a one-to-one correspondence between all elements in the proto-type and the analog network.

The advantage of the network model over the purely mathematical expression of the transfer function is that, while the latter does not provide any direct information about the structure of the system, the network model, if properly constructed, does allow the visualization of various interrelated components and their individual contributions as they make up the total system. Although it need not be so, the majority of network models are constructed as electrical networks as opposed to, say, mechanical networks. The reasons for this choice are that more investigators are familiar with electrical circuits than with other types, that it is easy to simulate the model, and that measurements on the simulated model can be made with great ease and accuracy. There is a direct correspondence between an acoustomechanical network and its electrical equivalent. This is because the differential equations that govern the operation of either type of network are in identical form. Consequently if one substitutes appropriate electrical variables and para-meters for acoustomechanical ones, the entire operation of the acoustic system can be described, quantitatively, in terms of the behavior of its electrical analog system. The most useful electrical analog is obtained if voltage is made to correspond to pressure and current to volume velocity in an acoustic system, while voltage and force, and current and velocity, are paired for a mechanical system. This type of analogy is designated as *impedance-type* analogy (Beranek, 1954). When one uses this type of analog, capacitors are substituted in place of acoustic compliances, inductors in place of acoustic mass, and electrical resistance in place of acoustic resistance. The following example (Fig. 3.2) shows how the electrical circuit analog

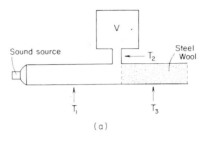

(a)

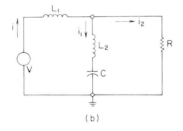

(b)

Fig. 3.2. (a) A simple acoustic circuit consisting of a sound source, two connecting tubes (T_1, T_2), a closed volume (V), and an open tube (T_3) filled with steel wool to provide acoustic resistance. (b) Electrical analog of the acoustic circuit.

can be drawn for an acoustic system. A loudspeaker generates a sound field into a tube (T_1), which branches into another tube (T_2) terminated in a large cavity (V). The first tube continues (T_3) beyond the branch and it is open at the far end. This tube section is filled with steel wool. Now, the loudspeaker is a pressure generator, and its electrical equivalent is a voltage source. An open tube acts as an acoustic mass, while a closed volume behaves as an acoustic compliance. The steel wool presents acoustic resistance to the passage of sound. The analog of volume velocity is electric current and, in constructing the electrical analog, the best guide is to consider how velocity changes from element to element. Thus the voltage source, which is equivalent to the loudspeaker, is in series with an inductor, which represents the first tube segment. At the branch point the pressure generates two sound velocities in tubes T_2 and T_3, but the sum of these volume velocities is equal to the volume velocity of the incoming sound field. Thus the analogs of tubes T_2 and T_3 should be connected in parallel. Tube T_2 and volume V represent a series combination of acoustic mass and compliance; this branch is modeled with a series inductance and capacitance, L_2 and C, respectively. The last branch T_3 is an acoustic resistance; its far end is open to atmospheric pressure, which is represented by ground potential in the analog. Thus the last branch is shown as a resistance connected between the junction point and ground. This one example is not intended to teach the reader how to set up these analogs in general, merely to give a taste of the method. For detailed treatment and other examples the books of Beranek (1954) and Olson (1943) should be consulted.

II. Toward the Derivation of the Middle Ear Transfer Function

A. THE PROBLEM OF LINEARITY

It should be clear from the foregoing discussion that the relatively straightforward description of a vibratory system with the aid of a transfer function is valid only if the system is linear. The general criterion for the linearity of a system is discussed in the introduction to Chapter 6.

The first task of an experimenter who is deriving a transfer function or network model is to show that his system is indeed linear and thus amenable to such description. This initial step of analysis was not generally taken in the past by designers of models for middle ear mechanics. Linearity was usually tacitly assumed. Some investigations, however, directly tested linearity. Mundie (1963) measured the acoustic impedance of guinea pig ears at 100 and 130 dB SPL and noted that there were differences between the functions obtained at the two levels. This indicates that the middle ear is nonlinear but gives no further information regarding the limit of linearity. Fischler et al. (1967) measured eardrum motion in cadaver ears with a capacitive probe and demonstrated that, at 250 Hz at least, the amplitude versus SPL function of the drum is linear between 64 and 104 dB SPL. Noticeable departure from linearity was seen at 114 dB. Dallos and Linnell (1966a, b) demonstrated that even-order subharmonics in the guinea pig ear arise from nonlinearities associated with the eardrum–malleus complex. These subharmonics appear above 110 dB SPL with real thresholds, indicating the presence of substantial nonlinear influences at these sound levels. Rubinstein et al. (1966) measured the displacement magnitude of the stapes footplate in cadaver ears as the function of sound level. They found proportional increase in amplitude up to 104 dB SPL at three frequencies. Guinan and Peake (1967) paid particular attention to linearity in their study of motion patterns of various components of the cat middle ear. With their method of direct observation under stroboscopic illumination they found that stapes displacement is proportional up to 130 dB SPL for frequencies below 1500 Hz

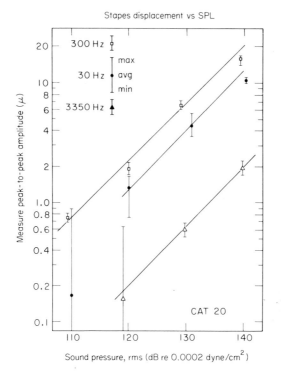

Fig. 3.3. Stapes displacement amplitude versus SPL at three frequencies for one cat. Each data point represents the average of 5–10 measurements; the range is shown by the vertical lines. (From Guinan and Peake, 1967, p. 1248.)

and that an even wider linear range might exist at higher frequencies. Their measurements at three frequencies are shown in Fig. 3.3.

The above-described observations indicate that it is fairly safe to assume that the middle ear operates as a linear system up to at least 100 dB SPL, and probably even higher in some species. Consequently linear modeling, that is, the use of transfer function descriptions, is probably a valid procedure at moderate intensity levels. Of course, it should be emphasized that, in the studies that supply the foundation for our conclusion, the middle ear muscle system was deactivated. It is almost certain that, in an awake animal whose acoustic reflex is intact, the middle ear system would not operate linearly above 60–70 dB SPL, which is the level of reflex threshold. It is known that the reflex mechanism is itself nonlinear (Dallos, 1964b). Consequently it is a safe assumption that, when active, it would cause the entire middle ear to operate nonlinearly. One should then be careful to limit the use of simple network and transfer function models to describe the operation of the middle ear without the contribution of the middle ear muscle reflex.

B. The Ideal Transformer Ratio of the Middle Ear

The evolutionary development of the middle ear as an impedance-matching structure is well known today. The outstanding treatment of middle ear properties by Wever and Lawrence (1954) is so complete and informative that it would be presumptuous to repeat much of it here. Instead, in the remainder of this chapter the more recent and more quantitative developments are presented.

The transformer mechanism of the middle ear is necessary to ensure efficient absorption of acoustic energy by the ear. Since the inner ear is fluid filled and the incoming sound waves are airborne, a great deal of reflection would occur at the air–fluid boundary if a matching mechanism were not interposed. The reason for this can be found in the characteristics of acoustic transmission at a boundary. Let us consider a plane progressive sound wave which propagates in a particular medium and approaches a boundary. Of great interest is the relative magnitude of the propagated and the reflected sound waves at the boundary. Because of the continuity of the boundary, both velocity and pressure must be the same on both sides. Symbolically,

$$\dot{x}_i + \dot{x}_r = \dot{x}_t \qquad \text{and} \qquad p_i + p_r = p_t \tag{3.8}$$

where the indices i, r, and t stand for incident, reflected, and transmitted quantities, respectively. However, in a propagating sound wave, pressure and velocity are related by the specific acoustic impedance of the medium, i.e., $p = Z\dot{x} = pc\dot{x}$, where Z is the impedance, c is the velocity of propagation, and ρ is the density of the medium. Substituting these relations, one obtains the following pair of equations:

$$p_i + p_r = p_t$$

$$\frac{p_i}{\rho_1 c_1} - \frac{p_r}{\rho_1 c_1} = \frac{p_t}{\rho_2 c_2} \tag{3.9}$$

Note that $\dot{x}_i = p_i/\rho_1 c_1$, the incident velocity; also $\dot{x}_r = -p_r/\rho_1 c_1$, the reflected velocity, which is taken with a negative sign because the reflected wave travels in the opposite direction; and finally $\dot{x}_t = p_t/\rho_2 c_2$, where $\rho_2 c_2$ is the acoustic impedance of the second medium. The above two equations can be combined to yield

$$\frac{p_i - p_r}{\rho_1 c_1} = \frac{p_i + p_r}{\rho_2 c_2} \tag{3.10}$$

or, if we denote the impedance of the air $\rho_1 c_1 = Z_a$, and $\rho_2 c_2 = Z_b$,

$$\frac{p_i - p_r}{Z_a} = \frac{p_i + p_r}{Z_b} \tag{3.11}$$

This equation can be solved easily for $p_r/p_i = (Z_b - Z_a)/(Z_b + Z_a)$, which is the relation of interest. If we now consider that acoustic intensity (I), which is energy per unit time per unit area, or power density, can be expressed as

$$I = p^2/\rho c \tag{3.12}$$

then acoustic intensity of the incident sound is $I_i = p_i^2/\rho_1 c_1$, while the intensity of the reflected sound wave is $I_r = p_r^2/\rho_1 c_1$. These expressions can be substituted in Eq. (3.11), resulting in

$$\frac{I_r}{I_i} = \left(\frac{Z_b - Z_a}{Z_b + Z_a}\right)^2 \tag{3.13}$$

Finally, the transmitted intensity I_t is obtainable as

$$I_t = I_i - I_r = \frac{4Z_b/Z_a}{(1 + Z_b/Z_a)^2} I_i \tag{3.14}$$

Consider that the specific acoustic resistance of air is 41.5 dynes second/cm^3, while the specific acoustic resistance of water is approximately 144,000 dynes second/cm^3. If one substitutes these resistance values into the above formula then the value of 1.08×10^{-3} obtains for the ratio of I_t/I_i. This means that at the air–fluid boundary only 0.1 % of the incident energy passes into the fluid and the remainder is reflected. Clearly, if airborne sound activated the cochlea directly a great transmission loss would have to be dealt with. The middle ear is an acoustic transformer that evolved to at least partially overcome this impedance disparity in matching the high impedance of the cochlear fluid to the low impedance of the air. The impedance match is mediated by two mechanisms. First, a force amplification exists in the middle ear as a consequence of the compound lever action of the malleus and the incus. The second mechanism, which is of more practical importance, is a pressure amplification afforded by the disparity between the areas of the drum and the stapes footplate. If there were no lever action, the force acting on the drum would be transmitted to the stapes (assuming lossless transmission). The arguments can be followed with the schematic sketch of the middle ear mechanism shown in Fig. 3.4. The force is expressible as pressure times area; thus in this situation

$$p_d A_d = p_s A_s \tag{3.15}$$

where the subscript d denotes the drum, and s denotes the stapes. If the lever action is also taken into account, this idealized (lossless) transformation can be described by

$$p_d A_d l_m = p_s A_s l_i \tag{3.16}$$

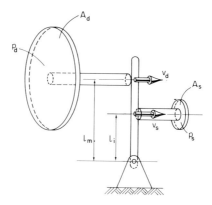

Fig. 3.4. Schematic diagram of the middle ear transformer. The force amplification is proportional to the level ratio l_m/l_i, while the pressure amplification is proportional to the area ratio A_d/A_s; v_d and v_s signify linear velocities, and p_d and p_s denote sound pressures.

where l_m and l_i are the lengths of the malleolar and incudal arms in the ossicular lever. The ratio of pressures at the drum and at the oval window can now be expressed as

$$\frac{p_d}{p_s} = \frac{A_s}{A_d} \frac{l_i}{l_m} \tag{3.17}$$

We can convert this relationship to one that describes the impedance transformation, if it is kept in mind that in general $Z = p/v$, where v is linear velocity, and also that a mechanical lever transforms not only displacement but also velocity,

$$v_d/v_s = l_m/l_i$$

Substitution yields

$$\frac{Z_d}{Z_c} = \frac{A_s}{A_d}\left(\frac{l_i}{l_m}\right)^2 \tag{3.18}$$

This expression relates the impedance transformation between the cochlea (Z_c) and the drum (Z_d) to the anatomical parameters of the middle ear. Using the values proposed by von Békésy and Rosenblith (1951) for human beings ($A_d = 0.55$ cm^2, $A_s = 0.032$ cm^2, $l_m/l_i = 1.3$), one can compute the transformer ratio as 0.0345. If the input impedance of the cochlea were assumed to be equal to the specific impedance of seawater, that is 144,000 dynes second/cm^3 (actually it is considerably smaller than this figure), then this resistance would appear at the drum as 4896 dynes second/cm^3. This is a significant reduction, but the value falls far short of the ideal magnitude of 41.5 dynes second/cm^3, which corresponds to perfect match and reflection-free transmission. The actually transmitted energy in the 4896 versus 41.5 dynes second/cm³ impedance disparity situation would amount to 3.4% of the incident energy. Using Zwislocki's (1965) estimate of 5600 dynes second/ cm³ for the cochlear impedance, one calculates that 60% of the incident energy is transmitted to the cochlea by the middle ear.

It is clear that in all of the above discussions the middle ear transformer is considered ideal, or lossless. In reality this transformer does contain frictional losses, as well as many reactive elements that render the transmission frequency dependent. One has to consider the acoustic properties of the middle ear air space, the elasticity of the drum, the ligaments, and the middle ear muscles, the inertia of the ossicles; and the imperfect coupling between the ossicles. All of these elements contribute to the overall transformer ratio, which in such a complex situation is better called the transfer function. The remainder of the chapter is devoted to the discussion of this transfer function.

C. THE MIDDLE EAR TRANSFER FUNCTION

1. A View from the Outside: Impedance of the Ear

Our first task is to select the most appropriate variables to appear in the transfer function of the middle ear. The input variable is relatively easy to dispose of, for clearly the quantity that activates the middle ear is sound pressure at the eardrum. This pressure is amplified by the middle ear, which acts as a pressure transformer, and the resultant pressure is delivered to the cochlear fluid by the footplate of the stapes. The actual sound pressure at the drum is determined by the incident pressure, which is generated by the sound source, and by the impedance characteristics of the drum membrane. Consider that a progressive sound wave with pressure p_i approaches the eardrum. At the boundary a certain portion of this wave is absorbed, and a certain portion is reflected. The sum of the incident and reflected waves is what one can measure at the eardrum, p_d. The ratio of reflected and incident pressure is determined by the impedances of the drum and of the earcanal or free field. Let us denote the impedance of the eardrum by Z_d and the impedance of air by Z_a; then the ratio of reflected and incident pressure is expressed as

$$p_r/p_i = (Z_d - Z_a)/(Z_d + Z_a) \qquad (3.19)$$

In general this is a complex ratio, indicating that, aside from a magnitude change, a phase difference also exists between the two waves at the boundary.

The acoustic impedance of the eardrum has been measured for cats, guinea pigs, and human beings. Specific acoustic impedance data for guinea pigs were obtained by Mundie (1963) and were analyzed mathematically by

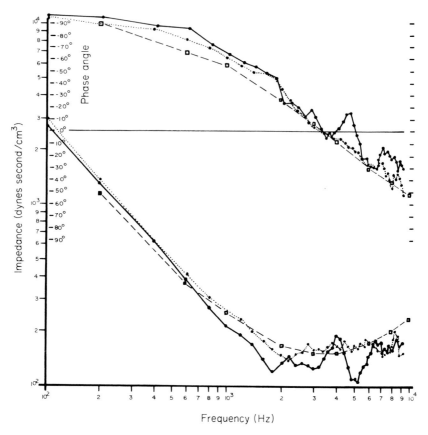

Fig. 3.5. Specific acoustic impedance of the guinea pig ear. Solid line represents one typical ear, the dotted line is the average of measurements on 10 ears, and the dashed line represents the response of a simple series acoustic circuit containing mass, compliance, and resistance. (From Mundie, 1963, p. 73.)

Zwislocki (1963). In Fig. 3.5 Mundie's data are shown, both for one specific animal and for the average of 10 ears. Note that the fine details that can be seen in the individual animal's data are "washed out" in the averaging process, even though the general characteristics are maintained. In this figure, instead of the real and imaginary parts of the impedance, its magnitude and phase are plotted as functions of frequency. The magnitude decreases from about 3000 rayls at 100 Hz to a flat minimum above 1500 Hz, while the phase goes from 90° lead at low frequencies toward 90° lag at high frequencies. Zero phase shift is seen in the vicinity of 3000 Hz. Information about the impedance characteristics of the cat eardrum was gathered by Møller (1963). His findings for one cat are shown in Fig. 3.6. Here again, amplitude

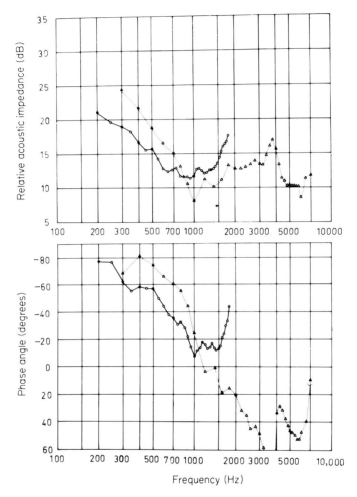

Fig. 3.6. Acoustic impedance (magnitude and phase) of a typical cat (△) and that of a typical human (○) subject. The reference for the logarithmic magnitude scale is 100 CGS units. (From Møller, 1963, p. 1531.)

and phase functions are given, with frequency being the independent variable. These plots are similar in overall appearance to the guinea pig data of Mundie. Note that the magnitude plot decreases from approximately 2000 acoustic ohms at low frequencies to a minimum of about 300 acoustic ohms at 1000 Hz. There is a resonance and antiresonance between 4000 and 7000 Hz, again similar to that found in the guinea pig. These high-frequency resonances are demonstrably due to the smaller cavity in the auditory bulla and to its opening in the bony septum. The phase versus frequency plot for the cat approaches 90° lead at low frequencies and it tends toward 90° lag at high frequencies, albeit with considerable undulations. The zero phase shift frequency is approximately 1500 Hz.

2. The Transfer Function

Up to this point our primary concern has been to assess input information about the middle ear. We noted that the most appropriate variable is sound pressure at the eardrum. The sound wave of course sets the drum in vibration and the motion is then transmitted to the stapes footplate. The next logical step might be to determine the transfer characteristic between stapes movement and drum movement, that is, to describe the magnitude and phase of stapes displacement as the function of drum displacement. However, before embarking on this course one should consider what the appropriate output variable from the middle ear might be. Asking the same question with a somewhat different emphasis, What is the appropriate input quantity to the cochlea? While details of the cochlear transduction process still elude us, it is now fairly widely accepted that the adequate stimulus to the hair cells is mechanical deformation. This deformation must be intimately tied in with local movements of the cochlear partition, which in turn depend on the overall motion pattern of the basilar membrane. The displacement of the cochlear partition is proportional to the pressure difference across it. This pressure differential, as we shall see in the following chapter, is a function of the pressure generated at the oval window by the movement of the stapes footplate. Thus it appears that the pressure at the oval window should be taken as the critical input variable to the cochlea. If one denotes the volume displacement of the stapes as X_s, the acoustic input impedance of the cochlea as Z_c, and the pressure at the oval window as p, then the following relationship applies:

$$p = \dot{X}_s Z_c \tag{3.20}$$

where $\dot{X}_s$ is the volume velocity of the stapes. As will be discussed in the following chapter, in many species the input impedance to the cochlea is resistive, and constant at least to a first approximation over the most important frequency range. With these relationships in mind one sees that the motion pattern of the cochlear partition is determined by the pressure at the oval window, which in turn depends directly on the stapes volume velocity. For sinusoidal signals $\dot{X}_s = j\omega X_s$. Thus in this case the input pressure is proportional to $j\omega X_s$; in other words, the magnitude of the pressure is directly proportional to the driving frequency and to stapedial displacement, while it leads the stapes motion by 90° in phase. These considerations indicate that the most appropriate input variable to the cochlea is *stapes volume velocity*.

Since velocity is somewhat difficult to measure, while displacement can be obtained with greater ease, stapes displacement is usually measured instead of stapes velocity in the process of obtaining the transfer function for the middle ear. In linear systems with harmonic inputs of course the two quantities contain the same information. Let us then denote the middle ear transfer function that relates stapes velocity to sound pressure at the eardrum by $H_2(j\omega)$ and the transfer function that connects stapes displacement with sound pressure at the drum by $H_3(j\omega)$. We immediately note that

$$H_2(j\omega) = j\omega H_3(j\omega) \qquad (3.21)$$

There is only one experiment reported in the literature in which the $H_3(j\omega)$, i.e., the stapes displacement/sound pressure at the drum transfer function,

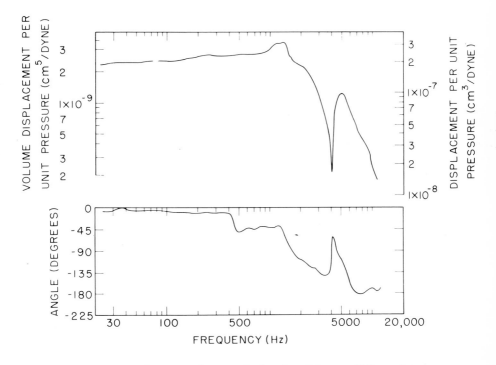

Fig. 3.7. Magnitude and phase of the transfer function of the cat middle ear. Intact ear, bulla closed, and septum in place. (From Guinan and Peake, 1967, p. 1252.)

was obtained with direct measurement of stapes motion. This is the 1967 experiment of Guinan and Peake in which anesthetized cats were the experimental animals, and visual, microscopic observation under stroboscopic illumination was the experimental method. Details of such a scheme for displacement measurement were discussed in Chapter 2. Other experimenters, notably Zwislocki (1963), Møller (1963, 1965), and Tonndorf and Khanna (1967), used a variety of more indirect measures to arrive at similar transfer functions. Their work will be discussed below in comparison with the more thoroughly treated Guinan–Peake data.

The important results of Guinan and Peake can be summarized with the help of Figs. 3.7 and 3.8. These plots give the magnitude and phase of the

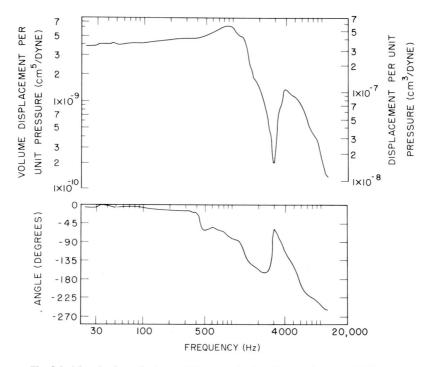

Fig. 3.8. Magnitude and phase of the transfer function of the cat middle ear. Bulla open, septum intact. (From Guinan and Peake, 1967, p. 1253.)

$H_3(j\omega)$ function for both open- and closed-bulla conditions. Clearly, the closed-bulla condition reveals more of the actual acoustic properties of the cat middle ear, but because many of the available electrophysiological data on this animal are gathered with the bulla widely opened, Guinan and Peake wisely chose to include transfer functions for this condition also.

These functions show the behavior of the "average" middle ear, which means that small individual variations are washed out, but the significant trends are maintained.

It might be instructive to discuss in some detail the method employed by Guinan and Peake in obtaining Figs. 3.7 and 3.8. A very important condition during the measurements was that both the bulla and the bony septum separating the bullar cavity into two volumes were widely opened in order to facilitate the microscopic observation of the middle ear structures. When data points from 25 cats were combined and smoothed by averaging within any 1-octave band, the middle ear transfer characteristics of Fig. 3.9 were derived. There are a number of outstanding features in the amplitude and

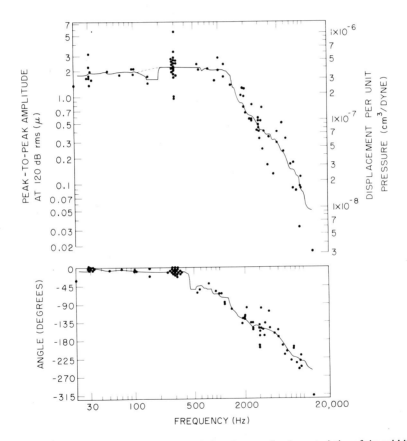

Fig. 3.9. Magnitude and phase data depicting the transfer characteristics of the middle ears of 25 cats (points). The curves were obtained by taking the average of all points within 1-octave bands of frequency. Bulla is open and the septum is removed. (From Guinan and Peake, 1967, p. 1248.)

phase plots of this figure. First, the magnitude plot is quite flat up to approximately 1200 Hz, and corresponding to this amplitude characteristic is the small phase shift observed at the low frequencies. At higher frequencies the magnitude of the transfer function decreases monotonically, and the phase seems to approach 270°. Quite clearly, with the middle ear wide open, the stapes displacement versus sound pressure at the drum transfer function appears to represent a simple low-pass filter than can be approximated by three reactive elements in combination with some dissipative elements. The average curves shown in this figure were used by Guinan and Peake to derive the transfer functions for the intact middle ear.

In order to obtain correction factors for the changed acoustic conditions imposed by the open bulla and septum, they measured the sound pressure at the eardrum that was required to produce a constant cochlear microphonic response from the vicinity of the round window, for conditions of bulla closed, bulla open and septum intact, and bulla and septum open. They reasoned that at any given frequency the constancy of the cochlear potential signified the constancy of stapes displacement. Thus the difference in sound level from one measurement to another could serve to correct for the difference in the acoustical properties of the middle ear system due to manipulations on the bulla and septum. These manipulations clearly have their most marked effect in the frequency range 2000–6000 Hz. The opening of the bulla produces a low-frequency advantage of about 5 dB and a pronounced antiresonance followed by resonance at approximately 3000 and 4000 Hz, respectively. The opening of the septum creates a strong resonance around 3000 Hz. It should be pointed out that the exact frequencies of the resonant and antiresonant peaks can change considerably from one animal to another. Evidently such individual variations can be somewhat in excess of 1000 Hz. It should also be mentioned, however, that averaging in this situation would not prove beneficial, because it would merely result in the complete washing out of the significant peaks and dips. The best strategy is to select a truly typical animal and use the correction factors obtained from it to make the appropriate adjustments on the average transfer function to be corrected. Not having such a "typical" animal for which complete data were available, Guinan and Peake shifted the resonant frequencies of their prototype animal to bring them in harmony with the group tendencies and then corrected the plots of Fig. 3.9 accordingly. The results are shown in Figs. 3.7 and 3.8.

The general character of these plots is again that of a low-pass filter. Transmission is quite flat up to approximately 1300 Hz, accompanied with small phase shift at the low frequencies. Above 1300 Hz the magnitude drops rapidly and the phase lag increases. It appears that the phase function approaches 270° at high frequencies for the open-bulla condition, indicating that middle ear transmission can best be approximated by a third-order system* (at least as far as the overall tendencies are concerned). The sharp dip at 4000 Hz in the transfer function of the intact middle ear is clearly due to the acoustic resonance of the bulla–septum cavity complex.

It might be quite instructive to consider how small-volumes such as that of the bulla or the middle ear cavity (beyond the septum) might exert their acoustic influence on the transmission and impedance properties of the middle ear transformer. Mundie (1963) has given an especially lucid demonstration of these effects in his studies of the impedance properties of the guinea pig ear. While the dimensions and shape of cat and guinea pig middle ears are quite different, the concepts of treating one apply equally well to the other. The guinea pig middle ear cavity is divided into two spaces by a septum with a small communicating hole, just as the cat's is. The larger of the two cavities has a volume of 0.2 cm^3, while the smaller is only 0.05 cm^3. At low frequencies the total volume of 0.25 cm^3 provides the dominant acoustic element that determines the input impedance of the guinea pig ear. The acoustic properties of such a compliance are indicated in Fig. 3.10 by the -6 dB/octave straight

---

* We use the term system "order" here in the following context. A transfer function for steady-state (sinusoidal) conditions can be generally expressed as

$$H(j\omega) = k \frac{(j\omega - s_1)(j\omega - s_2)\ldots(j\omega - s_n)}{(j\omega - s_a)(j\omega - s_b)\ldots(j\omega - s_m)}$$

The constants $s_1, s_2, \ldots, s_n$ are called the *zeros* of the transfer function, while the constants $s_a, s_b, \ldots, s_m$ are known as the *poles* of the function. Zeros and poles together comprise the singularities of the function; they represent the system's natural frequencies. The number of poles determines the system order. Most characteristic of the properties of a transfer function is its behavior at high frequencies. Consider that as ω approaches infinity the function $|H(j\omega)|$ approaches $k\omega^n/\omega^m$. This fraction can be zero, infinity, or can have a finite value depending on the ratio n/m. If $m > n$, which is the most common case of interest, then the magnitude of the transfer function approaches zero at high frequencies. The rate of this approach depends on the difference $m - n$. Every zero contributes an asymptotic 6 dB/octave *increase* in the magnitude of the transfer function at high frequencies, while every pole contributes an asymptotic 6 dB/octave *decrease*. The actual course of the function in the high-frequency region is then determined by the number of excess poles (or zeros). For example, the function

$$G(j\omega) = \frac{(j\omega - 5)}{(j\omega - 10)(j\omega - 3)(j\omega - 0.5)}$$

has two more poles than zeros. Thus at high frequencies its magnitude decreases at a rate of 12 dB/octave, 6 dB/octave for each excess pole. The difference $m - n$ describes the asymptotic high-frequency behavior. The high-frequency phase function is even more revealing than is the rate of change of the magnitude function. Each zero contributes 90° lead and each pole contributes 90° lag at high frequencies. Thus the ultimate phase portrait is determined by the difference between the number of poles and zeros. The high-frequency phase function approaches $(m - n) \pi/2$ radians. In the above example the high-frequency phase behavior is characterized by a lag of π radians or 180°.

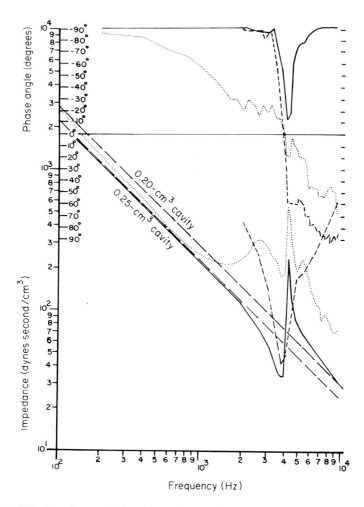

Fig. 3.10. Specific acoustic impedance (magnitude and phase) of the total middle ear of the guinea pig (dots), of the small cavity plus orifice (short dashes), and of the middle ear space (solid lines). The equivalent impedances of two volumes of 0.2 and 0.25 cm³ are also given. (From Mundie, 1963, p. 74.)

line, which represents the reactance of the cavity. At very high frequencies the acoustic mass that is comprised of the air in the opening between the two cavities possesses extremely high reactance; thus it effectively eliminates the small cavity. As a result at high frequencies the cavity impedance is determined by the large volume alone. The corresponding impedance is also plotted in Fig. 3.10. The transition between these two −6 dB/octave lines takes place between 3000 and 5000 Hz with a peak and a dip. One could consider the small cavity and the orifice to form a Helmholtz resonator* whose resonant frequency is at approximately 4000 Hz. The impedance characteristics of this resonator are also shown in the figure. Finally, the total measured impedance of the middle ear is also given by Mundie. It is very clear that at least for the guinea pig this impedance is primarily determined by the combined cavities at low frequencies and also that the effect of the small cavity–orifice resonator is definitely reflected in the overall impedance function. Similar arguments could be made for the cat, where as we have seen the dual cavity–orifice configuration is also present.

Let us now close the circle and obtain the transfer function of primary interest, that is, the relationship between stapes volume velocity and sound pressure at the eardrum. It is remembered that this function is $H_2(j\omega) = j\omega H_3(j\omega)$, where we now have $H_3(j\omega)$ as determined by Guinan and Peake. The simple operation of taking the derivative, or more precisely multiplying by $j\omega$ in the steady-state case, can be readily performed. The results of that computation for both the open- and closed-bulla situations are shown in Fig. 3.11. The most conspicuous feature of the magnitude plots is their band-pass filter characteristic. At the low-frequency end the absolute value of the transfer function rises at a rate of 6 dB/octave and reaches a maximum at approximately 1000 Hz. The pronounced midfrequency dip as we have seen is due to the resonance arising from the acoustic interplay of the middle ear cavity and the connecting hole in the bony septum. The high-frequency roll-off probably occurs at a rate of -12 dB/octave for the open-bulla and -6 dB/octave for the closed-bulla condition. The phase characteristic shows a 90° lead at low frequencies and it approaches a 180° lag for the open-bulla and 90° lag for the closed-bulla condition at high frequencies. Of course the effect of cavity resonance is clearly seen here also.

We have followed the development of the middle ear transfer function by using the experimental results obtained by Guinan and Peake (1967). The reason for choosing this set of data was that this study utilized the most direct method of measuring stapes motion and the largest number of experimental animals. Two other reports (Møller, 1963; Tonndorf and Khanna, 1967) also derived middle ear transfer functions for the cat, while Zwislocki's (1963) article presented such a function for the guinea pig. Transfer functions

---

* The approximate resonant frequency of a Helmholtz resonator can be computed as

$$f_0 = \frac{c}{2\pi}\left(\frac{S}{lV}\right)^{1/2}$$

where S is the area of the orifice, l is the length of the orifice, and V is the volume of the cavity.

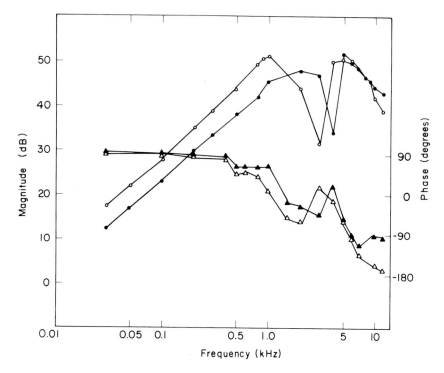

Fig. 3.11. Transfer functions (magnitude and phase) of the middle ear for open- and closed-bulla conditions. These functions express the relationship between stapes volume velocity and sound pressure at the eardrum. These plots are obtained from those of Figs. 3.7 and 3.8 on the basis of the operation $H_2(j\omega) = j\omega H_3(j\omega)$. Open bulla: magnitude, $\bigcirc$; phase, $\triangle$; closed bulla: magnitude, $\bullet$; phase, $\blacktriangle$.

or equivalent network models for the human ear were obtained by Zwislocki (1957), Møller (1960), and Glaesser *et al.* (1963). These models, which represent the behavior of normal human middle ears, are based on anatomical considerations and input impedance measurements. A number of investigators studied the input–output properties of the middle ear systems of human cadavers (von Békésy, 1960; Onchi, 1961; Fischler *et al.*, 1967; Rubinstein *et al.*, 1966). It appears, on the basis of impedance measurements of Zwislocki and Feldman (1963), that highly significant changes in the mechanical properties of the middle ear take place after death. As a result of these changes the transfer functions obtained in cadaver ears are generally not compatible with those representing the living system. The transfer function of the cadaver middle ear is much flatter, showing less than 20 dB variation in magnitude between 50 and 10,000 Hz. We are not going to treat cadaver data in any more detail; instead we shall give some consideration to the similarities and differences among the Guinan–Peake transfer function and others that can properly be compared to it.

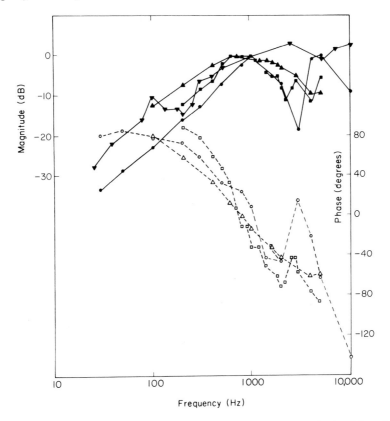

Fig. 3.12. Middle ear transfer function, $H_2(j\omega)$, computed on the basis of data from four investigators. Closed symbols, magnitude; open symbols, phase; ●, Guinan and Peake (1967); ■, Møller (1963); ▲, Zwislocki (1963); ▼, Tonndorf and Khanna (1967).

We have recomputed middle ear transfer characteristics on the basis of various data provided by four investigators. These data are included in Fig. 3.12. The plots show the degree of agreement among various investigators concerning the transfer characteristics of the middle ear. Strictly speaking only the Guinan and Peake, Møller, and Tonndorf and Khanna data are comparable, since these three sets are for the cat. However, the differences among their plots are not smaller than those between Zwislocki's data and, say, the median cat data. It is probably fair to say that data obtained in different laboratories with different techniques for a particular species are not homogeneous enough to show up species differences when compared to material obtained from a different species. The plots in Fig. 3.12 differ in detail quite significantly, especially at the higher frequencies, where measurements are more difficult and where the resonance properties of the middle ear are more prone to play havoc with any attempt at quantitative comparison. Nonetheless, these plots have a great deal in common. All four functions show approximately 6 dB/octave rising slope at the low frequencies. The functions appear to peak in the area of 1000 Hz and are probably quite unreliable at the high frequencies. Most likely, the correct high-frequency behavior corresponds to the Guinan and Peake plots, simply because, as stated before, they represent the most direct measurement method and the most extensive data. Accordingly, one can sum up these results by saying that the transfer properties of the middle ear are akin to those of a band-pass filter. On the low-frequency end of the audio spectrum the transfer function rises at a 6 dB/octave rate, simply because volume velocity is proportional to frequency, while the stapes displacement versus SPL relation is flat. Thus those who are used to describing middle ear mechanics in terms of stapes displacement versus SPL transfer ratios talk about a low-pass characteristic as the proper description. We feel that stapes volume velocity versus SPL is a more meaningful concept, and hence we champion the band-pass characteristic as the more appropriate description. The band-pass characteristic ensues, for at the high frequencies the efficiency of transmission drops rapidly, and as a consequence the volume velocity versus SPL function decreases at a rate of 6 dB/octave (for the closed-bulla condition). The corresponding phase characteristics are in harmony with the band-pass nature of middle ear transmission. At low frequencies the stapes volume velocity leads the sound at the drum by 90°, while at high frequencies a phase lag approaching 90° is seen. It is in fact this 90° lag, clearly obtainable from the Guinan and Peake data, that alerts us to assume a −6 dB/octave slope for the high-frequency end of the transfer function. It is almost invariably true that phase measurements can provide a more accurate estimate of the system order than can the slope of the magnitude function.

3. Network Models

Although we have accomplished the derivation of the transfer function of the middle ear, the aim of this chapter, it is important for us to go beyond the overall characteristics and discuss the contribution of individual elements within the middle ear complex. Actually, we started such a discussion in connection with the behavior of the transfer function around 4000 Hz. We described the approach that Mundie used to demonstrate the effects of the large and small bullar cavities and the connecting orifice between them (Fig. 3.10). With similar arguments, based on the functional anatomy of the middle ear, one can allocate various acoustic influences to the various middle ear structures. Zwislocki (1963) used such an approach to derive a transfer function of the guinea pig middle ear. His arguments are difficult to improve upon, and thus we shall present them essentially unchanged, although condensed.

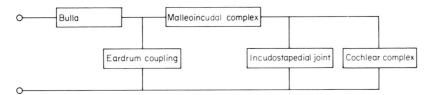

Fig. 3.13. Block diagram of the middle ear. (From Zwislocki, 1963, p. 1035.)

Figure 3.13 is a block diagram of the middle ear. To derive this diagram the following considerations are used. The volume velocity of the eardrum is the same as the rate of volume change of the air enclosed in the middle ear cavity. The equivalent quantity of volume velocity is current, and thus if an equivalent circuit is to be derived, a series element should be the first block representing the middle ear cavities. Since all energy must be transmitted by the malleus and the incus, and by the portion of the tympanic membrane that is firmly attached to the malleus, these elements are represented by a second series block. The portion of the eardrum that is not firmly attached to the manubrium of the malleus acts as an acoustic shunt; consequently it is represented by the first parallel block. It should be noted that in the guinea pig, and in rodents generally, the malleus and the incus are actually fused. Thus the vibratory motion of the malleus is transmitted to the incus *in toto*. This is why it is permissible to combine the acoustic contribution of these two ossicles in the second series block of Fig. 3.13. In the cat the malleus and incus exist as separate bones. While the majority of investigators agree that the coupling between them is extremely rigid, Guinan and Peake (1967) dissent, stating that there is relative motion between the malleus and incus. If this view is correct then, in block diagrams depicting the acoustic properties of the cat middle ear, a parallel block must be included between the now-separate series blocks of the eardrum–malleus and the incus. There seems to be fairly universal agreement that the incudostapedial joint is a loose one and that a transmission loss and phase shift must be attributed to this coupling. The joint is simulated by the last parallel block in Fig. 3.13. The last block represents the input impedance of the cochlea, and it should also include the acoustic properties of the oval and round windows.

The individual blocks can be simulated by simple electrical circuits in which capacitance stands for acoustic compliance (a closed volume), inductance is substituted for acoustic mass (a volume of air moving without compression), and resistance simulates acoustic dissipation. The actual circuit configurations can be derived on a semiintuitive basis from the anatomy and from the known effect of any portion of the middle ear that is modeled. Circuit values are chosen so that the frequency characteristic of a given bloc corresponds to that of the acoustic prototype.

The first block represents the auditory bulla. We already know that here the combined effects of two different volumes and the connecting orifice must be simulated. The easiest way to do this is to represent the two volumes with two capacitors, and if a series resistance and inductance are combined with the capacitance that represents the small volume, then the Helmholtz resonator which is present is adequately represented. Zwislocki derived this analog to match the input impedance that was obtained by Mundie for one guinea pig.

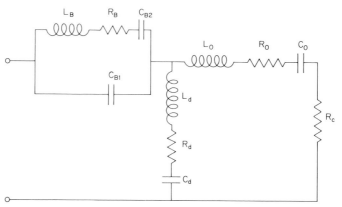

Fig. 3.14. Middle ear network analog based on the assumption that the input impedance of the cochlea is purely resistive. (From Zwislocki, 1963, p. 1037.)

The actual acoustic properties of the eardrum's shunting effect are completely unknown, but a series resonant circuit can probably serve as a first approximation. If one makes a very large opening in the bulla its acoustic effect is completely eliminated; thus under such a condition the first block can be ignored. If one makes one additional assumption, namely, that the impedance of the cochlea is much smaller than that of the incudostapedial joint, one can also eliminate the latter from the block diagram. With all these assumptions the network is reduced to one shunt branch and two series branches. The shunt branch is taken as a series resonant circuit, mainly because, as we have seen, so little is known about the actual acoustic behavior of the shunting effect of the eardrum. For largely similar reasons, the series eardrum–malleus–incus block, as well as the stapes–cochlea–round-window block, are assumed to comprise series resonant circuits. Direct determination of circuit values in this network is not possible (unless one specifically compiles data for it), but computations can be made by subtracting the acoustic effect of the bulla from Mundie's input impedance data.

The input impedance of the cochlea itself was determined by Mundie (1963), who found that the resistive component of this impedance is much greater than the reactive component. The value of the cochlear resistance is roughly constant with frequency, having a value of approximately 150 dynes second/cm^3. This being the case, the two reactive elements that together with R_c simulate the effect of the cochlea can be effectively ignored. Consequently the network that simulates the middle ear is in the form given in Fig. 3.14. To simulate Mundie's impedance data for one ear, Zwislocki chose the following set of electrical circuit values:

$$L_B = 50 \text{ mH} \qquad R_B = 190 \ \Omega \qquad C_{B1} = 0.155 \ \mu F \qquad C_{B2} = 0.038 \ \mu F$$

$$L_d = 20 \text{ mH} \qquad R_d = 700 \ \Omega \qquad C_d = 0.08 \ \mu F$$

$$L_0 = 40 \text{ mH} \qquad R_0 = 50 \ \Omega \qquad C_0 = 0.8 \ \mu F$$

$$R_c = 330 \ \Omega$$

To make his analog more general, Zwislocki also computed the parameters that are required for the same circuit configuration to represent not one particular animal, but the average impedance data obtained by Mundie on 10 guinea pigs. He arrived at the following array of circuit values:

$$L_B = 24 \text{ mH} \qquad R_B = 100 \ \Omega \qquad C_{B1} = 0.137 \ \mu F \qquad C_{B2} = 0.034 \ \mu F$$

$$L_d = 20 \text{ mH} \qquad R_d = 700 \ \Omega \qquad C_d = 0.04 \ \mu F$$

$$L_0 = 31 \text{ mH} \qquad R_0 = 100 \ \Omega \qquad C_0 = 0.8 \ \mu F$$

$$R_c = 350 \ \Omega$$

Figure 3.15 compares the input impedance of the analog network constructed with this set of parameters with that of the average input impedance of 10 guinea pig ears. The agreement is again found to be quite acceptable. The transmission characteristics of the network of Fig. 3.14 have already been shown. They were included in Fig. 3.12 for the sake of comparison with the transmission functions obtained by other investigators. The reader will recall that general agreement was noted among these functions.

It is of some interest to inquire which component or components are primarily responsible for the middle ear impedance and transmission proper-

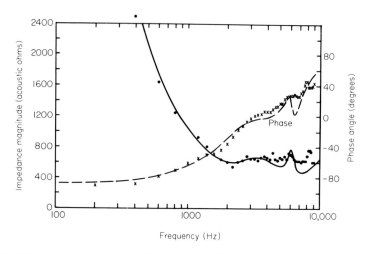

Fig. 3.15. Acoustic impedance of the eardrum. Data points indicate mean values of 10 guinea pig ears. Solid and dashed lines represent the response of the analog network when the parameters are adjusted to replicate an idealized middle ear. (From Zwislocki, 1963, p. 1037.)

ties in given frequency ranges. Mundie (1963) and Møller (1965) discussed this problem. Mundie concluded and Møller largely concurred that the low-frequency behavior is determined almost completely by the acoustic compliance of the bulla, that the midfrequency (between 2000 and 9000 Hz) properties are seemingly governed by the input impedance of the cochlea, and that at high frequencies the mass effect of the ossicular chain most likely dominates. Some reflection, and the review of data already presented, would show that this view is essentially correct. The reader's attention is first directed to Fig. 3.10, where Mundie's impedance data are compared to the impedance of two small cavities connected by a narrow passage. At low frequencies the middle ear input impedance is highly similar to the impedance of the cavities alone. In Fig. 3.5, which shows Mundie's average input impedance data for 10 guinea pig ears, we discover that, in the frequency range of approximately 2000–9000 Hz, the impedance of the ear is minimal, the magnitude is between 150 and 200 dynes second/cm^3, while the phase hovers around 0°. The cochlear impedance is resistive and of similar magnitude. It appears, then, that by good design in the very frequency range that is most important for communication, the middle ear simply reflects the input properties of the cochlea, and consequently it allows the effective transfer of sound energy with a relatively flat frequency response and negligible phase shift.

Lest it be misunderstood, I would like to emphasize that the approximately 150 dyne second/cm^3 acoustic resistance assigned to the cochlea is the resistance viewed at the drum.* In other words, this is an effective resistance as it appears at the input of the middle ear transformer. The actual cochlear resistance is of course much higher; impedances are transformed in proportion to the square of the transformer ratio. As we have already discussed, the ideal value of the impedance transformation is obtained as

$$\frac{Z_d}{Z_c} = \frac{A_s}{A_d}\left(\frac{l_i}{l_m}\right)^2 \tag{3.18}$$

where Z_d is the impedance at the drum, Z_c is the input impedance of the cochlea, A_s/A_d is the areal ratio of the stapes footplate and the drum, and l_m/l_i is the ossicular lever ratio. For the human being, Zwislocki (1965) gives the Z_d/Z_c ratio as 0.0345, which means that the real cochlear impedance of 5600 dynes second/cm³ is transformed so that it appears at the drum as 193 dynes second/cm³. The lever ratio l_m/l_i for cats is reported to be 2.5 by Wever and Lawrence (1954), 2.2 by Tonndorf and Khanna (1967), and 2.0 by Guinan and Peake (1967). The effective areal ratio is 0.047. Thus if a lever ratio of 2.0 is used, the impedance transformation by the cat middle ear is 0.012. Thus the cochlear impedance appears at the drum as 67 dynes second/cm³. This value is somewhat smaller than the midfrequency input impedance of the cat eardrum which was reported to be about 200 dynes second/cm³ by Møller (1963).

It is important to conclude that in the midfrequency range the ossicular chain performs its impedance matching function fairly adequately. In this range the system response is determined almost completely by the actual pressure transformation and mechanical advantage provided by the drum versus stapes footplate areal advantage and the ossicular lever ratio. The transformation here is very nearly without a phase shift, and it occurs with a loss only because the actual transformer ratio is not quite sufficient to overcome the fluid-to-air impedance disparity. In the human being, for example, the 193 dyne second/cm³ acoustic resistance is still considerably in excess of the characteristic resistance of air, which is approximately 41 dynes second/cm³. This impedance disparity allows only about 60% of the incoming sound to be absorbed at the drum even in this idealized case. The situation is more favorable for the cat, because of the greater transformer ratio. Theoretically only about 6% of the incident sound is reflected; however, in reality the conditions are somewhat less favorable. At low and high fre-

---

* The perceptive reader will notice that the input impedance value that can be obtained from Fig. 3.15 is approximately 600 acoustic ohms. The difference is simply due to differing units corresponding to acoustic impedance (dynes second/cm⁵) and specific acoustic impedance (dynes second/cm³). If the conversion is made by taking into account the approximate surface area of the guinea pig eardrum (0.2 cm²) then the specific impedance appears as 120 dynes second/cm³.

quencies the transmission efficiency of the middle ear is considerably poorer because the transformer action is degraded by the frequency-dependent acoustic properties of the middle ear, such as cavity effects at the low end of the spectrum and mass effects, probably combined with slippage of the incudostapedial joint, at the high end of the audio range.

Møller (1965) provided an especially illuminating demonstration of the effect of the inner ear on the properties of the middle ear. After showing that in cat between 400 and 4000 Hz the input admittance of the middle ear and the transmission characteristics of the middle ear (as measured by the CM at the round window at constant SPL) are extremely similar, he set out to see how the input impedance is modified by removing the cochlear load from the middle ear. He measured the input impedance both before and after disarticulating the incudostapedial joint. Clearly after the joint is interrupted the cochlea no longer affects the input impedance. His results are shown in Fig. 3.16. The important observation is that the reactive component of the

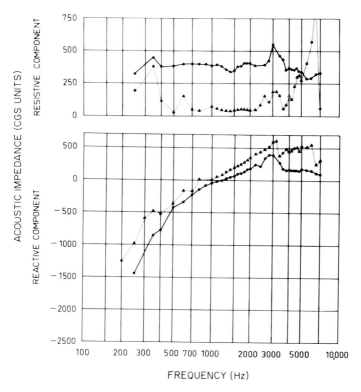

Fig. 3.16. Acoustic impedance of the eardrum of a cat before (●) and after (▲) interruption of the incudostapedial joint. (From Møller, 1965, p. 137.)

impedance is only very slightly affected, while the resistive component virtually disappears between 500 and 4000 Hz. It appears then that the ossicular chain itself possesses very little friction and that most of its damping originates from the resistive load presented to it by the inner ear. Between 500 and 4000 Hz the cochlea appears to be a pure resistance. The moderate influence of the disarticulation process on the reactance of the middle ear at the lowest frequencies seems to indicate that here the cochlear impedance might contain some reactive components. That this is indeed the case will be demonstrated in Section II,E of the next chapter.

4. Analytic Treatment

The final step in developing the transfer function of the middle ear is to examine the experimental data and derive analytical expressions that adequately fit the results. Several of the investigators who worked on middle ear transmission proposed such analytical formulations. Flanagan (1962) analyzed Zwislocki's circuit model and demonstrated that a third-order transfer function could reasonably well account for its major features. This is the case in spite of the fact that the analytical function that gives an exact description of the transfer properties of this circuit model (Fig. 3.14) is considerably more complex. Flanagan proposed the following function:

$$H_3(j\omega) = \frac{a(a^2 + b^2)}{(j\omega + a)[(j\omega + a)^2 + b^2]} \tag{3.22}$$

With the choice of $b = 2a = 2\pi \cdot 1500 \ \text{sec}^{-1}$, this function results in the amplitude and phase plots of Fig. 3.17. Note that this transfer function is given for stapes displacement versus sound pressure. To compute the more relevant volume velocity versus sound pressure function, we again have to multiply by $j\omega$. The amplitude and phase functions that result from this transformation are also given in Fig. 3.17; their general character conforms to the previously discussed salient behavior; namely, the function is band pass, the high-frequency slope is -12 dB/octave, the low-frequency slope is $+6$ dB/octave, and the phase changes from $90°$ lead at the low frequencies to $180°$ lag at the high frequencies. This type of function is quite adequate to describe the gross, overall behavior of the middle ear sound transmission; as derived it describes the open-bulla condition. Of course, with such few parameters as are allowed in a simple transfer function, which is further simplified by the $b = 2a$ choice, one cannot simulate the fine structure of the experimentally obtained functions, especially not those of single animals. It can be argued, however, that the local variations in the transfer functions, for example the 4000-Hz resonance, are incidental anyway, that they are a mere consequence of the acoustics of the system and are in no way essential from the teleological viewpoint.

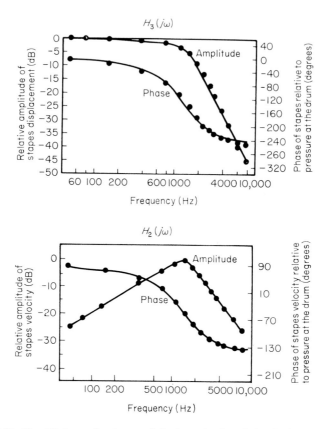

Fig. 3.17. Simplified transfer characteristics (magnitude and phase) of the human middle ear. Both $H_3(j\omega)$ and $H_2(j\omega)$ are shown. (Adapted from Flanagan, 1962, p. 966.)

Møller (1963) proposed a transfer function designed to fit his own data obtained on cats. Strictly speaking his analytical expression is not analogous to either our $H_2(j\omega)$ or $H_3(j\omega)$, for he derived his function to fit the experimental curve for the malleus displacement at a constant sound pressure level. This function was second order, in the form

$$G(j\omega) = \frac{a^2 + b^2}{(j\omega + a)^2 + b^2} \tag{3.23}$$

with the following parameters: $a = 2\pi \cdot 430 \text{ sec}^{-1}$; $b = 2\pi \cdot 1225 \text{ sec}^{-1}$.

Guinan and Peake (1976) suggested a second-order transfer function as a first approximation only, for their high-frequency data clearly show that one needs at least a third-order system to model the middle ear transmission properties. Nevertheless, at low and mid frequencies the second-order approximation is fairly adequate. They expressed the proposed transfer function in a slightly different form:

$$H_3(j\omega) = \frac{K}{1 - (\omega/\omega_0)^2 + j2\zeta\omega/\omega_0} \tag{3.24}$$

When expressed in this manner, the parameters are related to the natural (resonant) frequency of the system (ω_0) and to the damping factor (ζ). Guinan and Peake suggested the values of $\omega_0 = 2\pi \cdot 1300 \; \text{sec}^{-1}$, and $\zeta = 0.7$. One can compare the Møller and Guinan and Peake transfer functions by rewriting the former to make it correspond to the form of the latter. Thus,

$$\frac{a^2 + b^2}{(j\omega + a)^2 + b^2} = \frac{a^2 + b^2}{a^2 + b^2 - \omega^2 + 2ja\omega}$$

$$= \left(1 - \frac{\omega^2}{a^2 + b^2} + j2\frac{a\omega}{a^2 + b^2}\right)^{-1} \tag{3.25}$$

Clearly $(a^2 + b^2)^{1/2} = \omega_0$, while $a(a^2 + b^2)^{-1/2} = \zeta$. Hence the values for natural frequency and damping factor are $\omega_0 = 2\pi \cdot 1230 \; \text{sec}^{-1}$ and $\zeta = 0.35$. It seems that Møller modeled the system with a considerably less damped second-order system than did Guinan and Peake.

III. Comparisons with Behavioral Sensitivity

It is appropriate now to pause and compare the middle ear transfer characteristic discussed above with the behavioral sensitivity of the cat. While the properties of the middle ear obviously influence the characteristics of behavioral response, it is questionable whether the middle ear could be the sole determinant of sensitivity. It is certainly interesting and legitimate to ask to what extent the middle ear response dominates the overall sensitivity of the ear. In Fig. 3.18 the $H_2(j\omega)$ function for the closed-bulla condition is replotted, together with the average sensitivity curve as reported by Miller *et al.* (1963) for cats as obtained in a free-field testing situation. In order to facilitate comparison, the Guinan–Peake data are also plotted in the figure as sound pressure level/stapes volume velocity; that is, the reciprocal of the customary transfer function is shown. The similarities and differences between the two curves are quite interesting. Clearly there appears to be fair agreement at the high frequencies and great departures at the low frequencies. Both curves show a notch at 4000 Hz, but the reduction in sensitivity is much less pronounced in the behavioral response. We can make a meaningful comparison between these two curves only if we keep in mind the differences

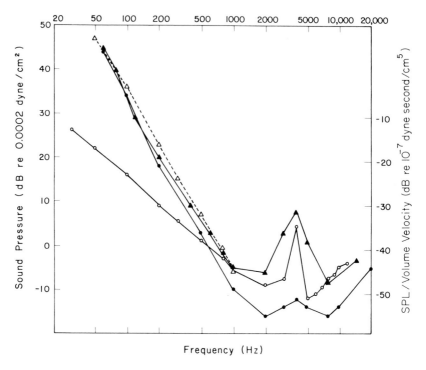

Fig. 3.18. Behavioral sensitivity response of the cat in free acoustic field, ● (adapted from Miller *et al.*, 1963, p. 21); $H_2(j\omega)$ with closed bulla, ○ (adapted from the data of Guinan and Peake, 1967, p. 1252); behavioral response data corrected on the basis of the Wiener *et al.* (1966, p. 261) data to show SPL at the drum at threshold, ▲; and $H_2(j\omega)$ corrected below 1000 Hz for the high-pass filter effect of the helicotrema, △ (from Dallos, 1970).

in experimental conditions. There are two major factors that can affect the experimental results that differ in the two testing situations. The Guinan and Peake data were obtained in a closed acoustic system and with anesthetized animals. In contrast the behavioral data were collected on awake, unrestrained animals and in a free-field acoustic environment. Let us first discuss the effects of anesthesia on middle ear function, and then scrutinize the influence of the acoustic environment.

Simmons (1964), in an elegant experiment, clearly demonstrated that active middle ear muscles significantly influence middle ear transmission, especially around the 4000-Hz antiresonance point. In Fig. 3.19, cochlear microphonic potentials, recorded at approximately 60 dB SPL from the cat round window, are shown for a number of experimental conditions. In one animal the middle ear muscles were cut on one side and were left intact in

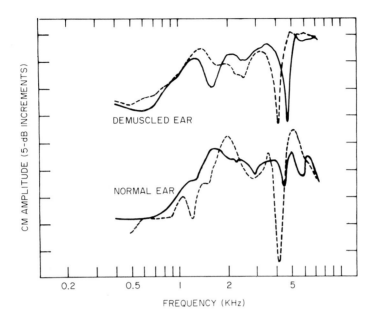

Fig. 3.19. Effect of the middle ear muscles on the transmission characteristics of the cat middle ear. The curves show round-window CM recorded at approximately 60 dB SPL. The four curves are for conditions when the animal is awake (solid lines) or asleep (dashed lines) and when the muscles are intact or severed. (From Simmons, 1964, p. 277.)

the other ear. Round-window electrodes were permanently implanted, and the animal was allowed to recover from surgery. Testing was done with the animal awake and under barbiturate anesthesia. Note that in the demuscled ear, whether the animal was awake or asleep, a pronounced notch is seen between 4000 and 5000 Hz. In the normal ear, the notch is very prominent in the anesthetized condition, but it almost completely disappears when the animal is awake. Simmons' interpretation of these findings is that, just as other striated muscles, the stapedius and the tensor tympani have a constantly fluctuating muscle tonus. In other words, from instant to instant there are slight contractions and relaxations in both muscles, resulting in constantly changing muscle tension. As the tension changes, the transmission properties of the middle ear change with it. Such alterations should be most noticeable in those frequency regions where the transmission characteristic is rapidly changing, in other words, at the resonant or antiresonant frequencies. When the muscles are normally active they shift the resonant and antiresonant points from frequency to frequency within a relatively narrow band; thus they effectively average out the sharp peaks of the function. This situation seems to occur for the normal, awake animal in Fig. 3.19, where the

4000-Hz dip is effectively eliminated. When the muscles are deactivated, either by surgery or anesthesia, the sharp antiresonance is unaffected. An alternate explanation is that the active muscles, attached to the ossicles, act as damping elements and through their internal friction provide a "dash-pot" effect in reducing resonant peaks. We can say then that the difference seen in Fig. 3.18 between the behavioral sensitivity and the middle ear transfer characteristic at 4000 Hz is at least partly due to the fact that the latter function was obtained from anesthetized preparations in which the middle ear muscles were inactive. Another contributing factor is that the behavioral curve represents an average, while the transmission curve was obtained from one animal. We have mentioned before that, because of the slight differences in the resonant points among animals, any averaging would flatten out the curve.

In order to make adjustments for the differences between testing in a closed acoustic system and in free field, we must make changes to account for two different factors. First, in the physiological experiments the sound was delivered to the animal's auditory meatus and it was monitored very close to the eardrum. Thus the reported SPL values are actually those that existed at the tympanic membrane during testing. In contrast, the values shown for the behavioral experiments were measured external to the pinna, and consequently the sound pressure at the eardrum was different than the reported values. Such differences are due to two separate factors. First, the auditory meatus, which is essentially a long and narrow tube, shows a peculiar acoustic resonance whereby certain frequencies are actually intensified at the eardrum. Second, the head and the pinna of the experimental animal act as an acoustic baffle in reflecting and diffracting the incident sound, so that it is different at the entrance to the meatus than it would be at the same point in space if the animal were not present. These effects were treated extensively for human beings (von Békésy, 1932; Wiener and Ross, 1946; Wiener, 1947; Zwislocki, 1958) and for cats (Wiener et al., 1966). The earcanal can be considered as a lossless acoustic transmission line in which plane waves propagate. The pressure at any one point is dependent on the input pressure, the frequency of the sound, the length of the meatus, and the nature of the terminating impedance (i.e., the impedance of the eardrum).

It is of some interest to derive an approximation for the magnitude of the pressure at different points within the meatus. In order to make the computations tractable, let us assume that the meatus is a tube of uniform cross section S of length l, which has rigid walls and is terminated in a rigid plate. The general solution of the acoustic wave equation* is written as

$$p(x,t) = f_1(t - x/c) + f_2(t + x/c) \qquad (3.26)$$

* Discussed further in the following chapter.

Here f_1 and f_2 are arbitrary functions, t is time, x is distance, and c is the velocity of propagation. Clearly this equation indicates that the total wave at any place and at any time is the sum of two waves, one traveling in the $+x$, the other in the $-x$, direction. The solution applies only to plane waves in a nondissipative medium. The most important case from our viewpoint is the situation in which the wave is studied in its steady state. For any given frequency component of the wave, one can write

$$f(x,t) = pe^{-j\omega x/c}e^{j\omega t} \tag{3.27}$$

provided it is clearly understood that this exponential shorthand is adopted as a computational convenience and that the actual numerical values can be obtained as the *real parts* of the function. This practice of using exponentials in the description of steady-state phenomena is extremely common in circuit theory, and it is a great notational simplification. The total pressure then can be expressed for the steady-state condition as

$$p(x,t) = p_+ e^{-j\omega x/c}e^{j\omega t} + p_- e^{j\omega x/c}e^{j\omega t} \tag{3.28}$$

In this expression p_+ and p_- are the amplitudes of the pressure waves traveling in the $+x$ and $-x$ directions, respectively. The equation can be simplified by factoring out $\exp(j\omega t)$ and by introducing the abbreviation of $k = \omega/c$.

$$p(x,t) = (p_+ e^{-j\omega x/c} + p_- e^{j\omega x/c})e^{j\omega t}$$

$$p(x,t) = (p_+ e^{-jkx} + p_- e^{jkx})e^{j\omega t} \tag{3.29}$$

In order to solve this general pressure equation for our particular acoustic configuration, we must establish boundary conditions. This can be done by assuming first that at the entrance of the tube the velocity is a known periodic function, thus at

$$x = 0 \qquad v(0,t) = v_0 e^{j\omega t} \tag{3.30}$$

In addition, since the terminating wall is rigid, the particle velocity must be zero at $x = l$, that is, $v(l,t) = 0$. The general equation for velocity can be patterned after the pressure equation (or could be derived following the same steps), for pressure and velocity are in general proportional: $p = Zv$. Thus

$$v(x,t) = (v_+ e^{-jkx} + v_- e^{jkx})e^{j\omega t} \tag{3.31}$$

Then at $x = 0$

$$v_0 e^{j\omega t} = (v_+ + v_-)e^{j\omega t}$$

or

$$v_0 = v_+ + v_- \tag{3.32}$$

At $x = l$

$$0 = v_+ e^{-jkl} + v_- e^{jkl} \tag{3.33}$$

These last two equations can be solved simultaneously, first to obtain v_+.

$$v_+(e^{jkl} - e^{jkl}) = v_0 e^{jkl} \tag{3.34}$$

Here one can make use of the identity $\sin y = (e^{jy} - e^{-jy})/2j$ to obtain

$$v_+ = v_0 \frac{e^{jkl}}{2j \sin kl}$$

Similarly,

$$v_- = v_0 \frac{e^{-jkl}}{-2j \sin kl} \tag{3.35}$$

These two expressions can be resubstituted to yield

$$v(x,t) = v_0 \frac{e^{jk(l-x)} - e^{-jk(l-x)}}{2j \sin kl} e^{j\omega t}$$

$$= v_0 \frac{\sin k(l-x)}{\sin kl} e^{j\omega t} \tag{3.36}$$

The pressure can be obtained from the just-computed velocity with the aid of the equation of motion, which in general is written as

$$\frac{\partial p}{\partial x} = \rho_0 \frac{\partial v}{\partial t} \tag{3.37}$$

In the steady state the equation can be written

$$\frac{\partial p}{\partial x} = j\omega \rho_0 v \tag{3.38}$$

Consequently,

$$p = j\omega \rho_0 \int v \, dx \tag{3.39}$$

Substituting for v

$$p = j\omega v_0 \rho_0 \int \frac{\sin k(l-x)}{\sin kl} e^{j\omega t} \, dx$$

$$= -j\rho_0 c v_0 \frac{\cos k(l-x)}{\sin kl} e^{j\omega t} \tag{3.40}$$

Our primary interest is the pressure transformation between the points $x = 0$ and $x = l$. The magnitude of this transfer function at any time can be expressed as

$$p(l,t)/p(0,t) = \left[-j\rho_0 v_0 c \, \frac{\cos k(l-x)}{\sin kl} \right]\Bigg|_{x=l} \bigg/ \left[-j\rho_0 v_0 c \, \frac{\cos k(l-x)}{\sin kl} \right]\Bigg|_{x=0}$$

$$= \frac{1}{\cos kl} \tag{3.41}$$

Assuming that for a human being $l = 2.5$ cm, one can compute a first approximation of the pressure transformation from the entrance of the meatus to the plane of the eardrum. In Fig. 3.20 the $p(l)/p(0)$ versus frequency plot is

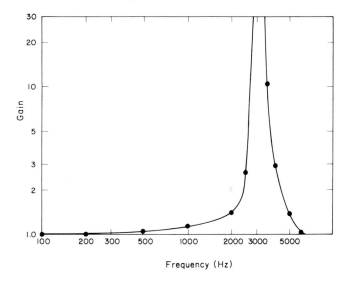

Fig. 3.20. Computed resonance characteristics of the straight earcanal.

shown. The interesting and important conclusion is that at approximately 3000 Hz there is a pressure resonance at the eardrum, meaning that in the midfrequency region the earcanal provides a considerable boost in sound pressure. In reality the canal does not have rigid walls, and more importantly it is not terminated in an infinite impedance. Because of these factors the resonance is greatly dampened, but it still provides a pressure amplification of approximately 10 dB. The actual pressure transformation in the human earcanal was measured by Wiener and Ross (1946); Zwislocki (1965) used a network analog to simulate the behavior of the meatus. The acoustic properties of the earcanal are those of a transmission line. Thus very accurate modeling could be accomplished by using an electrical transmission line for simulation purposes. The measurements and simulation show a resonance at 3500 Hz, with a peak gain of about 10 dB, much less of course than predicted by the theoretical treatment of the rigid-walled canal.

The auditory meatus of the cat is much more complex than that of a human being. In the cat the best approximation of the meatus can be obtained by using two tubes of different cross section and length in cascade. Wiener *et al.* (1966) on the basis of anatomical measurements proposed that one section should be 1.5 cm long, this to simulate that part of the canal between the drum and the abrupt bend in the canal, and the second section should be 0.5 cm long and twice the cross-sectional area as the first. This second section was designed to simulate the more peripheral portion of the canal. As a first approximation a rigid termination was assumed. The computation for obtaining the pressure ratio at a point x in the two-section canal relative to the entrance point ($x = 0$) is rather involved, but the general form of the result is very similar to that shown above for the simple straight-canal situation. The following was presented by Wiener *et al.*:

$$\frac{p(x)}{p(0)} = \frac{\cos k(l_1 + l_2 - x)}{\cos kl_1 \cos kl_2 - S_2/S_1 \sin kl_1 \sin kl_2} \tag{3.42}$$

Aside from the boost in sound pressure provided by the acoustic resonance in the meatus, there is a secondary effect that provides pressure amplification at the drum compared to the free-field pressure level. This secondary effect is due to the baffle properties of the pinna and the head. The computation of the amount of pressure increase at the entrance of the meatus which results from diffraction and reflection of sound waves by the head and the pinna is extremely difficult because of the irregular shapes of the active surfaces. Measurement of the effect, however, is possible, and has been done for the cat by Wiener *et al.* (1966). Their results for five animals are shown in Fig. 3.21. In this figure the ratios of sound pressure at the eardrum to free-field pressure are shown as the function of frequency. It is important to note that this figure depicts the combined effect of head baffle and meatus resonance, and it thus incorporates the pressure gain that was discussed above at some length. The additional boost in pressure at the eardrum is modest; the total maximum advantage over the free-field situation is about 20 dB at 3000 Hz. Approximately 15 dB of the total is due to the meatus resonance alone.

Before utilizing these eardrum versus free-field sound pressure data to make necessary corrections in the behavioral response curve of the cat, we must dispose of one more factor that might confound comparisons with the electrophysiological data. This additional factor is the so-called "closed ear effect" (Wever and Lawrence, 1954; Munson and Wiener, 1952). It has been observed that the loudness of a tone is greater when tested in a free field than under an earphone, even though in both cases the sound pressure

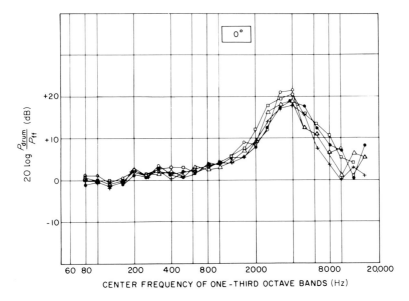

Fig. 3.21. Pressure transformation from free field to the cat eardrum for five animals. These curves show the combined effect of head baffle and meatus resonance. (From Wiener *et al.*, 1966, p. 261.)

is the same at the eardrum. The effect is particularly prominent at low frequencies. Tonndorf and Khanna (1967) measured this closed ear effect in cats by monitoring cochlear potentials when the sound stimuli were delivered in an open and closed acoustic system. They found highly consistent, but very small differences between the two testing situations; the effect is apparently much less significant in cats than in human beings. Because of the small numerical values involved (1–2 dB) we are not going to pay attention to the closed ear effect in making comparisons between behavioral and electrophysiological responses of the cat.

The behavioral response curve of Fig. 3.18 was plotted for sound pressure levels measured in the free field in the absence of the animal. The actual sound pressure at the eardrum can be approximated by using the Wiener *et al.* data, which were shown above to correct for meatus resonance and acoustic baffle effects. The corrected curve (filled triangles) is also included in Fig. 3.18. This plot is now directly comparable to the middle ear transfer function computed from the Guinan and Peake data, shown as open circles in Fig. 3.18. Such a comparison reveals the extent to which the cat's behavioral auditory sensitivity is determined by the middle ear itself. It would appear from a cursory comparison that the middle ear transfer function strongly dominates the overall sensitivity function for all frequencies above 500 Hz.

The departure between the two functions at low frequencies is significant because it is not merely a quantitative but a qualitative discrepancy. The middle ear transfer function changes at a 6 dB/octave rate at the low end of the audio spectrum, while the behavioral sensitivity curve changes at a 12 dB/octave rate, or even faster. It is very important to consider when making these comparisons that our middle ear transfer function simply describes the transformation from sound pressure to stapes velocity, whereas the pressure developed by the stapes in the oval window is proportional to the product of stapes velocity and the input impedance of the cochlea. If the input impedance were frequency independent then this would not matter; it can be demonstrated, however,* that in cat the input impedance is reactive. As a consequence of the reactive component of the input impedance, the pressure at the oval window decreases at a rate of 12 instead of 6 dB/octave at the low frequencies. If one corrects for this effect then below 1000 Hz the middle ear transfer function takes the shape that is indicated by open triangles in Fig. 3.18. It is clear that there is an excellent agreement between the behavioral sensitivity curve and this pressure at the oval window versus pressure at the drum transfer function. One can thus state that the combined properties of the middle ear and cochlear input impedance (which acts as a load on the middle ear) appear to be the primary determiners of the animal's behavioral sensitivity. It is interesting to mention parenthetically that the cochlear microphonic sensitivity function of the cat has a shape that is virtually identical with that of the behavioral sensitivity curve or the middle ear pressure transfer function curve. Thus both behavioral sensitivity and the CM obtained from the round-window region are determined largely by the properties of the middle ear.

* See Section II,E of Chapter 4.

Cochlear Mechanics

I. Some Acoustics and Hydrodynamics*

A. The Wave Equation and Its Solution

Our main interest in the sections that follow is to derive analytical expressions for the vibratory pattern of the cochlear partition. To give the reader an idea of the type of physical–mathematical arguments that are used in such derivations, it is appropriate to digress a little and present some of the basic mathematical background of sound propagation in fluids. Those familiar with the usual techniques of mathematical physics should skip this section and go directly to the derivation of equations for the motion pattern of the basilar membrane.

For simplicity we shall discuss events that occur in one dimension only, although the arguments can be easily generalized to the three-dimensional case. Consider that we disturb an elementary fluid volume by exerting a force on it in one direction. The effect of the disturbance is twofold. First, there is an alteration in the resting equilibrium pressure of the fluid and, second, there is a change in the equilibrium density. No matter what changes take place, however, no mass of fluid can be lost, and no new mass of fluid can be generated. In the physicist's jargon, the mass is conserved. These

---

* Lamb (1945), Lindsay (1960), Wood (1966), Zwislocki (1965).

relationships can be formalized in the equation of continuity of hydrodynamics. Consider the elementary volume dV and assume that there is fluid flow
in the x direction only. If v is the velocity of the flow, and if the fluid density
ρ can be expressed as the sum of a resting density (ρ_0) that characterizes the
undisturbed fluid and an excess density (ρ_e) that is due to the disturbance,
where the excess density is much smaller than the resting density, then one
obtains

$$\frac{\partial \rho_e}{\partial t} = -\rho_0 \frac{\partial v}{\partial x} \tag{4.1}$$

This equation is commonly known as the *equation of continuity*.

The force acting on the volume element dV is the difference of the forces
that act on the surface at x and at $x + dx$. The force on either of these surfaces is expressible as the area times the pressure on the surface. The net
force acting on the volume element dV can be written as $(\partial p/\partial x)dV$. Momentum is defined in physics as mass times velocity, and Newton's second law
states that force is equal to the time rate of change of momentum. We
assume here that the only force that resists the $(\partial p/\partial x)dV$ is the inertia term,
i.e., that there is no dissipation (friction, viscosity). We can write this by
considering that momentum is $(dV \rho)v$, and then the force is equal to

$$dV \rho_0 \frac{\partial v}{\partial t} \tag{4.2}$$

We can equate the two expressions for the force to obtain

$$\rho_0 \frac{\partial v}{\partial t} = -\frac{\partial p_e}{\partial x} \tag{4.3}$$

where p_e is the excess pressure over a resting pressure p_0. By definition the
sound velocity in the medium is related to excess pressure and excess density
by the expression

$$p_e/\rho_e = c^2 \tag{4.4}$$

where c is a constant. Then

$$\rho_0 \frac{\partial v}{\partial t} = -\frac{\partial}{\partial x}(c^2 \rho_e) = -c^2 \frac{\partial \rho_e}{\partial x} \tag{4.5}$$

This last equation for force balance and the continuity equation can be combined to yield

$$\frac{\partial^2 v}{\partial t^2} = c^2 \frac{\partial^2 v}{\partial x^2} \tag{4.6}$$

By eliminating other variables one can obtain a whole family of equations in exactly the same form

$$\frac{\partial^2 \theta}{\partial t^2} = c^2 \frac{\partial^2 \theta}{\partial x^2} \tag{4.7}$$

where the variable θ can be either pressure, velocity, displacement, or density. An equation in this form which relates the second time derivative of a variable with its second space derivative is called the one-dimensional *wave equation*. The solution of the wave equation in one dimension is

$$\theta = AF(ct - x) + BG(ct + x) \tag{4.8}$$

where A and B are constants, and F and G denote arbitrary functions. The correctness of this solution can be easily ascertained by substituting it back into Eq. (4.7). This solution to the wave equation is of utmost importance, and we should devote some time to a discussion of its properties. First, it should be emphasized again that the same functional form results whether the solution is for pressure, velocity, displacement, or density. Thus we might have

$$p = A_1 F_1(ct - x) + B_1 G_1(ct + x) \text{ or } v = A_2 F_2(ct - x) + B_2 G_2(ct + x) \tag{4.9}$$

No matter what the quantity of interest, the solution is always a function of both time and space, and moreover these independent variables (t and x) always appear in the functions together in the form of $ct - x$ or $ct + x$.

Let us now get acquainted with the properties of a function in the form of $F(ct \pm x)$. The dimensions of ct and x must be the same; that is, both are length. This is of course true because c is velocity, and thus ct is distance traveled during time t. Let us denote the value of the function F at time t_1 and distance x_1 as $F(t_1, x_1)$. Then at time $t_1 + t_2$ the disturbance will have traveled to a distance x_2. But x_2 can be written as $x_2 = x_1 + (x_2 - x_1)$, where the distance $x_2 - x_1$ is traveled during the time increment t_2. Thus $x_2 - x_1 = ct_2$. The value of the function F at time $t_1 + t_2$ and at distance x_2 is

$$F(t_1 + t_2, x_2) = F[(t_1 + t_2)c - x_2] = F\{(t_1 + t_2)c - [x_1 + (x_2 - x_1)]\} \tag{4.10}$$

After substitution of $ct_2 = x_2 - x_1$ one obtains

$$F[(t_1 + t_2)c - (x_1 + ct_2)] = F(t_1 c - x_1) = F(t_1, x_1) \tag{4.11}$$

We note the important conclusion that no matter what the functional form of F might be, this form does not change with time or distance. Consequently, the shape of the disturbance remains unchanged as the disturbance propagates with a velocity c. It was stated above that F can represent pressure, velocity, etc. Thus we can put our conclusions in a more concrete form by saying that the wave equation in the form derived above represents a pressure wave (velocity wave, etc.) that propagates without loss, without change in waveform. Recall that this wave equation was derived for the situation in which propagation occurs in the x direction only. The solution of this wave equation, $F(ct + x)$, represents a plane wave traveling in the x direction. It should be understood that this wave is not one dimensional. It is a wave traveling in space, i.e., in the x, y, and z dimensions, but at any $x = x_1$ the wave is the same for all y's and z's. That is, we have plane wavefronts in the y–z plane which travel along the x dimension.

We have not paid any attention to the meaning of the plus and minus signs in the solution of the wave equation. Consider first the partial solution $F(ct - x)$. We have shown that $F(t,x)$ remains constant for any t and x. Since F itself is not specified, this constancy can be satisfied only if the argument $ct - x$ itself stays constant for all t and x. Thus $ct - x = k$, and $ct = k + x$. This means that if t increases x must also increase. Consequently $F(ct - x)$ represents a disturbance that travels in the positive x direction, i.e., away from the source. The partial solution $F(ct + x)$ must also remain constant, and this implies that $ct + x = k$, or that $ct = k - x$. This means that as time (t) increases, x must decrease. Consequently, $F(ct + x)$ represents a wave moving toward the origin, toward the source. The general situation is then represented by two waves moving in the opposite direction with the same velocity.

For our purposes the most important wave propagation phenomena are described by periodic functions that represent steady-state conditions. Differently stated, we are most interested in the situation in which the waves have been established for some time so that transients have died out and a purely periodic propagation pattern prevails. Since according to Fourier's theorem a periodic wave can be resolved into the sum of sinusoids, it is sufficient to treat the behavior of one sinusoidal wave. The description of a steady-state wave as a sum of sinusoids implies that the functional form of F is expressible as $F(t,x) = F_i \cos(\omega_i t + \theta_i)$, where of course F_i is the amplitude of the ith member of the sum; $\omega_i = 2\pi f_i$, being the frequency; and θ_i is the phase angle of the wave. The amplitude function F_i is dependent on the distance x; thus $F_i = F_i(x)$. Let us now deal with only one member of the sum, and for convenience let us drop the index i. Then, since we know that the general solution of the wave equation is the sum of a forward and backward traveling wave, we can write

$$F_1(ct - x) + F_2(ct + x) = F_1(+x)\cos(\omega t + \theta) + F_2(-x)\cos(\omega t + \theta)$$

$$= [F_1(+x) + F_2(-x)]\cos(\omega t + \theta)$$

$$= [F_1(+x) + F_2(-x)]\operatorname{Re} e^{j(\omega t + \theta)} \qquad (4.12)$$

The exponential notation is familiar. We can drop the "real part" designation if we always keep in mind that the exponential designation is no more than a convenient shorthand and that for computations only the real part of the function should be used. Accordingly,

$$F_1(ct - x) + F_2(ct + x) = [F_1(+x) + F_2(-x)]e^{j(\omega t + \theta)} \qquad (4.13)$$

We can further simplify the above equation if we assume that the amplitude term $F_1 + F_2$ is a complex function, because in this case we can drop the phase angle θ without any loss of generality,

$$F_1(ct - x) + F_2(ct + x) = [F_1(+x) + F_2(-x)]e^{j\omega t} \qquad (4.14)$$

Consider further that in the steady state the wavefunction must be periodical in x as well as in t. We could thus write $F_1(+x) = F_1 \exp(-jkx)$ and $F_2(-x) = F_2 \exp(jkx)$ where k is a constant to be determined. Thus

$$
\begin{aligned}
F_1(ct - x) + F_2(ct + x) &= (F_1 e^{-jkx} + F_2 e^{jkx})e^{j\omega t} \\
&= F_1 e^{j(\omega t - kx)} + F_2 e^{j(\omega t + kx)} \qquad (4.15) \\
&= F_1 e^{jk(\omega t/k - x)} + F_2 e^{jk(\omega t/k + x)}
\end{aligned}
$$

This equation can be true only if

$$ct - x = \frac{\omega}{k}t - x \qquad \text{and} \qquad ct + x = \frac{\omega}{k}t + x \qquad (4.16)$$

or what is equivalent

$$c = \frac{\omega}{k} \qquad \text{or} \qquad k = \frac{\omega}{c} = \frac{2\pi f}{c} = \frac{2\pi}{\lambda} \qquad (4.17)$$

where k is designated as the wave number, while λ is the wavelength. It goes without saying that the exponential representation of the functions periodic in distance as well as those periodic in time is again the usual shorthand; for computational purposes the real part should be used.

Note that we did not specify the quantity represented by F. The functional form that we derived for a sinusoidal plane wave applies to particle displacement, velocity, pressure, or density in the wave. Thus if pressure is the quantity of interest then the general solution can be written as

$$p(x,t) = p_1 e^{jk(ct - x)} + p_2 e^{jk(ct + x)} \qquad (4.18)$$

We now clearly recognize the meaning of this description. The total pressure at x and t is the sum of a pressure wave traveling away from the source and one traveling toward the source with velocity c. Both waveforms are sinusoidal and have the frequency $\omega = kc$.

It might be a good idea to stop now and review some of the assumptions that were made in the derivation of the one-dimensional wave equation,

$$\frac{\partial^2 \theta}{\partial t^2} = c^2 \frac{\partial^2 \theta}{\partial x^2}$$

Recall that in order to obtain this equation we assumed that the change in density and the change in pressure due to the disturbance were much smaller than the resting density or resting pressure, respectively. That is, we wrote $\rho_0 \gg \rho_e$ and $\rho_0 \gg \rho_e$. These assumptions put a restriction on the intensity of the wave which under usual circumstances is not severe. Thus for wave propagation in the cochlea for moderate driving intensities one feels intuitively that the above inequalities are satisfied. At the upper limits of the intensity range for hearing, however, the assumptions of very small dynamic changes in pressure or density must be examined. Let us work with the inequality for density $\rho_e \ll \rho_0$. By definition $\rho = \rho_0 + \rho_e = \rho_0 + s\rho_0 = \rho_0 (1 + s)$. In this equation s is given the name condensation (strain); it expresses the increase in density per unit initial density. This is a dimensionless quantity, and it can alternatively be defined as the fractional deformation of the medium. That is, if the displacement of an elementary particle is denoted by ξ then by definition

$$s = -\frac{\partial \xi}{\partial x} \tag{4.19}$$

The inequality $\rho_e \ll \rho_0$ can be rewritten using the definition of condensation (s) as follows:

$$s \ll 1$$

Thus we can use this criterion for the acceptability of the simple wave equation in describing an acoustic phenomenon. Let us now test this criterion for the cochlea. At 140 dB SPL the approximate amplitude of the vibration of the stapes footplate is 10^{-3} cm. This is then equal to the amplitude of the fluid particles in the immediate vicinity of the footplate. If the stapes executes a harmonic motion, its displacement can be expressed as

$$x_s = A \sin(\omega t - kx) \tag{4.20}$$

Since $\xi = x_s$, we can obtain the condensation as

$$s = -\frac{\partial \xi}{\partial x} = -kA \cos(\omega t - kx)$$

The maximum condensation is then

$$s_{max} = kA = 2\pi A f/c \tag{4.21}$$

Assuming $f = 10^3$ Hz and a sound velocity in the cochlear fluid of 1.4×10^5 cm/second, and using $A = 10^{-3}$, we obtain $s_{max} = 4.5 \times 10^{-5}$, which is obviously much less than unity. It appears then that even at the highest sound levels the approximations involved in the derivation of the simple wave equation have validity. Note that s_{max} increases with frequency but that A decreases with frequency. Thus the above calculation is appropriate for testing the general validity of the small signal approximation for the cochlea.

B. The Effect of Viscosity

When the force equation [Eq. (4.5)] was derived, the tacit assumption was that the only internal force that resists the externally applied pressure is due to the inertia of the fluid element. This assumption yielded the wave equation as a final result, the solution of which, as we have seen, is satisfied by any function with argument $(ct \mp x)$. This solution implies a disturbance traveling in the $\pm x$ direction with a velocity of c and *without* a change in shape or magnitude. The implication is that a plane wave would propagate to an infinite distance without any decrease in magnitude. One feels that in general such a situation cannot arise and that such lossless propagation can only be an approximation of an actual physical situation. In reality sound waves in a liquid propagate with some loss, and the loss is due to a property of real liquids which is called viscosity. Viscosity expresses the friction that exists between layers of fluid that move with respect to one another. The magnitude of viscous force is proportional to fluid velocity. The coefficient of proportionality is called the coefficient of viscosity (μ), and its dimension is grams per centimeter second. The coefficient of viscosity depends on the nature of the fluid in question and on the temperature. For water at $10°C$, $\mu = 0.013$ CGS units.

One consequence of taking viscosity into account is that the relationship

$$c^2 = p_e / \rho_e$$

cannot be considered valid any longer. This relationship implies that a pressure change is followed by a density change instantaneously. In reality there is some time lag between such changes, and thus the relationship between p_e and ρ_e is more complex than a simple proportionality. The time lag can be taken into account if we write

$$p_e = c^2 \rho_e + R \dot{\rho}_e \tag{4.22}$$

With this relationship one can derive an equation for particle displacement as follows:

$$\frac{\partial^2 \xi}{\partial t^2} = c^2 \frac{\partial^2 \xi}{\partial x^2} + R \frac{\partial^2 \dot{\xi}}{\partial x^2} \tag{4.23}$$

Remember now that the simple wave equation for particle displacement has the form

$$\frac{\partial^2 \xi}{\partial t^2} = c^2 \frac{\partial^2 \xi}{\partial x^2} \qquad (4.24)$$

Clearly, Eq. (4.23) is a generalized form of the wave equation, where the expression

$$R \frac{\partial^2 \xi}{\partial x^2}$$

can be construed as a correction term, which takes the effect of viscosity into account. When we restrict our attention to the harmonic case, i.e., when $\xi = Xe^{j\omega t}$, the above equation can be written as

$$-\omega^2 X = c^2 \frac{d^2 X}{dx^2} + j\omega R \frac{d^2 X}{dx^2} = (c^2 + j\omega R) \frac{d^2 X}{dx^2} \qquad (4.25)$$

If we substitute

$$n^2 = -\omega^2 / (c^2 + j\omega R) \qquad (4.26)$$

then the equation is in the form

$$\frac{d^2 X}{dx^2} = +n^2 X \qquad (4.27)$$

The general solution of this differential equation is

$$X = Ae^{nx} + Be^{-nx} \qquad (4.28)$$

which represents the sum of two complex waves traveling in opposite directions with attenuation α and phase shift β per unit length, where

$$n = \alpha + j\beta \qquad (4.29)$$

The quantities A and B are complex and depend on the boundary conditions.

C. Deep-Water versus Shallow-Water Waves

It is now appropriate to discuss the conditions under which it is proper to assume that wave propagation takes place in one direction only. In other words, when is the one-dimensional wave equation an adequate description of the physical situation of interest? Probably the most instructive way to introduce this subject is to study, very briefly, the differences between so-called shallow-water waves and deep-water waves (Lamb, 1945; Ranke, 1950; Zwislocki, 1953).

Let us assume that we have a water surface of infinite extent. For simplicity, let us take the case in which wave propagation takes place in the x

direction only; i.e., we have wavefronts of infinite length parallel with the z axis propagating in the x direction. The y coordinate is perpendicular to the surface, which is taken at $y = 0$. We can write the continuity equation exactly as we did before if velocity in the x direction is u, and in the y direction is v.

$$\frac{\partial u}{\partial x} + \frac{\partial v}{\partial y} = 0 \qquad (4.30)$$

where the fluid is assumed to be incompressible, i.e., $\partial \rho / \partial t = 0$. Forces on an elementary liquid volume now act in both x and y directions. In the x direction the force due to a pressure difference is balanced by an inertial force. Thus

$$\rho \frac{\partial u}{\partial t} = - \frac{\partial p}{\partial x} \qquad (4.31)$$

In the y direction the gravitational force is also effective. Thus

$$\rho \frac{\partial v}{\partial t} = - \frac{\partial p}{\partial y} + g\rho \qquad (4.32)$$

where g is the constant of gravity. When these equations are solved together with appropriate boundary conditions, one can obtain the relationship

$$\omega^2 = gk \tanh k(h + y) \qquad (4.33)$$

where h is the depth of the fluid. At the surface $y = 0$, and thus

$$\omega^2 = gk \tanh kh \qquad (4.34)$$

In order to see some interesting relationships let us introduce the wavelength λ, by noting that

$$k = 2\pi / \lambda$$

Thus

$$\omega^2 = \frac{g2\pi}{\lambda} \tanh \frac{2\pi h}{\lambda} \qquad (4.35)$$

We are interested in two limiting cases. First, when the wavelength is much smaller than the depth of the fluid, i.e., when $2\pi h / \lambda \gg 1$, we can approximate $\tanh (2\pi h / \lambda)$ by unity. Then

$$\omega^2 = 2\pi g / \lambda = gk$$

By definition the velocity of propagation is equal to

$$c = \frac{\omega}{k} = \frac{(gk)^{1/2}}{k} = \left(\frac{g}{k}\right)^{1/2} = \left(\frac{g\lambda}{2\pi}\right)^{1/2} \qquad (4.36)$$

This implies the very important result that in deep water the velocity of propagation depends on the wavelength. Consequently, if a complex wavefront starts to propagate from a given point then its wave shape is not maintained, because its different frequency components propagate with different speeds. This is a condition of a *dispersive* wave. The opposite situation, that is, when $\lambda \gg h$, is also of great interest. This is the condition of wave propagation in very shallow water. When $\lambda \gg h$ we can approximate ω^2,

$$\omega^2 = gk \cdot kh = gk^2 h \qquad \text{or} \qquad c^2 k^2 = gk^2 h \qquad c = (gh)^{1/2} \qquad (4.37)$$

Such approximation is possible for $\tanh \theta \simeq \theta$ for $\theta \to 0$. We see that in this situation the propagation velocity no longer depends on the wavelength. It is, however, a function of the water depth.

One final comment concerns the vertical and horizontal velocity components that can now be shown to be

$$|v| = Ck \sinh k(h + y)$$

$$|u| = Ck \cosh k(h + y) \qquad (4.38)$$

In shallow water where $h + y$ is small, $\sinh k(h + y) \approx k(h + y)$ and $\cosh k(h + y) \approx 1$. Thus in this situation,

$$|v| \approx Ck^2(h + y) \approx 0$$

$$|u| \approx Ck \qquad (4.39)$$

This is a noteworthy result, for the facts that the vertical velocity component is negligible and the horizontal component is independent of the depth imply that in shallow water a one-dimensional treatment of the problem is adequate. This is of course a great simplification. All theoretical investigators except one (Ranke, 1942, 1950) made the assumption that the lengths of the waves traveling in the cochlea are sufficiently greater than the depth of the cochlear canal, so that a "long-wave" approximation is valid in this case. Such an assumption then implies that fluid movement perpendicular to the cochlear partition is ignored and the entire problem is treated as one dimensional. Aside from the saving afforded by the elimination of one variable from the partial differential equations, some further advantages also accrue from the one-dimensional treatment. The differential equations of fluid motion are solved by considering appropriate boundary conditions. In the case of one-dimensional treatment these boundary conditions simply describe the acoustic properties of the cochlear windows and that of the helicotrema. If two-dimensional treatment is necessary then, aside from these boundary conditions, one must also consider the acoustic properties of the cochlear partition, which in this case behaves as an elastic, moving boundary. It is intuitively felt that the mathematical treatment of such a case would be very difficult.

This is indeed the case, so much so that no complete solution of the two-dimensional problem is available as yet. In the one-dimensional case we can more easily include the properties of the cochlear partition in the solution, as will be seen below.

II. Analytical Treatment of Cochlear Dynamics

There are some common simplifications that were used by all who attempted to derive mathematical models for the operation of the cochlea. Two such common simplifications involve the shape of the cochlear canal and the nature of the cochlear partition. While the cochlea is actually coiled, in the mathematical treatment it is always* assumed to be a straight canal with rigid boundaries. The canal is divided into two compartments by the cochlear partition, which is commonly assumed to be one simple elastic sheet. In reality, of course, the cochlear partition is an extremely complex structure, roughly triangular, bounded by the basilar and Reissner's membranes, and filled with viscous fluid. In addition, the structures of the organ of Corti and the tectorial membrane contribute to the complexity. The reason that in the treatment of cochlear dynamics this entire partition is handled as a single unit is that, first, it would be mathematically untractable to do otherwise and, second, some experiments of von Békésy (1949) justify our doing so. Von Békésy observed under stroboscopic illumination that the basilar membrane and Reissner's membrane vibrate in phase at frequencies below 3000 Hz. This implies that the entire partition moves as one unit, and consequently one is justified in treating it as a single elastic layer.

A. Derivation of the Wave Equation

In the pages that follow, a standard analytic treatment of cochlear dynamics is given. The assumptions on which the derivation is based are those discussed above. That is, the cochlea is taken to be uncoiled and rigid walled, and the cochlear partition is assumed to be a single layer of tissue. Most important is the assumption that the wavelength of vibrations in the cochlea is large compared with the transversal dimensions of the cochlear canal. It is remembered that this hypothesis allows us to develop a one-dimensional treatment. Consequently the only dependence on space coordinates of any variable is restricted to one such coordinate along the long axis of the cochlea. In the initial derivation no additional simplifying restrictions are made. Thus we do not take the cochlear fluids as being incompressible; neither do we assume that viscous damping in the fluid is negligible. These

* The article of Huxley (1969) is an exception, for he considered, in fact emphasized, the curvature of the cochlear canal.

simplifications are made only after a general system equation is obtained.

One very important property of this derivation, in common with all others in the literature, is that an equation describing the properties of the cochlear partition is not derived in terms of a description for a vibrating membrane or plate. Instead, the interaction between membrane and fluid is taken into account by assuming that a balance of forces exists at the membrane–fluid interface. In other words, the physical properties of the partition are expressed by its acoustic impedance per unit length, and then a relationship between membrane motion and fluid dynamics is obtained through the well-known $p = Zv$ equation, where p is pressure acting on the impedance (i.e., fluid pressure), and v is volume velocity (i.e., membrane velocity). A more general treatment would use an equation of motion derived from the basic properties (anatomical and structural) of the partition. This equation of motion, combined with the equations describing the hydro-dynamic conditions of the fluid, would provide the solution.

Justified simplifications and assumptions will be explained as the deriva-tion proceeds. We shall start by setting up the fluid equations, one for the continuity condition and the other for the equilibrium of forces.

In Fig. 4.1 we find the geometrical configuration for the cochlear duct on the basis of which the equation of motion of the cochlear partition is derived.

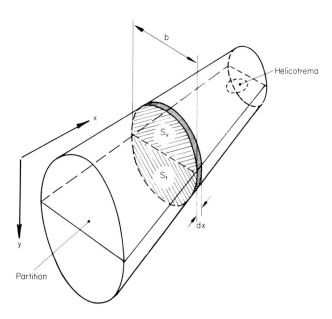

Fig. 4.1. Simplified geometry of the cochlea and volume elements in scalae vestibuli ($S_v\ dx$) and tympani ($S_t\ dx$).

Parameters such as S_v, S_t, and b are functions of x. Similar arguments apply to the volume elements $S_v \, dx$ and $S_t \, dx$. Let us now establish the mass flow conditions for the volume element shown in Fig. 4.2.

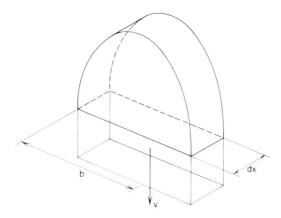

Fig. 4.2. Schematic showing the change in volume due to the up and down motion of the partition. For simplicity the partition is assumed to move without change in shape; that is, linear distention is used.

Assume that the velocity of a fluid element at distance x is u_v. Then the mass inflow per unit time is

$$u_v S_v \rho$$

where ρ is the fluid density at x. The outgoing mass per unit time through the surface at $x + dx$ is

$$\left(u_v + \frac{\partial u_v}{\partial x} dx \right) \left(S_v + \frac{\partial S_v}{\partial x} dx \right) \left(\rho + \frac{\partial \rho}{\partial x} dx \right) \tag{4.40}$$

because u_v, S_v, and ρ are all functions of the distance. This expression can be written as

$$u_v S_v \rho + \frac{\partial}{\partial x} (u_v S_v \rho) dx \tag{4.41}$$

if higher-order terms in dx are neglected. Then the net change of mass per unit time in this volume element due to fluid flow in the x direction is

$$-\frac{\partial}{\partial x} (u_v S_v \rho) dx \tag{4.42}$$

There is an additional change in mass in this volume element due to the

where u_v is the particle velocity in the x direction. Applying Newton's second law gives the inertial force

$$\frac{\partial}{\partial t} [(\rho S_v \, dx) u_v] \tag{4.54}$$

This is further equal to

$$S_v \frac{\partial (\rho u_v)}{\partial t} \, dx \tag{4.55}$$

Using $\rho = \rho_0 + \rho_e$ and the approximation $\rho \simeq \rho_0$, we obtain for the inertial force

$$S_v \rho_0 \frac{\partial u_v}{\partial t} \, dx \tag{4.56}$$

In a viscous fluid, force is exerted on moving particles in proportion to their velocity. The proportionality is expressed as

$$\text{Force} = (R_v S_v) u_v \, dx \tag{4.57}$$

where $(R_v S_v)$ is the resistance of the scala vestibuli per unit length; its dimensions are rayls/cm = dynes second/cm^4.

We can now write an equation for the balance of forces acting on the element $S_v \, dx$,

$$S_v \rho_0 \frac{\partial u_v}{\partial t} \, dx + S_v R_v u_v \, dx + \frac{\partial (p_v S_v)}{\partial x} \, dx = 0 \tag{4.58}$$

Let us consider the term

$$\frac{\partial (p_v S_v)}{\partial x}$$

Completing the differentiation, we obtain

$$S_v \frac{\partial p_v}{\partial x} + p_v \frac{\partial S_v}{\partial x} \tag{4.59}$$

While S_v is a function of x, it can be assumed that it varies slowly with distance, in which case

$$\frac{\partial S_v}{\partial x} \approx 0$$

Assuming this, the equation for the balance of forces can be simplified to

$$S_v \rho_0 \frac{\partial u_v}{\partial t} \, dx + S_v R_v u_v \, dx = -S_v \frac{\partial p_v}{\partial x} \, dx \tag{4.60}$$

which yields the following form:

$$\rho_0 \frac{\partial u_v}{\partial t} + R_v u_v = -\frac{\partial p_v}{\partial x} \qquad (4.61)$$

Consider now that the pressure p_v is the sum of the equilibrium pressure (p_0) and the excess pressure (p_{ve}) which is due to the disturbance:

$$p_v = p_0 + p_{ve}$$

This then results in

$$\frac{\partial p_v}{\partial x} = \frac{\partial p_{ve}}{\partial x} \qquad (4.62)$$

and further

$$\rho_0 \frac{\partial u_v}{\partial t} + R_v u_v = -\frac{\partial p_{ve}}{\partial x} \qquad (4.63)$$

We obtained the continuity equation before in the form

$$S_v \frac{\partial \rho_{ve}}{\partial t} + vb\rho_0 + \frac{\partial (u_v S_v)}{\partial x} \rho_0 = 0 \qquad (4.64)$$

Here again we are justified in substituting $S_v(\partial u_v/\partial x)$ in place of $\partial(u_v S_v)/\partial x$ because $\partial S_v/\partial x$ is assumed to be vanishingly small. Then we have the pair of equations for the scala vestibuli

$$\rho_0 \dot{u}_v + R_v u_v = -\frac{\partial p_{ve}}{\partial x} \qquad (4.65)$$

$$S_v \dot{\rho}_{ve} + \rho_0 vb + \rho_0 S_v \frac{\partial u_v}{\partial x} = 0 \qquad (4.66)$$

where the notational substitution $\dot{u}_v = \partial u_v/\partial t$ and $\dot{\rho}_{ve} = \partial \rho_{ve}/\partial t$ is made.

Let us now take the derivative of Eq. (4.65) with respect to x and the Eq. (4.66) with respect to t.

$$\rho_0 \frac{\partial \dot{u}_v}{\partial x} + \frac{\partial}{\partial x}(R_v u_v) = -\frac{\partial^2 p_{ve}}{\partial x^2}$$

$$\frac{S_v}{\rho_0} \ddot{\rho}_{ve} + b\dot{v} + S_v \frac{\partial \dot{u}_v}{\partial x} = 0$$

Then

$$\rho_0 \frac{\partial \dot{u}_v}{\partial x} + R_v \frac{\partial u_v}{\partial x} = -\frac{\partial^2 p_{ve}}{\partial x^2} \qquad (4.67a)$$

$$\frac{S_v}{\rho_0} \ddot{\rho}_{ve} + b\dot{v} + S_v \frac{\partial \dot{u}_v}{\partial x} = 0 \qquad (4.67b)$$

We can eliminate u_v and $\dot{u}_v$ from Eq. (4.67a), but first note that

$$\frac{\partial}{\partial x}(R_v u_v) \simeq R_v \frac{\partial u_v}{\partial x} \tag{4.68}$$

if we assume that R_v varies very slowly as a function of x, i.e., if

$$\frac{\partial R_v}{\partial x} \approx 0$$

This substitution was made in Eq. (4.67a).

$$\frac{\partial \dot{u}_v}{\partial x} = -\frac{1}{\rho_0}\ddot{p}_{ve} - \frac{b}{S_v}\dot{v} \tag{4.69}$$

This equation can be integrated to yield

$$\frac{\partial u_v}{\partial x} = -\frac{1}{\rho_0}\dot{p}_{ve} - \frac{b}{S_v}v \tag{4.70}$$

Then

$$-\rho_0\left(\frac{1}{\rho_0}\ddot{p}_{ve} + \frac{b}{S_v}\dot{v}\right) - R_v\left(\frac{1}{\rho_0}\dot{p}_{ve} + \frac{b}{S_v}v\right) = -\frac{\partial^2 p_{ve}}{\partial x^2} \tag{4.71}$$

A similar equation for the scala tympani is in the form

$$-\rho_0\left(\frac{1}{\rho_0}\ddot{p}_{te} - \frac{b}{S_t}\dot{v}\right) - R_t\left(\frac{1}{\rho_0}\dot{p}_{te} - \frac{b}{S_t}v\right) = -\frac{\partial^2 p_{te}}{\partial x^2} \tag{4.72}$$

If Eq. (4.72) is subtracted from Eq. (4.71) then we obtain

$$-(\ddot{p}_{ve} - \ddot{p}_{te}) - \rho_0 b\left(\frac{1}{S_v} + \frac{1}{S_t}\right)\dot{v} - \frac{1}{\rho_0}(R_v\dot{p}_{ve} - R_t\dot{p}_{te}) - b\left(\frac{R_v}{S_v} + \frac{R_t}{S_t}\right)v$$

$$= -\frac{\partial^2 p_{ve}}{\partial x^2} + \frac{\partial^2 p_{te}}{\partial x^2} \tag{4.73}$$

Let us now note that by definition

$$c^2 = p_e/\rho_e \tag{4.74}$$

Thus we can write

$$-\frac{1}{c^2}(\ddot{p}_{ve} - \ddot{p}_{te}) - \rho_0 b\left(\frac{1}{S_v} + \frac{1}{S_t}\right)\dot{v} - \frac{1}{\rho_0 c^2}(R_v\dot{p}_{ve} - R_t\dot{p}_{te}) - b\left(\frac{R_v}{S_v} + \frac{R_t}{S_t}\right)v$$

$$= -\frac{\partial^2 p_{ve}}{\partial x^2} + \frac{\partial^2 p_{te}}{\partial x^2} \tag{4.75}$$

In order to proceed we now make the reasonable (as it will be seen later) approximation of

$$R_v = R_t = R$$

Then our equation is in the form

$$-\frac{1}{c^2}(\ddot{p}_{ve} - \ddot{p}_{te}) - \rho_0 b\left(\frac{1}{S_v} + \frac{1}{S_t}\right)\dot{v} - \frac{R}{\rho_0 c^2}(\dot{p}_{ve} - \dot{p}_{te}) - bR\left(\frac{1}{S_v} + \frac{1}{S_t}\right)v$$

$$= -\frac{\partial^2 p_{ve}}{\partial x^2} + \frac{\partial^2 p_{te}}{\partial x^2} \qquad (4.76)$$

Introduce

$$p = p_{ve} - p_{te} \quad \text{and} \quad \frac{1}{S} = \frac{1}{S_v} + \frac{1}{S_t} \qquad (4.77)$$

Then

$$\frac{\ddot{p}}{c^2} + \frac{\rho_0 b}{S}\dot{v} + \frac{R}{\rho_0 c^2}\dot{p} + \frac{bR}{S}v = \frac{\partial^2 p}{\partial x^2} \qquad (4.78)$$

Let us now consider that we can obtain a relationship between p and v if we realize that pressure is equal to volume velocity times acoustic impedance. Thus

$$p = bvZ$$

where Z is the acoustic impedance of the cochlear partition per unit length, and bv is the volume velocity of a unit length of the partition. We can thus write

$$\frac{\ddot{p}}{c^2} + \frac{\rho_0 b}{S}\frac{1}{bZ}\dot{p} + \frac{R}{\rho_0 c^2}\dot{p} + \frac{bR}{S}\frac{1}{bZ}p = \frac{\partial^2 p}{\partial x^2} \qquad (4.79)$$

Collecting terms yields

$$\frac{\ddot{p}}{c^2} + \left(\frac{\rho_0}{SZ} + \frac{R}{\rho_0 c^2}\right)\dot{p} + \frac{R}{SZ}p = \frac{\partial^2 p}{\partial x^2} \qquad (4.80)$$

Assuming harmonic motion, i.e., $p = Pe^{j\omega t}$,

$$-\frac{\omega^2}{c^2}P + j\omega\left(\frac{\rho_0}{SZ} + \frac{R}{\rho_0 c^2}\right)P + \frac{R}{SZ}P = \frac{d^2 P}{dx^2} \qquad (4.81)$$

or, after rewriting,

$$-\left(\frac{\omega^2}{c^2} - j\omega\frac{\rho_0}{SZ}\right) + R\left(\frac{1}{SZ} + j\omega\frac{1}{\rho_0 c^2}\right) = \frac{1}{P}\frac{d^2 P}{dx^2} \qquad (4.82)$$

By using the relationship $p = Zbv$, we can obtain an equation in identical form that describes the velocity of the cochlear partition as a function of x and b.

$$\frac{\ddot{v}}{c^2} + \left(\frac{\rho_0}{SZ} + \frac{R}{\rho_0 c^2}\right)\dot{v} + \frac{R}{SZ}\,v = \frac{\partial^2 v}{\partial x^2} \tag{4.83}$$

and for the harmonic case, when $v = Ve^{j\omega t}$,

$$-\left(\frac{\omega^2}{c^2} - j\omega\,\frac{\rho_0}{SZ}\right) + R\left(\frac{1}{SZ} + j\omega\,\frac{1}{\rho_0 c^2}\right) = \frac{1}{V}\frac{d^2 V}{dx^2} \tag{4.84}$$

The ultimately desired solution of our problem is the displacement versus distance from the stapes: $y(x)$ function. This can be obtained by first solving the above differential equation for the partition velocity (v) and then integrating the solution with respect to time, since

$$y = \int_0^t v\,dt \tag{4.85}$$

Thus in the harmonic case,

$$Y = V/j\omega$$

Since R, S, and Z are all functions of distance, the differential equation has no general solution. One has two possible avenues of attack. Following Zwislocki (1950, 1965) it is possible to assume analytic functions for R, Z, and S and then simplify conditions so that an actual solution can be obtained, provided that only steady-state conditions are considered. Another possibility is to use numerical methods to obtain a solution.

We should consider first the effects of two possible simplifications which are often invoked. First, if we neglect viscosity effects of the cochlear fluids, then, since this implies $R = 0$, the equation has the form

$$-\frac{\omega^2}{c^2} + j\omega\,\frac{\rho_0}{SZ} = \frac{1}{P}\frac{d^2 P}{dx^2}$$

or

$$-\frac{\omega^2}{c^2}\left(1 - j\,\frac{\rho_0 c^2}{SZ\omega}\right) = \frac{1}{P}\frac{d^2 P}{dx^2} \tag{4.86}$$

This equation is essentially that which was obtained by Peterson and Bogert (1950). Another possible simplification is to assume that the cochlear fluid is incompressible; that is, $\partial\rho/\partial t = 0$. Looking back on the derivation we note that the terms $(\omega^2/c^2)P$ and $j\omega(R/\rho_0 c^2)P$ would have disappeared if the $\partial\rho/\partial t = 0$ assumption had been made early in the derivation. This can also be seen, for the $\partial\rho/\partial t = 0$ assumption implies infinite sound propagation velocity. Thus the two terms that contain c^2 in their denominators would vanish. The final equation in this case has the form

$$\frac{R + j\omega\rho_0}{SZ} = \frac{1}{P}\frac{d^2P}{dx^2} \tag{4.87}$$

This equation is like that derived by Zwislocki (1948, 1950, 1965). If one neglects both the viscosity and compressibility of the cochlear fluid then the equation assumes the particularly simple form

$$j\omega\frac{\rho_0}{SZ} = \frac{1}{P}\frac{d^2P}{dx^2} \tag{4.88}$$

This is essentially the equation that was considered, and solved numerically, by Fletcher (1953).

Note that the general equation, as well as all its simplified forms, is in the familiar form

$$\frac{d^2P}{dx^2} = n^2P \tag{4.89}$$

Clearly n^2 is a complex function of x, but if for a moment we assume that n^2 is *not* dependent on the distance, then we have an inkling of the type of solution that might satisfy this equation. In such a situation the solution is

$$P = Ae^{nx} + Be^{-nx} \tag{4.90}$$

which is the sum of two propagating waves suffering both attenuation and phase shift. Intuitively we feel that in the actual situation when $n^2 = n^2(x)$ we still will have two waves as the solution. Again these would travel in opposing directions and their attenuation and phase shift would be dependent on the distance x. Whether both of these waves contribute to the final wave pattern is determined by the boundary conditions that are applicable to the system.

Probably the most profitable way to proceed from this point is to follow the solution of one of the above simplified wave equations. The most complete solutions are those of Zwislocki and Peterson and Bogert. We shall study Zwislocki's solution because he utilized various physical measurements of von Békésy in order to affix functional and numerical values to the parameters in the equations, so as to provide the most realistic solutions. It should be noted in addition that Zwislocki did not use a curve fitting technique in obtaining the solution to the cochlear vibration problem. Instead he used basic physical considerations and actual measurements of parameters to establish quantitative relationships and then compared his results to experimental observations on the pattern of vibrations made by von Békésy (1947, 1949). He then made small final adjustments of some parameters to achieve good harmony between the theoretical and experimental results. Another approach would be to set up the general equation and adjust its parameters so that the solution should agree with experimental observations. An example of the latter approach of deriving cochlear models is the work by Klatt (1964). A third approach, less physically oriented, is straight curve fitting. According to this method the experimental results, such as von Békésy's displacement versus place versus frequency curves, are taken as input–output functions, where the output is partition displacement and the input is stapes displacement. A transfer function is then fitted to the curve, the inverse Laplace transform of which can provide the time function of cochlear partition displacement. This approach was used by Flanagan (1962), Siebert (1962), and Laszlo (1968).

After discussing Zwislocki's approach quite thoroughly, we shall briefly treat some interesting ideas set forth by Peterson and Bogert. The latter authors studied two wave patterns; one was compressional wave motion in the cochlear fluid, the other being the usual transversal vibration of the cochlear partition. The comparison of these two patterns is quite illuminating.

B. PARAMETERS OF THE WAVE EQUATION

The reader will recall that if the cochlear fluid is assumed to be incompressible and if viscosity is taken into account, the following equation for the harmonic pressure difference across the cochlear partition results:

$$\frac{R + j\omega\rho_0}{SZ} = \frac{1}{P}\frac{d^2P}{dx^2} \tag{4.91}$$

In this equation the parameters R, S, and Z are all functions of x, and consequently a general solution is not available. The first task is to obtain the functional relationships $R = R(x)$, $S = S(x)$, and $Z = Z(x)$ in analytic form so that after substitution into the original equation a solution can be attempted. In the derivation of these analytic functions we shall closely follow the arguments of Zwislocki, particularly his 1965 treatment of the problem.

1. Cross-Sectional Area of the Scalae

The easiest parameter to obtain is the cross-sectional area of the cochlear duct. In Fig. 4.3 some data are shown for the dependence of $S_v + S_t$ on the distance from the stapes, x. Aside from the data points, a straight-line approximation is shown; this has the form $S_v + S_t = 0.05e^{-0.5x}$. If for simplicity one assumes that $S_v = S_t$ (which is clearly a crude approximation), then from the definition $S = S_v S_t/(S_v + S_t)$ one obtains $S = (S_v + S_t)/4$. Consequently

$$S = 0.0125e^{-0.5x} = S_0 e^{-ax} \tag{4.92}$$

This expression is in the appropriate form for substitution into Eq. (4.91).

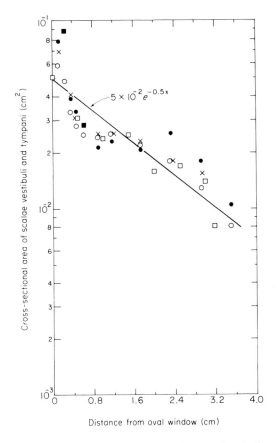

Fig. 4.3. Cross-sectional area of scalae vestibuli and tympani as the function of distance from the oval window. The straight line is a mathematical approximation. (From Zwislocki, 1965, p. 28.)

2. Resistance of the Scalae

Note that the functional form of S was established by fitting an analytic function to data points obtained from anatomical measurements. In contrast, the frictional fluid resistance (viscosity) can be obtained on theoretical grounds.

The derivation is fairly involved and it would not be of great interest to most readers. The result of the appropriate derivation is

$$\frac{1}{U}\frac{\partial P}{\partial x} = -\left\{\frac{(2\mu\rho\omega)^{1/2}}{a} + j\left[\rho\omega + \frac{(2\mu\rho\omega)^{1/2}}{a}\right]\right\} \tag{4.93}$$

where μ is the coefficient of viscosity and a is the radius of the cochlear canal. Note that the expression in braces is a term expressing specific acoustic impedance per unit length, that is, pressure gradient per particle velocity. This impedance describes the opposition to a sound wave that travels in a relatively narrow tube filled with viscous fluid. It is interesting to note that the effect of viscosity is manifested by both resistive and reactive terms. It is the frictional term that is of great interest to us. This resistance per unit length then is written as

$$R = (2\mu\rho\omega)^{1/2}/a \tag{4.94}$$

or, alternatively, if the surface area $S = \pi a^2$, then

$$R = (2\pi\mu\rho\omega/S)^{1/2} \tag{4.95}$$

We need to determine the viscous resistance for both cochlear scalae. It is probably permissible to assume equal cross-sectional areas for scala tympani and scala vestibuli, which leads to equal frictional fluid resistance functions for both scalae. We can see from Eq. (4.75) that

$$\frac{R}{S} = \frac{R_t}{S_t} + \frac{R_v}{S_v}$$

and

$$S = S_v S_t/(S_v + S_t) \simeq S_t/2 \simeq S_v/2$$

Consequently

$$R = S\left(\frac{R_v}{S_v} + \frac{R_t}{S_t}\right) \simeq S \cdot 2\frac{R_v}{S_v} \simeq S \cdot 2\frac{R}{S_t} \simeq \frac{S_v}{2}2\frac{R_v}{S_v} \simeq R_v \simeq R_t \tag{4.96}$$

Then R can be obtained from Eq. (4.95) if we assume that the closest approximation of the cross-sectional area can be obtained as the average area of the scala vestibuli and scala tympani, i.e., if we substitute $S = S' = (S_v + S_t)/2$,

$$R = \left(\frac{4\pi\mu\rho\omega}{S_v + S_t}\right)^{1/2} \tag{4.97}$$

We already obtained an expression for $(S_v + S_t)/4$ in Eq. (4.92). After substitution we get the final result,

$$R = \left(\frac{\pi\mu\rho\omega}{S_0 e^{-ax}}\right)^{1/2} = \left(\frac{\pi\rho\mu}{S_0}\right)^{1/2}\omega^{1/2}\,e^{ax/2} \tag{4.98}$$

The coefficient in this equation can be computed if one considers that the coefficient of viscosity (μ) was measured by von Békésy (1960) and was found to have a value of 0.02 gm/cm second; the density of perilymph is very much like that of seawater, numerically $\rho = 1$ gm/cm^3; finally, we have already obtained $S_0 = 0.0125$. After substitution we obtain for the constant 2.24 gm/cm^3 second$^{1/2} = R_0$.

$$R = R_0 \omega^{1/2} \, e^{ax/2} \qquad (4.99)$$

where $a = 0.5$ cm^{-1}.

3. The Membrane Impedance

Now that expressions for $S = S(x)$ and $R = R(x)$ have been obtained the remaining task is to determine the membrane impedance $Z = Z(x)$. This is the step where the assumptions made by various model builders have been the most divergent. In general one can start by stating that any membrane element should possess equivalent mass, elasticity, and friction. If these quantities are denoted by $M = M(x)$, $C = C(x)$, and $R_m = R_m(x)$, and if steady-state conditions are assumed, then

$$Z(x) = R_m(x) + j[\omega M(x) - 1/\omega C(x)] \qquad (4.100)$$

This general form for the membrane impedance was assumed by almost all investigators, but considerable disagreement exists as to the relative importance of the various factors. Thus Kucharski (1930) and Peterson and Bogert (1950) considered the damping R_m as negligible, Reboul (1938) neglected both mass and friction, and Zwislocki (1948, 1953, and 1965) neglected the mass. Fletcher (1953), Ranke (1950), and Wansdronk (1962) took all three parameters into account.

a. Compliance. An analytic expression for the compliance function $C(x)$ was derived by Zwislocki (1965) on the basis of von Békésy's (1960, pp. 473–476) measurements of static elasticity of the cochlear partition. Von Békésy prepared fresh temporal bones for the measurement of static elasticity by affixing a slim rubber tube into the round window after opening the round-window membrane. The rubber tube was connected to a jar containing water. By raising or lowering the jar various fluid pressures could be exerted on the contents of the cochlea. Before measurements commenced, von Békésy closed the helicotrema with an agar–gelatine stopper in order to prevent static pressure equalization, that is, in order to be able to set up a pressure differential across the cochlear partition. After this maneuver pressure was exerted on the perilymph and the shape of deformation of the partition was carefully measured at various points along its length. From the shape of the deformation von Békésy calculated the volume displacements of individual sections of the cochlear partition having a length of 1 mm under 1 cm water pressure condition. His results along with a straight-line approximation to the data points made by Zwislocki are shown in Fig. 4.4. This is

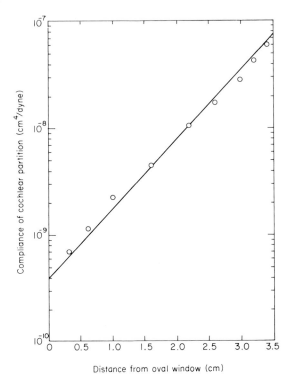

Fig. 4.4. Compliance of cochlear partition as the function of distance from the oval window. The points are from von Békésy's data, and the straight line is a mathematical approximation. (From Zwislocki, 1965, p. 30.)

a very significant plot, because it is the changing elasticity of the cochlear partition that is primarily responsible for the form of the vibratory patterns sustained in the cochlea. We see that the membrane elasticity is low at the stapes end and that it increases rapidly toward the helicotrema. The overall change in elasticity is over a hundredfold. The straight line in this semilogarithmic plot can be expressed analytically as follows:

$$C = C_0 e^{hx}$$

where $C_0 = 4 \times 10^{-10}$ cm^4/dyne, and $h = 1.5$ cm^{-1}.

Von Békésy's measurements of the coefficient of elasticity were static measurements; in other words, they determined the value of this coefficient at a number of points along the cochlear partition, but in all cases the determination was for static loading conditions. There is considerable evidence (McElhaney, 1966) that the coefficient of elasticity (Young's modulus) is dependent on the rate of loading in biological tissues. This simply means that at any point along the partition Young's modulus is frequency dependent. On the basis of McElhaney's measurements for muscle tissue, Allaire (1972) computed that the average Young's modulus over one cycle of a sinusoidal excursion is expressible as $E_0(1 + 2.3f^{0.14})$, where E_0 is the static value. The basilar membrane compliance C is related to the Young's modulus, and thus in precise calculations the above frequency-dependent expression should be utilized. Actually, the frequency dependence is relatively mild; between 100 and 10,000 Hz the change in Young's modulus is about twofold. Because of this, in the subsequent computations the frequency dependence of the partition stiffness is not taken into account.

b. Resistance. The resistive component of the membrane impedance, $R_m(x)$, was assumed to be independent of the distance by Zwislocki, again on the basis of some data that were gathered by von Békésy. Von Békésy (1960, pp. 459, 560) measured the speed of decay of the vibration of the cochlear partition when subjected to brief acoustic pulses or to tones switched on and off abruptly. He measured the ratios of two successive deflections of the partition in the same direction, and from these ratios he computed the so-called logarithmic decrement. This quantity is defined as $\delta = \log_e (A_1/A_2)$, where A_1 and A_2 are the two amplitudes in question. The logarithmic decrement of a decay process is characteristic of the magnitude of damping that is present in the oscillating system. The greater the damping, the larger the logarithmic decrement. Damping of course arises from dissipative forces, and consequently resistance in the system can be assessed with the aid of the logarithmic decrement.*

In von Békésy's measurements δ ranged from 1.4 to 1.8 for the entire frequency range and for all positions along the cochlear partition where measurements were made. The constancy of the logarithmic decrement implies that the damping does not change spatially in the cochlea. Thus it appears reasonable to take the resistive component of the membrane impedance (R_m), which is responsible for the damping, as independent of the distance x. Zwislocki assumed that $R_m = $ constant and adjusted its value so that his results would fit von Békésy's experimental data. The intuitively correct assumption that constant damping implies constant resistance is not

---

* The logarithmic decrement has the physical significance that it represents the number of periods of the decaying oscillation that are required for the amplitude to decrease to $1/e$ times its initial value. In terms of the damping constant (δ) of the system, the logarithmic decrement can be expressed as $\delta = 2\pi\zeta/(1 - \zeta^2)^{1/2}$.

completely proper on a theoretical basis. As a matter of fact, one can derive that

$$R_m = R_{mo}e^{-0.35x/2} = R_{mo}e^{-0.175x} \tag{4.101}$$

This expression indicates that the resistance decreases from base to apex. If a cochlear length of 3.0 cm is assumed then the change in resistance is approximately 1.25-fold. Considering that the change in elasticity over this same length is about 100-fold, the assumption that R_m is approximately constant over the length of the cochlear partition appears to be an excellent one.

c. Mass. Zwislocki considered the magnitude of the mass component as exceedingly small and he neglected it completely in his calculations. This maneuver should again be considered as a reasonable first approximation, made in order to render the mathematical expressions tractable. The following example will show that neglecting the mass does indeed appear to be a permissible procedure. In the impedance expression the imaginary component was written as

$$\omega M - 1/(\omega C)$$

The mass can be neglected if it can be shown that

$$\omega M \ll 1/(\omega C)$$

Let us take the arbitrary frequency of 4000 Hz and compute the values of ωM and $1/(\omega C)$ at the point where the 4000-Hz tone would create maximal disturbance in the cochlea. This point is at a distance of $x = 1.0$ cm from the stapes. Using Fletcher's (1953, p. 239) formula for the mass component, one can calculate that $\omega M = 16$ gm/cm^3 second at this point. Using the compliance value from von Békésy's experiments (Fig. 4.4) one computes that $1/(\omega C) = 2 \times 10^4$ gm/cm^3 second. Clearly in this case ignoring the mass is a perfectly justified procedure. At the beginning of the basilar membrane, i.e., at $x = 0$, the discrepancy between the mass and compliance components is even more pronounced, 0.5 versus 10^5. Thus the example indicates that it is the compliance of the cochlear partition that dominates the reactive component of that structure's impedance.

C. SOLUTION OF THE WAVE EQUATION

It is now possible to combine the various functional expressions obtained above for $R(x)$, $S(x)$, and $Z(x)$ with the pressure equation and to attempt a general solution of the resulting partial differential equation. To catalog the distance-dependent parameters

$$R(x) = R_0 \omega^{1/2} e^{ax/2}$$

$$S(x) = S_0 e^{-ax}$$

$$R_m(x) = R_{mo} e^{0.175x} \approx R_{mo}$$

$$M(x) \approx 0$$

$$C(x) = C_0 e^{hx} \tag{4.102}$$

After substituting these expressions into Eq. (4.91) we obtain

$$\frac{1}{P}\frac{d^2 P}{dx^2} = \frac{R + j\omega\rho_0}{SZ} = \frac{R_0 \omega^{1/2} e^{ax/2} + j\omega\rho_0}{S_0 e^{-ax}(R_m - je^{-hx}/\omega C_0)} \tag{4.103}$$

This differential equation is still too complex to yield an analytical solution. Of course, it would be relatively easy to obtain numerical (computer) solutions but, if at all possible, closed form, analytical solutions are preferable because of the physical insight they usually provide. As Zwislocki showed, an analytical solution can be obtained for the above equation, provided that further simplifications can be made. Specifically, it is assumed that $R_m \ll 1/\omega C$ in all regions of the cochlea where the amplitude of vibrations is substantial. That this approach is permissible can be shown with an example. We have already computed that at $f = 4 \times 10^3$ Hz, and at the location where the vibratory amplitude corresponding to this frequency is maximal, i.e. at $x = 1$ cm, $1/\omega C$ has the value of 2×10^4 CGS units. It can be shown that the actual expression for R_m is

$$R_m = 0.5 (M_0/C_0)^{1/2} e^{-0.175x} = 1.1 \times 10^2 e^{-0.175x} \tag{4.104}$$

Then at $x = 1$, $R_m = 92$ CGS units. This magnitude is clearly much smaller than the 20,000 CGS unit value of the reactive component. Thus the move to neglect the resistance as a first approximation appears to be justified.

The expression $1/[R_m + 1/(j\omega C)]$ can be written as $j\omega C/(1 + j\omega R_m C)$. Considering the above arguments on the relative size of R_m and $1/\omega C$, it is clear that $\omega R_m C \ll 1$. This allows us to expand $1/(1 + j\omega R_m C)$ into a series as follows:

$$\frac{j\omega C}{1 + j\omega R_m C} = j\omega C[1 - (j\omega R_m C) \pm \ldots] \tag{4.105}$$

As a first approximation, the above series can be truncated after its first two terms, yielding $j\omega C + \omega^2 R_m C^2$. This expression can now be substituted back into the differential equation:

$$\frac{1}{P}\frac{d^2 P}{dx^2} = \frac{R + j\omega\rho_0}{SZ} = \frac{R + j\omega\rho_0}{S}(j\omega C + \omega^2 R_m C^2)$$

$$= \frac{1}{S}\omega^2 \rho_0 C\left[\left(\frac{RR_m C}{\rho_0} - 1\right) + j\left(\frac{R}{\omega\rho_0} + \omega R_m C\right)\right] \tag{4.106}$$

In this equation the term $RR_m C/\rho_0$ is generally negligible compared to unity (at our usual frequency of 4000 Hz and point in the cochlea of $x = 1$ cm, the value of this term is 2.5×10^{-5}); thus as a further simplification we shall neglect it. Then our equation is in the form

$$-\frac{1}{P}\frac{d^2P}{dx^2} = \frac{\omega^2\rho_0 C}{S}\left[1-j\left(\omega R_m C + \frac{R}{\omega\rho_0}\right)\right] \tag{4.107}$$

In this form the equation is still troublesome, but if Zwislocki's arguments are heeded then the bracketed term can be considered as independent of x, in which case the solution is straightforward. The justification for assuming that the bracketed term is independent of the distance lies in the observation that, for the important regions of x where the vibratory amplitude is significant, one can show that $(\omega R_m C + R/\omega\rho_0) \ll 1$. To give a numerical value, we shall again use $f = 4000$ Hz and $x = 1$ cm. Then the above expression assumes a value of 7.2×10^{-3}, clearly much smaller than unity, which justifies ignoring the small effect on the magnitude of the bracketed term that is due to variation with distance. Let us then denote the bracketed term by a constant K

$$K = 1 - j\left(\omega R_m C + \frac{R}{\omega\rho_0}\right) \tag{4.108}$$

With this substitution the differential equation takes the form

$$-\frac{1}{P}\frac{d^2P}{dx^2} = K\omega^2\rho_0\frac{C}{S} \tag{4.109}$$

After substituting the proper expressions for C and S, we arrive at the final form,

$$-\frac{1}{P}\frac{d^2P}{dx^2} = K\omega^2\rho_0\frac{C_0}{S_0}e^{hx}e^{ax} = \frac{KC_0\omega^2\rho_0}{S_0}e^{(h+a)x} = D^2 e^{(h+a)x} \tag{4.110}$$

This equation can be solved by first utilizing a series of appropriately chosen substitutions of variables. Let us first make the substitution $x = [2/(h+a)]u$. Then our final differential equation takes the form

$$\frac{d^2P}{du^2} + \left(\frac{2D}{h+a}\right)^2 e^{2u}P = 0 \tag{4.111}$$

Let us now make a second change in variable by designating $[2D/(h+a)]e^u = z$. Then the equation assumes the form

$$\frac{d^2P}{dz^2} + \frac{1}{z}\frac{dP}{dz} + P = 0 \tag{4.112}$$

Since this equation is the well-known Bessel differential equation, its solution can be written by inspection. One appropriate complete solution utilizes Hankel functions:

$$P = A_1 H_0^{(1)}(z) + B_1 H_0^{(2)}(z) \qquad (4.113)$$

Hankel functions are also called Bessel functions of the third kind. They are related to Bessel functions of the first and second kind by the relationships

$$H_0^{(1)}(z) = J_0(z) + jY_0(z)$$
$$H_0^{(2)}(z) = J_0(z) - jY_0(z) \qquad (4.114)$$

Note that these relationships are analogous to those existing between circular functions (sine and cosine) and exponential functions. Clearly the Hankel functions are complex quantities. They appear frequently in the solution of problems of traveling wave propagation. Unfamiliarity with these functions and the associated nomenclature should not prevent the reader from going on and assimilating the necessary concepts by doing so. The important consideration when dealing with these functions is that they are simply a shorthand notation for describing the solutions of a particular differential equation, that of Bessel. This approach is not unusual in applied mathematics, some such shorthand notations have become truly familiar. The complete solution of the differential equation

$$\frac{d^2 y}{dt^2} + \omega^2 y = 0$$

is denoted as $y = A \cos \omega t + B \sin \omega t$. The symbols sin and cos are merely the descriptions of a functional relationship that relates certain numbers to any combination of the pair of numbers ω and t. These relationships are of course very well known. This is because many common problems have solutions that involve these so-called circular functions, the sine and cosine. The problems whose solutions are satisfied by Bessel functions of various kinds are somewhat more esoteric than the usual trigonometric problem. Nevertheless, the method of treatment is similar. When we wish to find the magnitude of one side in a right triangle if one of the other angles and sides are known, we simply look up the sine or cosine of the angle in a table and proceed with the calculation. When computations are to be performed with Bessel functions, we do the same thing. We go to an appropriate table and look up the necesary magnitude. Thus at least conceptually the use of Bessel functions does not present any more difficulty than the use of circular functions. Of course, the factor of familiarity can be a stumbling block. Good treatment of Bessel functions can be found in McLachlan (1934), Goldman (1949), and Watson (1922). A comprehensive table of values is given in Jahnke and Emde (1945).

Let us now retrace our various substitutions and obtain the solution in terms of the original independent variable, x.

$$z = \frac{2D}{h+a} e^u = \frac{2}{h+a} \left(\frac{\omega^2 K C_0 \rho_0}{S_0} \right)^{1/2} \exp\left(\frac{h+a}{2} \right) x$$

$$= \frac{2\omega}{h+a} \left(\frac{K C_0 \rho_0}{S_0} \right)^{1/2} e^{(h+a)x/2} \quad (4.115)$$

Thus the argument of the Hankel functions is this rather involved function of x. It is remembered that K denotes a complex number, a function of distance x and of ω, which as a first approximation is taken as constant. If we keep the approximation then clearly the argument of the solution (z) is a real number. If more accuracy is desired, the frequency and distance dependence of K must be taken into account, and under those circumstances z is a complex number. The solution of our differential equation in terms of Hankel functions was chosen because these functions have the property of approaching zero at very large complex arguments. In physical terms this means that if no approximations are to be used then we need a solution that is defined for complex arguments. Moreover, since the helicotrema acts as a quasi-short-circuit for the pressure, we need a solution that tends toward zero at large distances, that is, in the region of the helicotrema. Hankel function solutions have these properties. If one considers the argument z somewhat further, it becomes clear that the solution can be simplified. Note that the complex number $K^{1/2}$ is equal to

$$\left[1 - j \left(\omega R_m C + \frac{R}{\omega \rho_0} \right) \right]^{1/2} \quad (4.116)$$

The imaginary part of this number was shown to be quite small compared to the real part. Under such circumstances, if $Z = A + jB$, with $B \ll A$, then with a good approximation we can write $Z^{1/2} = A + jB/2$. Consequently $K^{1/2}$ can be approximated by

$$1 - j \cdot \tfrac{1}{2} \left(\omega R_m C + \frac{R}{\omega \rho_0} \right) \quad (4.117)$$

The expression for the argument then becomes

$$z = \frac{2\omega}{h+a} \left(\frac{C_0 \rho_0}{S_0} \right)^{1/2} \left[1 - j \cdot \tfrac{1}{2} \left(\omega R_m C + \frac{R}{\omega \rho_0} \right) \right] e^{(h+a)x/2} \quad (4.118)$$

Let us now consider the behavior of the two functions $H_0^{(1)}$ and $H_0^{(2)}$ at very large values of the complex argument z. The $H_0^{(1)}$ vanishes if the magnitude of the argument increases without bound, provided that the imaginary part of the argument is positive. In contrast, $H_0^{(2)}$ disappears at large values of z if the imaginary part of z is negative. The physical constraint provided by the helicotrema, which comprises a virtual short circuit for pressure at large values of the distance x, dictates that we cannot have solutions for the pressure that do not diminish at large arguments. This consideration necessitates that the coefficient A_1 be identically zero. Thus the solution should be written as

$$P = B_1 H_0^{(2)} \left\{ \frac{2\omega}{h+a} \frac{(C_0\rho_0)^{1/2}}{S_0} \left[1 - j \cdot \tfrac{1}{2} \left(\omega R_m C + \frac{R}{\omega\rho_0} \right) \right] e^{(h+a)x/2} \right\} \quad (4.119)$$

In the simplified case in which K can be considered a constant, the solution is

$$P = B_1 H_0^{(2)} \left\{ \frac{2\omega}{h+a} \frac{(KC_0\rho_0)^{1/2}}{S_0} e^{(h+a)x/2} \right\} \quad (4.120)$$

When the argument of a Hankel function is large, it can be approximated by an exponential function with good accuracy. If the argument is complex, i.e., $z = re^{j\phi} = \xi + j\eta$, then the approximation takes the following form (Jahnke and Emde, 1945):

$$H_0^{(2)}(z) = \frac{e^{\eta}}{(\pi r/2)^{1/2}} \exp[j(-\xi - \phi/2 + \pi/4)] \quad (4.121)$$

Let us first concern ourselves with approximating the magnitude of the pressure response. Clearly, $|H_0^{(2)}(z)| = e^{\eta}(\pi r/2)^{-1/2}$. Let us then determine η and r. From the expression given for z, with the realization that $\omega R_m C + R/\omega\rho_0 \ll 1$, we can write

$$r = \frac{2\omega}{h+a} \frac{(C_0\rho_0)^{1/2}}{S_0} e^{(h+a)x/2} \quad (4.122)$$

Furthermore,

$$\eta = - \frac{\omega}{h+a} \frac{(C_0\rho_0)^{1/2}}{S_0} \left(\omega R_m C + \frac{R}{\omega\rho_0} \right) e^{(h+a)x/2} \quad (4.123)$$

Consequently $|P(x,\omega)|$ can be approximated as

$$|P(x,\omega)| = B_1 \frac{\exp\left[- \dfrac{\omega}{h+a} \left(\dfrac{C_0\rho_0}{S_0} \right)^{1/2} \left(\omega R_m C + \dfrac{R}{\omega\rho_0} \right) e^{(h+a)x/2} \right]}{\left[\dfrac{\pi}{2} \dfrac{2\omega}{h+a} \left(\dfrac{C_0\rho_0}{S_0} \right)^{1/2} e^{(h+a)x/2} \right]^{1/2}}$$

$$= B_1' \omega^{-1/2} \exp\left[- \frac{(h+a)x}{4} - \frac{\omega}{h+a} \left(\frac{C_0\rho_0}{S_0} \right)^{1/2} \right.$$

$$\left. \left(\omega R_m C + \frac{R}{\omega\rho_0} \right) e^{(h+a)x/2} \right] \quad (4.124)$$

After the functional values for C and R are substituted, the following expression is obtained

$$|P(x,\omega)| = B'_1\omega^{-1/2} \exp\left[-\frac{(h+a)x}{4} - \frac{Q}{2}\omega^2 R_m C_0 e^{(3h+a)x/2} \right.$$

$$\left. -\frac{Q}{2}\frac{R_0\omega^{1/2}}{\rho_0} e^{(h+2a)x/2} \right] \quad (4.125)$$

where

$$Q = \frac{2\rho_0^{1/2} C_0^{1/2}}{(h+a)S_0^{1/2}} \quad (4.126)$$

To make this expression a little easier to understand, the available numerical values are now substituted:

$$|P(x,f)| = B'_1 f^{-1/2} \exp[-\tfrac{1}{2}x - 1.5 \times 10^{-10} f^2 e^{2.5x}$$

$$-5 \times 10^{-4} f^{1/2} e^{1.25x}] \quad (4.127)$$

The following values were substituted: $R_0 = 2.24$, $C_0 = 4 \times 10^{-10}$, $S_0 = 0.0125$, $a = 0.5$, $Q = 1.79 \times 10^{-4}$, $h = 1.5$, $R_m = 1.1 \times 10^2$. All are in CGS units. We note that the pressure monotonically decreases with an increase in both f and x. At a constant frequency then, the pressure wave gradually decreases from the stapes toward the helicotrema, becoming negligible at a particular distance. The greater the frequency, the earlier the pressure magnitude diminishes to a negligible value. At a constant distance from the stapes the pressure magnitude depends on frequency; the greater the frequency, the smaller the pressure. To really bring these points home, let us assume that the pressure at the stapes ($x = 0$) is P_0. Then

$$|P_0| = B'_1 f^{-1/2} \exp[-1.5 \times 10^{-10} f^2 - 5 \times 10^{-4} f^{1/2}] \quad (4.128)$$

The relative pressure magnitude at any point x and at any frequency f is then written as follows:

$$\left|\frac{P}{P_0}\right| = \exp[-\tfrac{1}{2}x - 1.5 \times 10^{-10} f^2(e^{2.5x} - 1)$$

$$-5 \times 10^{-4} f^{1/2} (e^{1.25x} - 1)] \quad (4.129)$$

The phase of the pressure wave can be determined if one considers that $\phi = \angle z = 0$, provided that the usual approximation of $\omega R_m C + R/\omega\rho_0 \ll 1$ is again used. Furthermore, $\mathrm{Re}(z) = \xi$ is obtained as

$$\xi = \frac{2\omega}{h+a}\left(\frac{C_0\rho_0}{S_0}\right)^{1/2} e^{(h+a)x/2} = \omega Q e^{(h+a)x/2} \quad (4.130)$$

The phase function of the pressure wave is then written as

$$\angle P = -\omega Q e^{(h+a)x/2} + \tfrac{1}{4}\pi = -1.12 \times 10^{-3} f e^x + \tfrac{1}{4}\pi \quad (4.131)$$

The reference phase $\angle P_0 = -\omega Q + \frac{1}{4}\pi = -1.12 \times 10^{-3} f + \frac{1}{4}\pi$ can now be subtracted to yield the relative phase of the pressure wave

$$\angle P - \angle P_0 = -1.12 \times 10^{-3} f(e^x - 1) \tag{4.132}$$

A plot of this function is given in Fig. 4.5. Clearly the phase lag monotonically increases with both frequency and distance from the stapes.

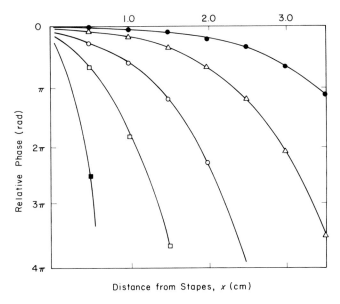

Distance from Stapes, x (cm)

Fig. 4.5. Relative phase shift (lag) between pressure difference at point x and at the oval window, computed from Eq. (4.132). The abscissa is distance from the oval window, and frequency is the parameter ($\bullet$, 100 Hz; $\triangle$, 300 Hz; $\bigcirc$, 1 kHz; $\square$, 3 kHz; $\blacksquare$, 10 kHz).

The quantity of greatest interest to us is the displacement pattern of the cochlear partition. This pattern can be obtained from the pressure function with relative ease if it is considered that $p = Zv = j\omega Zy$. Consequently,

$$y = p/j\omega Z$$

Let us first consider the magnitude of the displacement $|y|$. As we have seen [Eq.(4.105)], $1/Z$ can be written as $j\omega C + \omega^2 R_m C^2$. Consequently the magnitude of the impedance takes the form

$$(\omega^2 C^2 + \omega^4 R_m^2 C^4)^{1/2} = \omega C(1 + \omega^2 R_m C^2)^{1/2} \tag{4.133}$$

It is remembered that $\omega^2 R_m C^2 \ll 1$ for the values of frequency and distance of interest, and consequently we are justified in approximating $|1/Z|$ by $\omega C =$

$2\pi f \cdot 4 \times 10^{-10} e^{1.5x}$. Let us now substitute this value of $|1/Z|$, and our equation for $|P(x,f)|$, into the formula for membrane displacement $|y|$.

$$|y| = \frac{\omega CP}{\omega} = B_1'' f^{-1/2} \exp[x - 1.5 \times 10^{-10} f^2 e^{2.5x}$$
$$- 5 \times 10^{-4} f^{1/2} e^{1.25x}] \qquad (4.134)$$

This expression can also be normalized by noting that $|y(0,f)| = B_1'' f^{-1/2} \exp[-1.5 \times 10^{-10} f^2 - 5 \times 10^{-4} f^{1/2}]$. Finally,

$$\left| \frac{y(x,f)}{y(0,f)} \right| = \exp[x - 1.5 \times 10^{-10} f^2 (e^{2.5x} - 1)$$
$$- 5 \times 10^{-4} f^{1/2} (e^{1.25x} - 1)] \qquad (4.135)$$

The phase of the partition displacement is the same as the phase of the pressure wave, provided that we maintain the approximation $\omega R_m C \ll 1$. Under these circumstances the displacement function can be written as

$$y = \frac{p}{j\omega Z} = \frac{p}{j\omega} (j\omega C + \omega^2 R_m C^2) = \frac{pj\omega C}{j\omega} (1 - j\omega R_m C) \simeq pC \quad (4.136)$$

Consequently, as stated,

$$\angle y \simeq \angle pC = \angle p \qquad (4.137)$$

The function that describes the theoretical shape of membrane displacement (to be precise, the amplitude of membrane displacement as the function of distance, which should not be confused with the instantaneous value of membrane motion) reveals that for most frequencies a distinct point of amplitude maximum exists. This maximum moves away from the stapes as the driving frequency decreases. At very low frequencies there is no maximum in that the magnitude of vibrations monotonically increases toward the apex. Since the maxima are quite shallow, the distance between the 3dB-down points is a relatively constant 1.25 cm, which is of course about one-third of the entire cochlear length. Nevertheless, the most conspicuous property of the amplitude distribution is that points of maximal vibration are correlated with individual frequency components. These points line up in a base-to-apex succession with decreasing input frequency. Together with changes in amplitude the partition vibration also exhibits a gradually accumulating phase shift. It is clear that phase changes are more rapid at higher frequencies than at the lower ones and also that close to the stapes the phase changes much more slowly than in a more apical region. One could summarize by saying that as a result of harmonic excitation a pressure wave of monotically decreasing magnitude and increasing phase shift travels in the cochlear fluid from base toward the apex. This pressure wave decreases to a negligible magnitude at a given point removed from its origin. The location of this point depends on the driving frequency; the lower the frequency the greater the spatial extent of the pressure wave. This pressure wave is developed *across* the cochlear partition and is directly responsible for setting the latter in vibration. In contrast with the monotonically decreasing fluid pressure differential, the vibratory amplitude of the partition shows an extremum, that is, a point of maximal vibration. The maximum is located at a point that is determined by the frequency of the stimulus; high frequencies create a peak in the basal region, and the lower the frequency the closer the peak moves to the apex. Very low frequencies do not elicit a clear-cut maximum. As a first approximation the phase of the fluid pressure differential across the partition and the phase of the partition displacement are the same. The theoretical results indicate that the cochlea acts as a mechanical frequency analyzer in rendering a point of vibration maximally sensitive to a particular frequency.

D. Comparison of Solutions with Experimental Data

1. Introduction

The natural question now arises, How well do our computations fit whatever experimental evidence is available on the vibratory pattern of the cochlear partition? There have been only three sets of measurements made on the vibrations of the basilar membrane: the classic experimental observations of von Békésy (1942, 1943, 1947) and the recent measurements of Johnstone and Boyle (1967) and of Rhode (1971). We shall review these data in detail, but before doing so it might be well to obtain a quick answer to the previous question: How good is our theoretical structure? The fastest comparison can be made between the obtained locus for vibratory maxima and the observed ones. Zwislocki (1965) made such comparisons, and our data are superimposed on his plot in Fig. 4.6. Our points are obtained by differentiating the $y = y(x)$ function with respect to x, setting the resultant function equal to zero, and solving for x at various values of the frequency. It is clear that the agreement between the present results and the experimental data is meager indeed. Our displacement functions do not produce vibratory maxima for frequencies below approximately 300 Hz, and all maxima occur too far toward the apex. This comparison appears to be quite discouraging at first glance, but it need not be so. Consider that our results were derived strictly on a theoretical basis, without any adjustment of parameters to better the fit. Moreover, a very large number of simplifying assumptions were made in practically all stages of the derivation. Considering these facts, it is rather promising that at least a good qualitative agreement could be obtained. It seems that with some appropriate readjustment of parameters in the equations the fit to the experimental data could be improved without any change in the actual mathematical form of the equations; in other words without any reassessment of the basic physical considerations on the basis of which the derivation proceeded. This possibility will be investigated in some detail below, but first the experimental evidence concerning the vibratory motion pattern of the cochlear partition is reviewed.

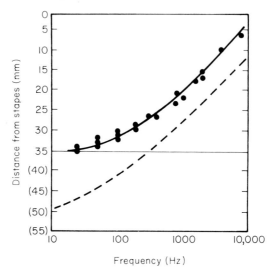

Fig. 4.6. Maxima of the $y(x)/y(0)$ functions at different frequencies. Dashed line results from taking the maxima based on Eq. (4.135); the data points were obtained by Zwislocki from von Békésy's experimental observations (Zwislocki, 1965, p. 33); and the solid line is based on maxima from computations with Eq. (4.139). These latter computations are to be discussed later in the text.

Von Békésy's (1928, 1942, 1943, 1947, 1960) observations on scale models, cadaver ears, and live specimens provide us with the experimental basis on which our current views on the motion patterns of the cochlear partition are founded. The reader should learn about these experiments first hand by reading the original versions. Here a mere synopsis is given of the salient findings. Von Békésy's technique of direct observation of cochlear vibrations consisted of opening the cochlear capsule under water, sealing the opening with a glass window, and viewing the apical portion of the cochlear partition with a stereoscopic microscope under stroboscopic illumination. As a first step he ascertained that at the high intensity levels that were necessary for visualization of the partition motion, nonlinear effects were insignificant. He noted that the amplitude of vibrations changed in proportion with the stimulus strength, and thus nonlinearities contributed second-order effects at the most. He noted that for input frequencies of 30 Hz and less the entire visible portion of the cochlear partition vibrated in phase and there was no discernible place of amplitude maximum. At higher frequencies the vibrations moved toward the stapes, with a clear-cut point of maximum amplitude correlated with the driving frequency. Above 800 Hz the vibratory pattern moved too far basally to be visible through the opening, which uncovered only the highest turn of the cochlea. In Fig. 4.7, sketches of the vibratory

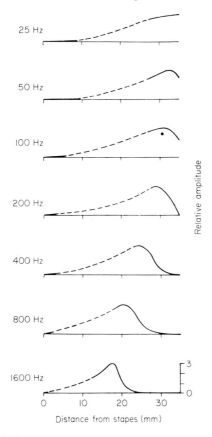

Fig. 4.7. Patterns of vibrations of the cochlear partition in a human cadaver at various frequencies. Abscissa is distance from the stapes. (From von Békésy, 1960, p. 448.)

amplitude (relative magnitudes) are shown. Solid lines indicate the results of actual measurements, while the dashed lines are von Békésy's extrapolations. In order to study the vibratory pattern above 800 Hz von Békésy gradually ground off more and more of the cochlear capsule as he increased the stimulus frequency. Since apical portions of the membrane do not participate in the vibration at high frequencies, this process of shortening the cochlea did not significantly affect the high-frequency vibratory patterns.

It is clear that the cochlea performs a frequency analysis function in that a given position along the cochlear partition is maximally sensitive to a certain input frequency. At any given frequency the amplitude of vibrations builds up to a shallow maximum located at a particular distance from the stapes; beyond this point the vibration decays relatively fast and portions of the membrane that are far apically from the maximum are in rest.

In a later experiment von Békésy (1947) measured the relative phase of the cochlear partition along with its amplitude variations at various low driving frequencies in the apical region of the cochlea. His amplitude and phase plots are reproduced in Fig. 4.8. The amplitude plots in this later

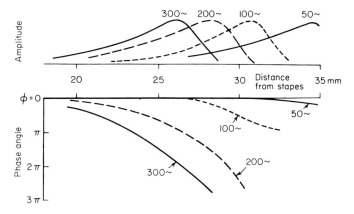

Fig. 4.8. Magnitude and phase plots of the vibratory pattern of the cochlear partition at four low-frequency sinusoidal stimuli. Abscissa is distance from stapes. (From von Békésy, 1960, p. 462.)

measurement series are similar to those he obtained previously. The phase angles are given in reference to the phase of the stapedial motion. As pointed out by Siebert (1962) and Flanagan (1962) these amplitude and phase plots are not internally consistent; it is almost certain that von Békésy did not take into account a constant 90° phase difference between stapes and partition displacement. His plots seem to extrapolate to zero phase difference between stapes and partition movement at the stapedial region, whereas theoretical considerations (as we shall discuss in detail later) dictate that the partition displacement lead the stapes displacement by at least 90°.

The phase shift at the point of maximum vibrations is between π and 2π from von Békésy's measurements. It is important to emphasize that the phase apparently accumulates well beyond the values seen at the maximum. This is an important proof that the traveling wave maximum is not due to a resonance phenomenon. More up to date coordinated amplitude and phase information has been obtained by two groups of experimenters with the use of the Mössbauer technique. Johnstone and Boyle (1967) reported the first use of the method, and later more data were provided by Johnstone and Taylor (1970), Johnstone *et al.* (1970), and Rhode (1971). Johnstone and colleagues measured basilar membrane vibrations in the guinea pig approximately 1.5 mm from the stapes, while Rhode's measurements were made in the squirrel monkey in the apical end of the first turn. These investigators obtained both amplitude and phase measurements. Johnstone and co-workers, provide their data with reference to stapes displacement, while Rhode used the displacement of the malleus as the base line. Since the shapes of the amplitude plots obtained by these investigators are strikingly similar, only one set of data, that of Rhode, is shown here (Fig. 4.9). There is a low-frequency rise in the amplitude at a rate of approximately 6 dB/octave. Somewhat below the best frequency the slope increases to about 24 dB/octave while beyond the point of maximum the decrease in amplitude is of the order of 100 dB/octave. The best frequencies of Rhode and of Johnstone and co-workers are quite different from one another and very different from those of von Békésy. The qualitative similarity of the data indicates that at any point along the basilar membrane the vibratory patterns are quite similar for the appropriate range of frequencies. Thus near the stapes and near the helicotrema the cochlea performs the same type of frequency analysis. There are apparent quantitative differences, especially between von Békésy's curves and the later results. We shall discuss some of these below but first let us compare the available phase information.

In all Mössbauer results the low-frequency phase asymptotes to a 90° lead; in other words, the basilar membrane leads the stapes (malleus) by this amount of phase. As we recall from Flanagan's (1962) argument this phase behavior is necessary for consistency with the amplitude data. The 90° low-frequency phase lead of course means that the displacement of the basilar membrane is proportional to the *derivative* of the stapes displacement, that is, to its velocity. All investigators agree that as frequency increases a gradually accumulating phase lag of the basilar membrane motion becomes evident. There is however, some disagreement about the amount of phase shift. We recall that from von Békésy's observations it appears that at the point of maximum the phase lag is between π and 2π. The data of Johnstone and colleagues tentatively place this figure at $\pi/2$ rad, while Rhode consistently obtains phase shifts of the order of 5π. It is interesting to note, parenthetically, that cochlear microphonic data are more in line with small phase accumulation, while 8th nerve unit discharge data apparently exhibit phase shifts commensurate with those obtained by Rhode. These discrepancies are yet to be resolved and explained. The most important, and common, observation is that beyond the point of maximum the phase does not asymptote to

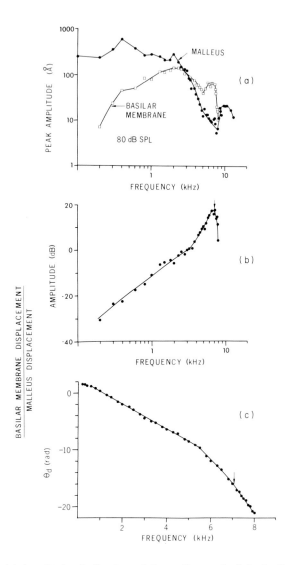

Fig. 4.9. (a) Amplitude of vibration of the malleus and of the basilar membrane as the function of frequency. (b) Input–output ratio, in decibels, for the malleus and the basilar membrane. (c) Phase differences between the motion of the basilar membrane and the motion of the malleus. Negative numbers signify that the motion of the basilar membrane lags behind the motion of the malleus. The arrows indicate the values of the curves at the maximally effective frequency. Note that the value of the phase difference is 1.6 rad, about 90°, at frequencies less than 300 Hz. (From Rhode, 1971, p. 1222.)

a small integer multiple of π, thus contradicting the possibility of a dominant resonance in the cochlea.

The greatest differences among the various tuning curves are seen in their width and in the high-frequency slope. The von Békésy curves are generally shallower and their cutoff rate is less. It is likely that the more sensitive experimental method (Mössbauer technique versus visual observation) allows an investigator to better assess the quantitative features of the vibratory motion. It is also possible that the tuning curves actually differ in their quantitative features at different locations along the basilar membrane. Thus Tonndorf and Khanna (1968c) showed that even within von Békésy's data there is a gradation in that the width of the tuning curves becomes less as measurements move toward the stapes. They replotted von Békésy's tuning curves in a normalized fashion to demonstrate this narrowing (Fig. 4.10).

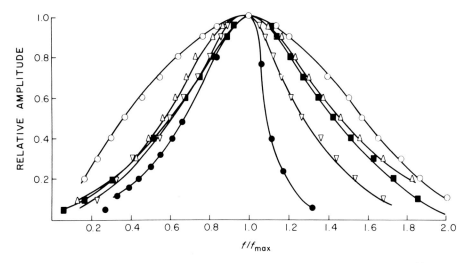

Fig. 4.10. Normalized tuning curves at various cochlear locations that are identified by the best frequencies ($\bigcirc$, 200 Hz; $\triangle$, 300 Hz; $\blacksquare$, 675 Hz; $\triangledown$, 950 Hz; $\bullet$, 18,000 Hz). (From Tonndorf and Khanna, 1968c, p. 1139.)

The effects are very systematic and quite sizable. It is interesting to consider that even our theoretical results seem to indicate a trend toward narrower tuning curves in the basal region of the cochlea. When normalized tuning curves are plotted on the basis of Eq. (4.139) for various locations, these curves, as well as those prepared by Tonndorf and Khanna (Fig. 4.10), are very similar in that the low-frequency slope is largely independent of location but that significant effects on the high-frequency slopes are seen.

One way to describe the sharpness of a tuning curve is to compute the so-called Q or quality factor. This is obtained by dividing the best frequency with the half-power bandwidth. Von Békésy's tuning curves have Q values ranging between 1.2 and 2.5, while the Q of the Johnstone–Boyle curve is approximately 3.3 (Tonndorf and Khanna, 1968c). In fact there appears to be a systematic increase in Q with increasing best frequency (or more precisely with decreasing distance toward the stapes), as was pointed out by Tonndorf and Khanna (1968c). They prepared a plot based on the available data which does indicate a definite trend for the narrowing of the tuning curve. This graph is reproduced in Fig. 4.11. I have modified this plot by

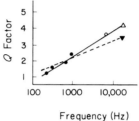

Frequency (Hz)

Fig. 4.11. Relation of Q and best frequency of cochlear tuning curves. Dashed line is after Tonndorf and Khana (1968c, p. 1140), who based their plot on the data of (●) von Békésy (1947) and (▼) Johnstone and Boyle (1967). Solid line indicates a better fit between von Békésy's data points and the more recent data of (△) Johnstone and Taylor (1970) and (○) Rhode (1971).

adding some newer data. One can compute from Rhode's tuning curves that his Q is of the order of 3.5, while the newer results of Johnstone and Taylor (1970) yield a quality factor of approximately 4.2. When these points are added to the graph it becomes evident that they provide a better extrapolation of the von Békésy data than do the originally considered Johnstone and Boyle material. One can thus conclude that there appears to be a systematic trend for the narrowing of the tuning curves with increasing best frequency.

There are two electrical indices of activity in the cochlea that can yield information related to these tuning curves. One of these is the spread of the cochlear microphonic potential along the length of the cochlea. The other is the so-called response area obtained by plotting the intensity and frequency relationship at threshold for a single auditory nerve fiber. A revealing comparison can be made with the response areas of single auditory nerve fibers. Kiang (1965) obtained a measure akin to the conventional Q factor by computing the ratio best frequency/bandwidth at 10 dB above threshold for a large number of first-order neurons. The absolute values of his figures are not directly comparable with the more conventional Q, but an interesting trend emerges. His Q values show a gradual increase with increasing best frequency. This observation of course appears to be in line with the trend noted for the mechanical tuning curves. Comparison of actual tuning curves at critical frequencies approximating those of the available mechanical tuning curves reveals that the neural plots are somewhat sharper (having higher Q) than the corresponding mechanical tuning curves.

An interesting comparison was prepared by Evans (1970), who compared some 8th nerve tuning curves from the guinea pig with a schematized mechanical tuning curve. His picture is presented in Fig. 4.12. It is apparent that

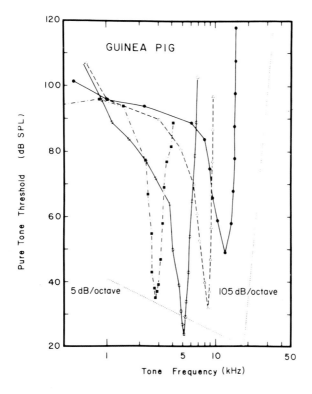

Fig. 4.12. Threshold response area curves (tuning curves) for four auditory nerve fibers of a guinea pig compared with low- and high-frequency slopes of 5 and 105 dB/octave. Sound pressure was measured at the tympanic membrane. (From Evans, 1970, p. 14P.)

while the high-frequency slope of the neural tuning curves is apparently steeper (up to 500 dB/octave versus about 100 dB/octave) the main difference is on the low-frequency side. Below the maximum the mechanical tuning curves seem to be quite uniform and they possess relatively shallow slopes, as we have discussed above. In contrast there is apparently a great variety of low-frequency slopes that can be seen in the neural tuning curves, and these slopes are almost always considerably steeper. Some recent arguments of Rhode (1971) could bring the high-frequency slopes in harmony, but apparently the mechanical tuning cannot account for the sharpness of the low-frequency side of the neural response curves. Rhode noted that in the immediate vicinity of the best frequency the mechanical response is nonlinear (see details in Section IV,B,1). If compensation is made for this nonlinearity the high-frequency slopes of the mechanical tuning curves are of the order of 200 dB/octave, certainly commensurate with most neural responses.

Before we return to our derivation of the displacement pattern of the basilar membrane, one more set of von Békésy's observations should be presented. His tuning curves were given in a normalized form, and thus they contained no information about the relative magnitudes of vibrations, say, at the points of maxima at various frequencies. To remedy this shortcoming von Békésy also provided information on this aspect of cochlear function, and his data are reproduced in Fig. 4.13. The stapes displacement

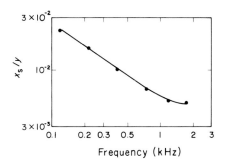

Fig. 4.13. Ratio between the volume displacement of the stapes (x_s) and the maximum amplitude of the cochlear partition (y) as a function of frequency. (Adapted from von Békésy, 1960, p. 455.)

amplitude given in this plot was measured when the amplitude of the maximally vibrating basilar membrane segment was kept constant. The measurements imply that, if stapes amplitude had been kept constant, then at any frequency the amplitude of the maximally vibrating segment would have increased with increasing stimulus frequency. This rate of increase is somewhat less than 6 dB/octave.

Now that we have become acquainted with the experimental data that describe the tuning characteristics of basilar membrane vibrations, it is appropriate to pick up the thread of our derivation. When the place of maximum vibrations of the basilar membrane as determined by visual observations is plotted as the function of stimulus frequency, one obtains the graph of

Fig. 4.6. The data points show that all frequencies, except for the very lowest, have their definite place of maximum along the cochlear partition. Our model must satisfy this condition, and it must give good agreement with the observed form of the cochlear resonance curves. It is remembered that the results of our computations provided at least a qualitative agreement with the experimental observations in that definite vibratory maxima were predicted for most frequencies. The location of these maxima depended on the input frequency in the appropriate way; that is, the maxima moved toward the stapes with the increase in the driving frequency.

As we have mentioned before, the quantitative agreement between the results of the theoretical arguments set forth above and the experimental observations is not very impressive, even though the general qualitative features are the same. In discussing the apparent differences, let us keep in mind that, in the choice of the system parameters, we attempted to use only anatomical, experimental, and physical considerations. Peterson and Bogert (1950) also obtained theoretical results without curve fitting procedures, and their agreement with the experimental data is also only qualitative. Fletcher (1953) obtained better quantitative agreement on the basis of his calculations, which again utilized experimental and physical constants only (no curve fitting techniques). Zwislocki's results are the closest to the experimental observations, but he had to modify certain parameters to bring the solution in harmony with von Békésy's observations. Specifically, the two resistance parameters, viscosity and membrane damping, were both adjusted so that agreement between experimental and theoretical work could be obtained.

2. Adjustment of Parameters

We can follow Zwislocki's example in adjusting the resistance parameters in order to better the fit of the model to the experimental data. The choice of altering the resistance parameters as opposed to some other system parameter is logical. Of all the numerical values that were utilized in our computations the values for viscous resistance and membrane resistance were based on the most meager foundation. It is remembered that the value of viscous damping was obtained on a theoretical basis and that approximations were clearly involved in the computational process. The membrane damping was indirectly determined from von Békésy's measurements of decay times in the cochlea. This computation necessitated the knowledge of membrane mass, which is not a well-established quantity. All in all, it is quite legitimate to adjust these parameters to obtain a better fit, provided that the adjustments do not have to be of such magnitude that they would be inconsistent with the physical nature of these parameters. Fortunately, relatively modest adjustments of the resistance parameters can bring the analytical and experimental results into harmony. Specifically, our expression for viscous fluid resistance was

$$R = R_0 \omega^{1/2} e^{ax/2} = 2.24 \omega^{1/2} e^{0.25x}$$

If we change R_0 from its originally computed value of 2.24 gm/cm^3 second$^{1/2}$ to 8.15 gm/cm^3 second$^{1/2}$, then this change is adequate in readjusting the value of this parameter.

The membrane resistance R_m was previously expressed as

$$R_m = R_{mo} e^{-0.175x} = 110 e^{-0.175x} \simeq 110$$

If we assume that the membrane resistance is constant and that its value is $R_m = 468$ CGS units, then this change is appropriate to readjust the value of this parameter. If these two proposed changes are incorporated, the expression for the relative magnitude of pressure in the cochlea takes the form

$$\left| \frac{P}{P_0} \right| = \exp[-\tfrac{1}{2}x - 6.7 \times 10^{-10} f^2 (e^{2.5x} - 1) $$
$$-1.84 \times 10^{-3} f^{1/2} (e^{1.25x} - 1)] \qquad (4.138)$$

The expression for relative membrane displacement amplitude is as follows:

$$\left| \frac{y}{y_0} \right| = \exp[x - 6.7 \times 10^{-10} f^2 (e^{2.5x} - 1) $$
$$-1.84 \times 10^{-3} f^{1/2} (e^{1.25x} - 1)] \qquad (4.139)$$

The parameter changes do not affect the phase; it is remembered that the phase of the pressure wave and that of the membrane displacement are approximately the same:

$$\angle P - \angle P_0 = \angle y - \angle y_0 = -1.12 \times 10^{-3} f(e^x - 1) \quad \text{rad} \qquad (4.140)$$

The values computed from the above expressions for $|y/y_0|$ are shown in Fig. 4.14, and the maxima of the vibratory amplitude that can be obtained from the $|y/y_0|$ function by differentiation are shown in Fig. 4.6. In the latter figure the various experimental values plotted by Zwislocki on the basis of von Békésy's data are also shown for comparison. Clearly the agreement is now excellent. This is, of course, not surprising since the new parameter values were so chosen to provide such agreement.

It is well to state again that we needed changes of less than an order of magnitude in two parameters to achieve this fit. This indicates that the original assumptions and approximations that were made in deriving the analytic model of the cochlea were probably quite appropriate and permissible.

While our equations now predict the positions of the traveling wave maxima with good precision, a simple inquiry reveals that there are some discrepancies between the shapes of the tuning curves that can be computed

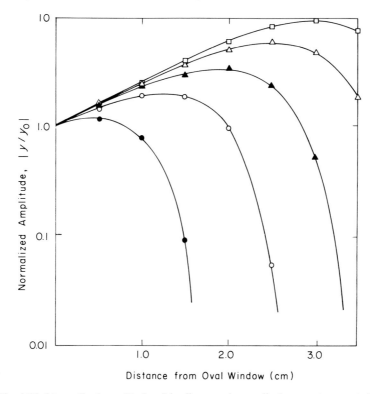

Fig. 4.14. Normalized amplitude of basilar membrane displacement computed from Eq. (4.139). The ordinate is logarithmic, the abscissa is the distance from the oval window, and frequency is the parameter. The fit of the locations of the maxima of these curves to that of experimental data is shown with the solid line in Fig. 4.6. Frequencies (hertz): □, 100; △, 300; ▲, 1000; ○, 3000; ●, 10,000.

with their aid and the experimental observations. If one plots some of the normalized tuning curves based on Eq. (4.139), then it is seen that these tuning curves are generally wider than the experimental plots; their Q ranges between 0.4 and 0.8. We recall that even the relatively shallow curves that were reported by von Békésy were sharp enough that their quality factor ranged up to 2.5 and of course the newer data of Johnstone and Taylor provided a Q of 4.2. Our computations [and apparently those of Zwislocki (1948) as well (Allaire, 1971)] consequently do not yield the correct shape for the frequency dependence of the vibration amplitude of a given basilar membrane site. In spite of this shortcoming the computations do provide many excellent results, as we are to see below.

Armed with the model, we can now compute some additional functions that are of interest in cochlear mechanics—specifically, the phase velocity of membrane displacement and the input impedance of the cochlea. As before, in these derivations we follow Zwislocki's steps (1965) to a large extent.

3. Phase Velocity and Travel Time*

The phase velocity of the partition displacement is by definition expressed as dx/dt. We can obtain the phase velocity if we keep in mind that the instantaneous phase of the partition displacement can be expressed as

$$\angle y = \omega t - \omega Q e^{(h+a)x/2} + \tfrac{1}{4} \tag{4.141}$$

Then

$$\frac{d\angle y}{dt} = -\frac{a+h}{2} Q\omega e^{(h+a)x/2} \frac{dx}{dt} + \omega \tag{4.142}$$

For points that are one cycle apart the phase is constant; then $d\angle y/dt = 0$, and we can express dx/dt from the above expression,

$$\frac{dx}{dt} = \frac{2}{(h+a)Q} e^{-(h+a)x/2} \tag{4.143}$$

After substitution of our numerical values the following formula obtains:

$$\frac{dx}{dt} = 5.6 \times 10^3 e^{-x} \quad \text{cm/second} \tag{4.144}$$

This expression clearly shows that the velocity of the disturbance that travels along the cochlear partition diminishes exponentially as it gets farther and farther away from the stapes. The velocity of propagation is independent of the frequency of the stimulation. The travel time of a particular disturbance from the stapes to a point on the partition can be obtained by integrating the reciprocal of the above expression for the phase velocity between $x = 0$ and $x = x_0$, where x_0 is the point of interest. The computation yields

$$T = 1.79 \times 10^{-4} (e^{x_0} - 1) \quad \text{second} \tag{4.145}$$

Thus the total travel time between stapes and helicotrema is 5.7 mseconds. This computed result is in acceptable agreement with von Békésy's measurements of the travel times of impulses in the cochlea. Von Békésy (1949) measured the travel time on the cochlear partition by placing very small mirrors at various successive points along the apical end of the basilar membrane and stimulating the ear by sharp clicks generated by spark discharges. By reflecting light from the mirror he could observe the instant when the disturbance arrived at the point on the membrane where the mirror was located by a deflection of the light beam. Our theoretical results give transit times of the same order of magnitude as his experimental observations.

* Zwislocki (1965).

E. INPUT IMPEDANCE

1. Theoretical Considerations

Now, again following Zwislocki's arguments (1965), we can address ourselves to the determination of the input impedance of the cochlea. Specific acoustic impedance is obtained as the ratio of pressure and particle velocity. Thus these quantities must first be determined at $x = 0$, that is, at the stapes, We can start by repeating the two force balance equations for the cochlear scalae [Eq. (4.65)].

$$\rho_0 \dot{u}_v + R_v u_v + \frac{\partial p_{ve}}{\partial x} = 0 \tag{4.65a}$$

$$\rho_0 \dot{u}_t + R_t u_t + \frac{\partial p_{te}}{\partial x} = 0 \tag{4.65b}$$

It is expedient to neglect the viscous resistance effects as a first approximation. Thus we can work with the equations

$$\rho_0 \dot{u}_v + \frac{\partial p_{ve}}{\partial x} = 0$$

$$\rho_0 \dot{u}_t + \frac{\partial p_{te}}{\partial x} = 0 \tag{4.146}$$

After subtracting these equations, and with the reasonable assumption that $\dot{u}_t = -\dot{u}_v$ and the substitution $(p_{ve} - p_{te}) = p$, we obtain

$$2\rho_0 \dot{u} + \frac{\partial p}{\partial x} = 0 \tag{4.147}$$

For the harmonic case this equation reduces to

$$2j\rho_0 \omega U + \frac{dP}{dx} = 0 \tag{4.148}$$

From Eq. (4.120) we can obtain the pressure gradient by differentiation if we note that $dH_0^{(2)}(z)/dz = -H_1^{(2)}(z)$. Of course, $dH_0^{(2)}(z)/dx = -H_1^{(2)}(z) \, dz/dx$. Performing the differentiation of Eq. (4.120) we obtain

$$\frac{dP}{dx} = -B_1 \omega \left(\frac{KC_0\rho_0}{S_0}\right)^{1/2} e^{(h+a)x/2}$$

$$H_1^{(2)}\left[\frac{2\omega}{h+a}\left(\frac{KC_0\rho_0}{S_0}\right)^{1/2} e^{(h+a)x/2}\right] \tag{4.149}$$

It is realized that if the argument of the Hankel function is large (as we have already shown) then, approximately, $H_1^{(2)}(z) \simeq j H_0^{(2)}(z)$. It is recognized, however, that $B_1 H_0^{(2)}(z) = P$; consequently we can write

$$\frac{dP}{dx} = -j\omega \left(\frac{KC_0\rho_0}{S_0}\right)^{1/2} e^{(h+a)x/2} P \tag{4.150}$$

This result can be substituted into Eq. (4.148) to yield

$$2j\rho_0\omega U - j\omega \left(\frac{KC_0\rho_0}{S_0}\right)^{1/2} e^{(h+a)x/2} P = 0 \tag{4.151}$$

From this the input impedance Z_c can be obtained as the ratio of P and U with the substitution $x = 0$.

$$Z_c = 2\left(\frac{\rho_0 S_0}{C_0}\right)^{1/2} K^{-1/2}$$

$$= 2\left(\frac{\rho_0 S_0}{C_0}\right)^{1/2} \left[1 - j \cdot \tfrac{1}{2}\left(\omega R_m C + \frac{R}{\omega\rho_0}\right)\right]^{-1} \tag{4.152}$$

For most frequencies of importance $K^{1/2} = 1$, in which case the input impedance of the cochlea is real and has a value of $2(\rho_0 S_0/C_0)^{1/2} = 11{,}200$ dynes second/cm^3 = Z_{co}.

To obtain the exact functional dependence of Z_c on frequency, let us substitute the numerical values of the parameters ρ_0, S_0, C_0, R_0, C, and R, keeping in mind that, where appropriate, the $x = 0$ substitution must be used.

$$Z_c = Z_{co} \left[1 - j\left(5.86 \times 10^{-7} f + \frac{1.62}{f^{1/2}}\right)\right]^{-1} \tag{4.153}$$

The first term in the parentheses does not become significant at any of the audio frequencies. Consequently we can write

$$Z_c = Z_{co}\left(1 - j\frac{1.62}{f^{1/2}}\right)^{-1} \tag{4.154}$$

The absolute value of the impedance

$$|Z_c| = Z_{co}\left(1 + \frac{2.6}{f}\right)^{-1/2} \tag{4.155}$$

The phase of the impedance

$$\angle Z_c = tg^{-1}\frac{1.62}{f^{1/2}} \tag{4.156}$$

Plots of the magnitude and phase of the impedance are given in Fig. 4.15. These amplitude and phase plots of the cochlear input impedance can be

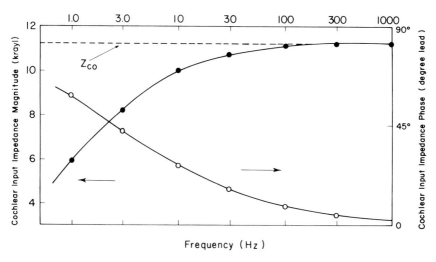

Fig. 4.15. Input impedance of the cochlea (phase and magnitude) as the function of stimulus frequency, computed from Eqs. (4.155) and (4.156).

compared to similar functions that are derived in the following section on the basis of cochlear microphonic data. The comparison indicates that the theoretical impedance plots break at too low a frequency to explain the 12 dB/octave low-frequency slope and the 180° low-frequency phase lead that was observed for the CM functions of cat and chinchilla. The theoretical impedance function is much more in line with the guinea pig data, which showed 6 dB/octave slope and 90° phase lead above 20 Hz. Of course, it should be realized that species-dependent parameter changes would shift the corner frequency of the theoretical plot upward in frequency and thus could allow the reactive component of the input impedance to exert its effect on the measurable, low-frequency portion of the CM sensitivity curve. Stating it somewhat differently, it is eminently clear from the derivation that the cochlear input impedance does have a significant reactive component at the low frequencies. The only question is, in what frequency region would this reactive component be large enough to affect the transmission characteristics of the middle ear–cochlea pathway? The theoretical plot indicates that the reactive component is significant below 3 Hz and certainly negligible above 10 Hz. As shown in the following section, this behavior correlates well with the CM measurements on the guinea pig, where the apparent cochlear input impedance is resistive above 10 Hz. In the cat and chinchilla, however, we can expect that the theoretical values do not represent the real-life situation, for our CM measurements for these species indicate the presence of a significant reactive component in the cochlear input impedance in the frequency range 10–100 Hz.

*2. Comparison with CM Data: The Effect of the Helicotrema** *

In the previous section we examined the input impedance of the cochlea as obtained from our general hydrodynamic considerations. It appears that except at the very lowest frequencies the cochlea presents a pure resistance to the ossicular chain. The computation showed that below 3 Hz the input impedance contains a reactive component due to which the magnitude of the impedance approaches zero and its phase $+90°$ as frequency diminishes. This result indicates that if different computational parameters had been used then conceivably the reactive component could have been of importance at higher frequencies also. The presence or absence of a significant reactive component in the cochlear input impedance has considerable bearing on the energy transfer into the cochlea by the ossicular chain (Khanna and Tonndorf, 1969). Specifically, the pressure developed by the stapes footplate in the oval window is proportional to the product of stapedial velocity and cochlear input impedance, $p = \dot{x}_s Z_c$. It is quite commonly assumed that the displacement of the cochlear partition is proportional to stapes velocity or, to phrase it another way, that the input impedance is constant and resistive (Zwislocki, 1948; Flanagan, 1960; Weiss et al., 1969). Since it is known from the observations of von Békésy (1951) that the cochlear microphonic potential (CM) is proportional to the displacement of the cochlear partition, and since at low frequencies the partition displacement is proportional (in the basal region) to the pressure at the oval window, the measurement of CM sensitivity functions affords a means of investigating cochlear input impedance. An added incentive to study these functions is the apparent lack of agreement in the literature concerning their shape and characteristics (Dallos, 1970). In the following some experimental data are presented on the low-frequency properties of CM sensitivity functions obtained from four species of laboratory animals, and inferences about the cochlear input impedances are drawn.

The data shown were collected with identical experimental techniques. The details are inconsequential and only two items are mentioned: The CM were recorded with differential electrodes from the basal turn, and the sound pressure was carefully measured at the eardrum. Four species were studied: cat, chinchilla, guinea pig, and kangaroo rat.

The results are presented in the form of median magnitude and phase versus frequency functions. For any species the median data were obtained from three animals. The variation from animal to animal within a given group was small. The magnitude data are expressed as the sound pressure level that is required to elicit a cochlear potential of 3 μV rms. In other words, the microphonic was kept constant and the sound pressure was adjusted at every test frequency. Strictly speaking this method generates a sensiti-

* Based on Dallos (1970).

vity function instead of a magnitude function. We did demonstrate the actual equivalence of the magnitude and sensitivity functions at the sound levels used by showing the equivalence of plots of the SPL required to elicit the standard 3-μV CM, and the CM measured at constant 60 dB SPL.

The phase data are given as the phase of the microphonic referred to the phase of the sound field at the eardrum. Thus, a positive phase means that the CM leads the sound. The actual measurements were taken while keeping the CM approximately constant at 10 μV. Our experience was that the phase was little affected by up to tenfold changes in CM.

In Fig. 4.16 the median sensitivity and phase functions are given for chinchilla and guinea pig. Other data show that plots for cats are virtually identical with those for chinchillas, while the kangaroo rat data are a replica of the guinea pig results. All the plots have been approximated by two straight-line segments between 20 and 1000 Hz. The higher-frequency straight-line approximations are drawn with a slope of -6 dB/octave for *all* four species; these lines provide adequate representation of the sensitivity curves between the frequency limits of 200 and 1000 Hz. The most important finding concerns the slope of the lower-frequency straight-line segment. Guinea pigs and kangaroo rats show sensitivity functions whose approximate low-frequency straight-line representation consists of segments having -6 dB/octave slope, while the slopes of these lines for cat and chinchilla are -12 dB/octave. If these functions represent the transfer characteristics of linear, minimum phase systems, then the phase characteristics should be in conformity with the amplitude characteristics (Bode, 1945). This is indeed the case. The low-frequency phase for the animals whose sensitivity function changes at a 6 dB/octave rate is 90° lead, while 180° low-frequency lead clearly corresponds to the 12 dB/octave change in sensitivity. The phase characteristics themselves demonstrate two segments.

Before starting these experiments it was assumed that some, and probably all, of the differences in the low-frequency characteristics of CM functions that can be discerned from plots appearing in the literature would be due to differing experimental procedures among studies. The data clearly indicate that this is not the case. In the present experiments particular care was taken to insure that all measurement procedures were the same from one animal to another and from one species to another. In spite of the identical experimental procedures, significant differences were found at very low frequencies in the cochlear microphonic sensitivity functions. The characteristics of our sensitivity functions are in general agreement with those found in the literature. Thus our 6 dB/octave low-frequency slope for guinea pig is similar to that found by Eldredge (cited by Zwislocki, 1963). In addition, the steeper slope for cat agrees with the findings of Møller (1963), Tonndorf and Khanna (1967), and Weiss *et al.* (1969).

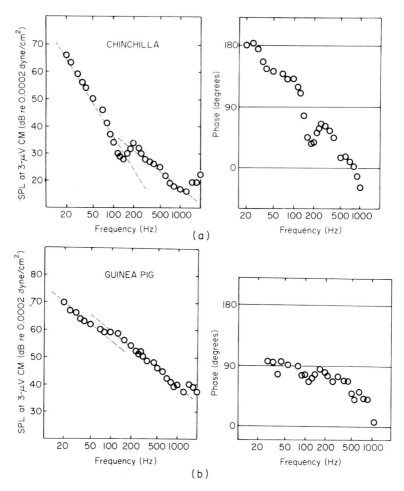

Fig. 4.16. (a) Median sensitivity and phase functions for chinchilla: $N = 3$. The straight-line approximations have slopes of -12 and -6 dB/octave. (b) Median sensitivity and phase functions for guinea pig: $N = 3$. The straight-line approximations have slopes of -6 dB/octave. (From Dallos, 1970, pp. 491, 492.)

Since procedural differences have been ruled out, one can conceive that one or more of the following factors have contributed to the observed differences in transfer characteristics. (*a*) The transfer characteristics might be the same, but a high-pass filtering effect is introduced in cat and chinchilla due to the electrical pickup characteristics of the electrodes in their interaction with the electroanatomy of a particular species. (*b*) The middle ear transfer characteristics of the two groups of animals are different. (*c*) The inner ear characteristics of the two groups of animals are different. The first two possibilities can be ruled out (Dallos, 1970), but the third is of interest here.

Elementary considerations of middle ear mechanics (see Chapter 3) indicate that the stapes displacement versus sound pressure at the eardrum transfer function should have low-pass character for all species considered; moreover in the frequency range of interest ($f < 100$ Hz) these functions should be flat. In other words, at low frequencies $x_s \propto p_d$, where x_s is stapes displacement, and p_d is sound pressure at the drum. It is also notable that in the steady state $CM \propto j\omega p_d Z_c$, or the transfer function CM/p_d is proportional to $j\omega Z_c$. This final relationship is of great importance. It means that the magnitude of the CM versus p_d transfer function is proportional to frequency *and* to the input impedance of the cochlea. Only if the cochlear input impedance is resistive will the CM versus p_d transfer function have unity slope (i.e., 6 dB/octave low-frequency configuration) accompanied by 90° phase lead of the CM over the sound field at the drum. These conditions have been tacitly assumed by most authorities writing on the subject (Zwislocki, 1965; Flanagan, 1960; Weiss *et al.*, 1969).

It is clear from our experimental results that for guinea pig and kangaroo rat the cochlear input impedance can indeed be considered resistive. It is equally clear that in cat and chinchilla the experimental data do not agree with an assumption of purely resistive cochlear input impedance. In fact, in these two species the input impedance of the cochlea appears to contain a significant reactive component at low frequencies. This reactive component is manifested by a high-pass filter characteristic. It can be shown (Dallos, 1970) that the primary cause of the filter effect is the acoustic behavior of the helicotrema. At low frequencies the pressure difference across the cochlear partition equilibrates through the motion of the partition and through the helicotrema. It is clear that, as more equilibration takes place through the helicotrema, less pressure difference is available to move the cochlear partition. Thus for all purposes the helicotrema and the cochlear partition form a parallel acoustic circuit. It appears intuitively clear that the larger the helicotrema the more effective acoustic shunt it represents. We have made measurements on the size of the helicotrema two ways, either by reconstructing the helicotremas from serial sections, or directly in osmium-fixed preparations. These measurements are rather difficult, and not very accurate, due to the fact that the helicotrema is a very complex three-dimensional structure, especially in cat and chinchilla. It is possible that our measurements might be off as much as 30%. Even without extremely accurate measures, it is quite striking that the helicotremas of cat and chinchilla have cross-sectional areas that are approximately ten times as large as those of guinea pig and kangaroo rat. Thus the possibility of explaining the dichotomy seen in the CM functions by the acoustic shunting effect of the helicotrema does exist.

The acoustic impedance of a circular opening of radius a and length l is (Beranek, 1954, p. 135)

$$Z_h = R_h + j\omega M_h = \frac{8\mu l}{\pi a^4} + j\frac{4\rho_0 l}{3\pi a^2}\omega \tag{4.157}$$

where μ is the coefficient of viscosity of the fluid in the opening and ρ_0 is its density. We assume that this impedance shunts some acoustic resistance R_c, which represents the input impedance of the cochlea, *without* the contribution of the helicotrema. Zwislocki (1948) computed this value and obtained approximately 10,000 dynes second/cm^3. The area of the scala vestibuli at $x = 0$ is approximately 2 mm^2; thus we shall use the value of $R_c = 5-10^5$ dynes second/cm^5. The total input impedance is computed as

$$Z_c = \frac{R_c Z_h}{R_c + Z_h} = \frac{R_c(R_h + j\omega M_h)}{R_c + R_h + j\omega M_h} \tag{4.158}$$

The absolute value of the input impedance Z_c can be obtained from Eq. (4.158). It is easiest to treat in the form of Eq. (4.159).

$$Z_c = \frac{R_c R_h}{R_c + R_h}\frac{[1+\omega^2(M_h/R_h)^2]^{1/2}}{\{1+\omega^2[M_h/(R_c + R_h)]^2\}^{1/2}} \tag{4.159}$$

Inspection of Eq. (4.159) reveals that the dc value of the impedance is $R_c R_h/(R_c + R_h)$, while at high frequencies the impedance tends toward R_c. Thus the high-frequency input impedance is independent of the helicotrema, while the low-frequency value is strongly dependent on it. Between the low-frequency asymptote $[R_c R_h/(R_c + R_h)]$ and the high-frequency asymptote (R_c) the function is frequency dependent. The value of the low corner frequency is $\omega_1 = R_h/M_h$, while the value of the high corner frequency is $\omega_2 = (R_c + R_h)/M_h$. By substituting the appropriate expressions from Eq. (4.157), we obtain the two cutoff frequencies

$$f_1 = \frac{3\mu}{\pi\rho_0 a^2} \quad \text{and} \quad f_2 = \frac{3}{8\pi}\left(\frac{8\mu}{\rho_0 a^2} + \frac{R_c \pi a^2}{l\rho_0}\right) \tag{4.160}$$

The important conclusion can be drawn from Eq. (4.160) that the lower cutoff frequency is independent of the depth of the helicotrema (l), and it changes in inverse proportion with the square of the equivalent radius. The higher cutoff frequency is related to the radius and the depth in a more complex manner. For comparison, numerical values are computed for guinea pig and chinchilla with the assumption that $l = 0.1$ mm, $\mu = 0.02$ gm/cm second, and $\rho_0 = 1$ gm/cm^3. The following values result: $f_1^{gp} = 298$ Hz, $f_1^{ch} = 30.5$ Hz, $f_2^{gp} = 890$ Hz, $f_2^{ch} = 5820$ Hz. Thus the cutoff frequencies are relatively close together for the guinea pig and far apart for the chinchilla. The low-frequency asymptotes can also be computed for these two species to yield $|Z_c^{ch}(0)| = 1.3 \times 10^3$ dynes second/cm^5, while $|Z_c^{gp}(0)| = 10^5$ dynes second/cm^5. The high-frequency asymptote of course is the same for both species, $R_c = 5 \times 10^5$ dynes second/cm^5. Clearly there is a much more pronounced frequency-dependent effect in the chinchilla's input impedance than in the guinea pig's. In the former a change in impedance magnitude of approximately 77-fold takes place between the approximate frequencies of 30 and 6000 Hz. In the latter only a fivefold change occurs within the narrow frequency band from 300 to 900 Hz. Both the magnitude and the phase of

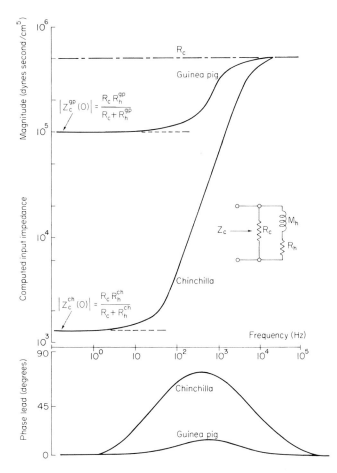

Fig. 4.17. Theoretical plot of cochlear input impedance magnitude and phase for guinea pig and chinchilla. The plots are based on Eq. (4.159) and our anatomical data. (From Dallos, 1970, p. 498.)

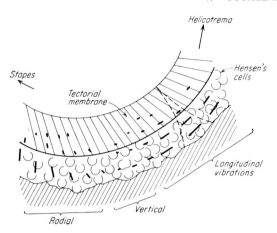

Fig. 4.19. Positions of radial and longitudinal vibrations of the organ of Corti during tonal stimulation. The partition is viewed through Reissner's membrane. (From von Békésy, 1960, p. 497.)

Von Békésy (1953) noted that the longitudinal displacement of a cell would be proportional to the derivative of the traveling wave, and Khanna *et al.* (1968a) studied the distribution of the longitudinal vibrations in the cochlea. These authors programmed a computer to calculate the spatial

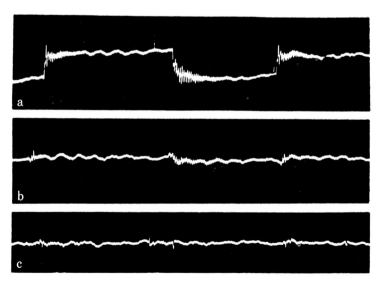

Fig. 4.20. Microphonic potentials in the guinea pig cochlea obtained by the vibrating electrode when the direction of electrode movement was (a) radial, (b) longitudinal, and (c) vertical relative to the basilar membrane. (From von Békésy, 1960, p. 684.)

distribution of these longitudinal "shear waves"; some of their results are shown in Fig. 4.21. Note that in this figure the envelopes of both the traveling wave and the shear wave are given for a number of frequencies. It is very clear that the shear wave is more localized than the traveling wave. The increase in sharpness is especially pronounced at the lower frequencies. The shear wave is displaced toward the apex from the peak of the traveling wave. The significant constriction of the longitudinal shear wave as opposed to the traveling wave, and the fact that this constriction is primarily on the low-frequency side, where it is most needed, seem to provide a very plausible basis of sharpening. Higher order derivatives of the traveling wave displacement function show ever-increasing sharpness, in that they occupy narrower and narrower segments of the basilar membrane. At least one theory (Huggins

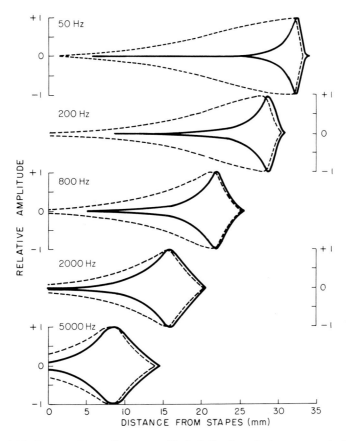

Fig. 4.21. Computed traveling wave (dashed lines) and shear wave (solid lines) envelopes at various frequencies as the function of distance along the cochlear partition. (From Khanna *et al.*, 1968a, p. 1081.)

1953) attributes major importance to the fourth derivative of the membrane displacement function. In Huggins' model the appropriate stimulus to the external hair cells is a force wave that is proportional to the fourth derivative.

B. Energy Transfer in the Cochlea: Fluid or Membrane?

Let us consider some implications of the prior treatment of membrane dynamics. In the derivation a force balance is assumed, through the $p = Zv$ relationship, for an elementary membrane segment of width dx. No coupling terms are introduced between adjacent membrane segments, which implies that all energy transfer is between individual segments of the membrane and the surrounding fluid, and that there is no energy transfer from one membrane element to the next. The distinction between "driving" the membrane from one element to the next and from the surrounding fluid to each independent element can be illustrated by the following examples. If a rope is anchored at one end and is being shaken at the other end, then in this familiar situation we know that a periodic up and down motion of the free end creates waves that move along the rope. This is a clear case of energy transfer from element to element within the vibrating structure itself. The surrounding medium has no effect on the movement of the rope. The converse arrangement can be described by a more artificial situation. Assume that little balls are placed in cylinders so that they can freely move up and down in them. All cylinders communicate with one another at the top and the bottom through a common space. The entire structure is filled with fluid. Under stationary conditions all balls float at the same height. If harmonic pressure differences are created between the top and bottom chambers then the balls are going to be displaced about their equilibrium positions, and under appropriate circumstances they will be displaced so that, visually at least, one would see a wave pattern traveling along the row of balls. In this situation of course the individual balls are not directly connected, and thus no energy can be transferred from one to another. They all are, however, within the same medium, and it is the interaction of the medium and the individual elements that creates the wave motion.

It is intuitively clear that neither of these simple models is adequate to describe the type of vibrations that exist in the cochlea. In the first model the effect of the surrounding medium is ignored, while in the second model the mutual coupling of adjacent elements within the vibrating structure is ignored. In the cochlea the fluids surrounding the partition certainly exert their influence on whatever vibratory patterns develop, but one must keep in mind that the cochlear partition is not made up of completely independent segments. Thus to some degree coupling must exist both between the membrane and the surrounding fluid and between adjacent membrane elements. The usual derivation of analytic expressions for wave motion of the partition ignores the interaction between membrane elements and places all emphasis on the energy transfer between membrane and fluid. Consequently such derivations are only approximate. The question is, how good is the approximation, and what is the justification for using it? Conversely, one should inquire whether the opposite simplification might not be appropriate; that is, could one obtain an appropriate mathematical model by completely ignoring the fluid dynamics of the cochlea and considering only the membrane properties? This last possibility can be easily discarded, for one of von Békésy's model experiments (1960, p. 446) is directly addressed to this question. In a cochlear model von Békésy closed the helicotrema, drained out the fluid, and introduced airborne stimulating sound into the cochlear canal. He argued that if the fluid load on the membrane were unimportant, that is, if the characteristics of the vibratory pattern were determined solely by the mechanical properties of the cochlear partition, then the pattern of vibrations in a dry cochlea would be similar to that in a normal, fluid-filled model. He noted that this was not the case: In the dry model the entire partition vibrated in the same phase and there was no displacement of the maximum of the vibration with a change in frequency. One can conclude on this basis that the surrounding fluid is indispensable for the development of the usual frequency-sensitive vibratory pattern in the cochlear partition. Consequently, any mathematical model of cochlear dynamics must take the hydrodynamic properties of the cochlea into account.

To investigate the relative contributions to membrane motion of energy transmission via the fluid and via the membrane, von Békésy (1960, pp. 526–532) constructed some simple and ingenious models; one of these consisted of a rigid cylinder rotated around its axis by a heavy pendulum. From the cylinder he suspended many smaller pendulums, varying in length, but all having the same bob mass. Between each adjacent pendulum von Békésy suspended a small coupling mass. These coupling masses could be adjusted in height. In the first experiment he pushed all coupling masses all the way up to the driving cylinder, which of course is a situation in which there is no effective coupling between adjacent pendulums. Consider that this situation is analogous to the hypothetical case for the cochlea in which all energy to the membrane is communicated through the fluid (modeled by the driving rod, which in this case provides the same driving force to all the individual pendulums) and no energy is transmitted from one membrane element to the next. Von Békésy noted that when his pendulum system was disturbed by an initial displacement and then left free, all pendulums started to vibrate together, but due to their different lengths (and consequently to their different natural periods) phase differences rapidly developed between successive pendulums and the observer could see a wavelike displacement pattern travel from the short toward the long pendulums. The striking observation was made that as time passed the wavelengths of the oscillation decreased. Von Békésy commented that in actual cochleae such diminution of wavelength with time is not observed, and thus it is unlikely that the coupling between adjacent membrane elements would be completely negligible.

In his next experiment von Békésy arranged the coupling weights so that the coupling between pendulums gradually decreased from shorter to longer pendulums. This he achieved by placing the coupling weights at different heights. This situation is analogous to a cochlea in which part of the energy to a given membrane segment is supplied by the surrounding fluid (the cylinder) and part of it by the adjacent membrane segments (the coupling weights). Von Békésy noted that when this system was driven with a constant input, waves traveled from the short pendulum end toward the long pendulum end. Various experiments with this system implied that, while the cochlear fluid and the energy transmission from the fluid to the cochlear partition are absolutely necessary for the establishment of a traveling wave pattern, the coupling between neighboring segments of the partition is significant.

It should be mentioned that the approximation imposed by neglecting membrane coupling might not be as severe as one would think on the basis of von Békésy's pendulum experiments. The reason is that while the pendulum system is a very illuminating analog of the cochlea it certainly does not mimic all properties of the cochlea to such a degree that extremely close quantitative conclusions could be drawn from its use. For example, the use of a rigid driving cylinder implies infinite sound velocity in the fluids and would mean that all segments of the cochlear partition are subjected to the same driving force, namely, that the pressure difference across the membrane is the same magnitude and is in the same phase at all points. A study of the fluid equations indicates that this is not the case; in fact the pressure difference decreases significantly from stapes toward the apex (Zwislocki, 1965; Peterson and Bogert, 1950; Fletcher, 1953). The reader will undoubtedly recognize that the above is a somewhat circular argument, because the mathematical models did not assume mutual coupling between membrane elements. Thus these results, showing significant changes in fluid pressure, are not completely adequate to disprove von Békésy's conclusions. The only safe conclusion at this time is that coupling effects are more likely than not to be of some significance but probably are not as dominant as the pendulum experiments suggest. Consequently, mathematical models that ignore cross coupling in the membrane are probably adequate approximations, even though better results could be obtained if the actual membrane equations were introduced into the solution of the cochlear vibration problem.

Strong proponents of the idea that the membrane receives its energy from the fluid are Wever and Lawrence (1954) and Tonndorf (1959). The former authors used electrophysiological methods to study energy balance in the cochlea under conditions in which sound was simultaneously delivered at the oval window and through a fenestra in the apical end of the cochlea. By measuring cochlear potentials with electrodes placed on the bony capsule of the cochlea, Wever and Lawrence noted at that low frequencies these potentials could be nulled simultaneously at all electrode positions by adjustment of the two sound inputs. At higher frequencies, in order to maintain a null for basal versus apical electrodes, slight amplitude and phase adjustments were necessary. The authors interpreted their findings as evidence that the membrane receives its energy by a rapidly traveling pressure wave in the fluid and that the actual vibratory pattern is determined by the properties of the membrane itself. In an article jointly authored with von Békésy, Wever and Lawrence (1954) present a very clear statement of their views. To them, the term "traveling wave" implies energy transfer by the wave in the vibrating medium, in this case within the cochlear partition. They are in full accord with von Békésy's findings on the wave pattern in the cochlea, but they feel that the term used to describe this pattern is a misnomer. If it is understood that by traveling wave one means simply a temporal sequence of events without implying any form of energy transfer by the wave, then they are willing to accept the term. The same point concerning terminology was also emphasized by Davis (1957) and Tonndorf (1959).

One of the most compelling arguments in favor of the fluid energy transfer hypothesis comes from correlated clinical and histological evidence. It has been noted in human temporal bones that calcification of the basalmost portion of the basilar membrane often occurs without any appreciable low-frequency hearing loss (Crowe *et al.*, 1934). If the low-frequency, apical portion of the membrane received its energy from the more basal portion of the membrane, this finding could not be easily accepted. If, however, each membrane segment is supplied by the surrounding fluid, there is no contradiction, for defects of the high-frequency segment of the membrane should then have no significant influence on the function of the low-frequency region. One can summarize the prevailing view by quoting Tonndorf (1959).

> . . . traveling waves . . . are only produced in the transfer of energy from one perilymphatic scala to the other across the partition. There is no sense in considering the basilar membrane as an isolated system *within* which energy is being propagated from one end to the other. The partition, together with the fluids of both scalae, forms one complex system. On the one hand, properties of the membrane, viz. (a) its absolute value of stiffness, and (b) its gradient of stiffness, are responsible for the travelling wave *pattern* as such, its *extent*, the *rate* of accumulating phase shift, and its frequency *discrimination.* . . . On the other hand structural continuity of the membraneous partition does not seem to be absolutely mandatory for the existence of traveling waves. For the waves are seen to travel right across small discontinuities.

IV. Fine Motion Patterns in the Cochlea

A. Transformation of Motion from Basilar Membrane to Cilia

As we have seen in the extensive discussions above, the gross motion pattern of the cochlear partition is reasonably well understood. By using general hydrodynamic principles and known anatomical data we were able to derive analytic expressions that could be shown to fit the available experimental facts. Thus the traveling wave pattern of the cochlear partition as described by von Békésy, and as approximated by computations, can be accepted as an entity whose properties are fairly well known and which most certainly plays an important, although probably not exhaustive, role in the peripheral transmission of energy. Much less understood is the process whereby the vibration of the basilar membrane is transduced into neural responses. An incredible number of theories have been promulgated in the past, all aimed at explaining this step of the transducer process. As von Békésy (1966) rightly objected, most of these theories have no experimental basis whatsoever. Some more interesting ideas are discussed in the next chapter in connection with the theories of cochlear microphonic generation. Here we shall confine ourselves to the treatment of some ramifications of the most generally accepted scheme, and we shall discuss simple mechanical processes only.

It is widely conceded that the hair cells and their stereocilia must be intimately involved in the transduction chain. This conclusion is almost inescapable if one considers the fine anatomy of the organ of Corti, specifically the fact that it is the hair cell with which the neural connections are made. The role of the cilia themselves is not so clear-cut, but they seem to assume considerable importance in all theories formulated thus far. The cells or the cilia can be alternately construed to play primary roles. Thus if the cell is assumed to be the site of the final transduction from mechanical motion to electrical potentials or chemical substances, then the cilia are usually relegated to the role of mechanical transducers between the cell and its surrounding. If, however, the cilia are assumed to be the primary transducers, then the cell is merely assigned metabolic or conductive functions. The most common view is that the cell itself is the transducer and that the cilia act as mechanical linkages.

In discussing the transduction of mechanical energy by the hair cell one must first resolve the issue of adequate stimulus. The vibrations of the basilar membrane are transmitted to the hair cells in some form, with an eventual modification of the cell. The question is what this modification might be. Some possibilities can be discounted rather quickly; a few others are equiprobable. The most obvious first possibility is that the pressure in the cochlear fluid itself stimulates the cell. Von Békésy (1966) discussed and dismissed this possibility on the basis of comparisons with other mechano-receptors and by showing experimental evidence that pressure itself does not produce a sensation on the skin. He demonstrated that sensations can be elicited only by pressure gradients that set up shearing forces in the skin. Loewenstein (1965) has clearly shown that both the Lorenzinian ampulla and the Pacinian corpuscle are insensitive to static pressure, no matter how high the pressure is. In contrast both of these receptors are highly sensitive to distortional strain. It is probably a valid generalization that all mechano-receptors are stimulated by distortion and not by hydrostatic stress. Thus when dealing with the hair cell we must seek a mechanism that is capable of dis-torting the cell body or some surface of the cell to provide adequate stimula-tion.

One of the most attractive such mechanisms is comprised of the numerous cilia protruding from the top surface of the cells. If these cilia were bent or

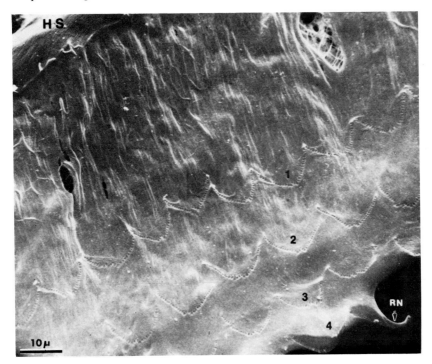

Fig. 4.22. Scanning electron microgram of the underside of the tectorial membrane. Indentations left by the tallest rows of cilia belonging to the four rows of outer hair cells (rows numbered) are clearly distinguished by their characteristic W pattern. There is no sign of indentations for the inner hair cell cilia in the area of Hansen's stripe (HS). Marginal net (RN) probably provides attachment between the tectorial membrane and the upper surface of Corti's organ, squirrel monkey. (Courtesy of Dr. D. Lim, 1972.)

deflected by some mechanism they would undoubtedly exert some lateral force on the surface from which they emerge. Such lateral force could distort the surface and thus give rise to stimulation (von Békésy, 1960). It is also conceivable that, instead of bending, the hairs would push down on the hair-bearing surface of the cell, causing a deformation in this manner (Crane, 1966). Some quantitative work is available on the relationship between basilar membrane displacement and the corresponding change in hair angle. The treatment assumes that the bending of the hair is facilitated by a relative sliding motion between the tectorial membrane and the reticular lamina. It is now quite safe to assume that at least the tallest cilia of the external hair cells are in actual contact with the bottom surface of the tectorial membrane (Kimura, 1966; Spoendlin, 1966). In Fig. 4.22 a scanning electron micrograph of the bottom surface of the tectorial membrane is shown. The picture clearly shows shallow indentations or pits corresponding to the tallest rows of cilia of the outer hair cells. There is no sign of similar pits for the inner hair cell cilia. The connection between the cilia of the outer hair cells and their pits on the tectorial membrane is probably secure enough to anchor the hair during a lateral relative displacement between the reticular lamina and the tectorial membrane. As von Békésy (1960) and Davis (1958) argued, such a lateral displacement could develop between the two membranes because of the structural geography of the organ of Corti.

The easiest way to explain this is by referring to a sketch by Davis, reproduced in Fig. 4.23. Here the basilar membrane, arch of Corti, and reticular

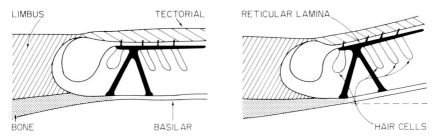

Fig. 4.23. Probable pattern of shearing action between tectorial membrane and reticular lamina resulting in the bending of hairs. (From Davis, 1958, p. 369.)

lamina, which form a complex, are assumed to move together or, more precisely, to rotate around a flexible suspension at the osseous spiral lamina. In contrast, the tectorial membrane is assumed to rotate about another pivot point located at the edge of the spiral limbus. Clearly, if two parallel planes are rotated about displaced centers, then points on the planes that were opposite to one another in the planes' resting positions, would no longer be so situated. A line (a hair) between two such opposing points would be rotated as the consequence of the lateral sliding of the two opposing points. This type of shearing motion, set up by the relative displacement between tectorial membrane and reticular lamina, on the hairs is the most commonly assumed distorting stimulus on the hair cell. It is immediately evident that the type of shear that is provided in the above scheme is a radial shear. In other words, in this process the hairs are bent in a radial direction when referenced to the spatial orientation of the cochlear spiral. It is remembered that von Békésy (1953) noted this type of shear to be evident on the proximal slope of the traveling wave envelope. There is apparently another, longitudinal shear pattern that could provide a different mode of stimulation via the longitudinal bending of the hairs. The two types of shear arise due to the dominant modes of curvature of the basilar membrane at the region of maximal vibrations and somewhat toward the base from that segment.

Tonndorf (1960a) gives a very clear demonstration of the genesis of these shear patterns. In Fig. 4.24 we reproduce the schematic on which his argument is based. Panel (a) of the figure shows the traveling wave in a situation where the basilar membrane is *not* fixed at its two edges. In this case all curvature,

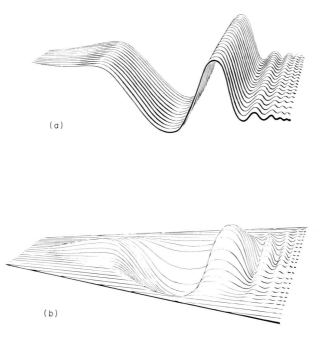

Fig. 4.24. Traveling wave patterns: (a) executed by a hypothetical ribbonlike partition; (b) observed along the single-layer partition of a cochlear model. Here the partition is anchored along its edges. Scales are arbitrary in both drawings, and magnitudes are exaggerated. (From Tonndorf, 1960a, p. 241.)

and consequently all shear, is in the longitudinal direction. Panel (b) shows the real situation, in which the basilar membrane is depicted at rest all along its attached edges. In this case in the region where the wavelength is long (much longer than the width of the membrane) the dominant curvature, and shear, is radial. Beyond the maximum, where the wavelength becomes short and the amplitude small, the dominant curvature assumes a longitudinal character. It is noteworthy that almost all considerations, qualitative or quantitative, of hair bending in the stimulation process have been directed at radial bending. There is no a priori reason why this would constitute the right approach. In fact the observation that the spatial extent of the longitudinal shear wave is more restricted might favor the study of this phenomenon. The quantitative treatments that have been developed apply to radial shear only.

The two quantitative studies that were addressed to relating basilar membrane motion to hair angle change or to the magnitude of the displacement of the two opposing points on the two parallel membranes are those of Johnstone and Johnstone (1966) and Rhode and Geissler (1967). The former model will be discussed in the next chapter, since its originators intended to explain with it the production of summating potentials in the cochlea. Suffice it to say here that this model derives a nonlinear hair motion pattern associated with linear basilar membrane vibrations. A direct consequence of the nonlinear hair displacement is a strong dc bending component, which is of opposite polarity for inner and outer hair cells and thus presumably provides the genesis for positive and negative summating potentials. As we shall discuss later in detail, one flaw in this model is that it assumes that there is a resting angle associated with the hairs which is different for hairs emanating from the two types of hair cell. With zero resting angle (which is the actual situation, substantiated by all electron microscope evidence) there is no nonlinear interrelationship between hair and basilar membrane motion. Of course, the actual geometrical model of Johnstone and Johnstone is valid in this case and can be useful in computing the magnitude of angular displacement of the hairs that correspond to a given up or down motion of the basilar membrane. The model of Rhode and Geissler was designed to quantify this latter relationship or, more precisely, to relate the magnitude of displacement between two quiescently opposing points to the displacement of the basilar membrane. Their assumptions are that the tectorial membrane is rigid and pivots around the edge of the limbus, that the complex consisting of the reticular lamina, the arch of Corti, and the portion of the basilar membrane between the pillars of Corti is rigid, and that the entire complex rotates around a pivot at the foot of the inner pillars. For small values of basilar membrane deflection they derived that opposing point displacement is proportional to basilar membrane displacement. The proportionality factor was computed by Rhode and Geissler for both the exact and approximate solutions, at various points along the basilar membrane and at various magnitudes of basilar membrane displacement.

They found that at least for the cat, for which the anatomical data apply, the opposing point displacement is a linear function of the basilar membrane displacement up to about 10 μ. This implies that nonlinearities in the mechanical transduction are most likely not due to distortion occurring between basilar membrane and hair motion. It is interesting to note that for a given basilar membrane displacement (0.1 μ) the opposing point displacement is not constant at all points along the basilar membrane; it is smaller as the distance from the stapes increases. This implies that to provide the same degree of stimulation at the low- and high-frequency regions of the cochlea, one must increase the amplitude of the basilar membrane.

While the opposing point displacement is apparently a linear function of basilar membrane displacement, it is important to remember some peculiarities of hair cell anatomy before we assume that this linearity implies that the hair cells are stimulated by a linear deformation pattern. All electron microscope evidence indicates that only one row of cilia on any given outer hair cell actually makes contact with the tectorial membrane (see Fig. 4.22). This W-shaped row is the one closest to the opening on the cuticular plate (farthest away from the modiolus). All other rows of cilia are shorter and they do not contact the tectorial membrane. If the bending of the hairs is the crucial stimulus then the anatomical considerations indicate that stimulation will be unequal when the hairs are bent toward or away from the modiolus. To explain, consider that the basilar membrane is moving down (toward scala tympani). Under this condition the relative sliding motion between reticular lamina and tectorial membrane is such that the latter is displaced toward the modiolus, and as a consequence the hairs are bent toward the central axis of the cochlea. Since the outermost hairs are anchored by the tectorial membrane, during their bending they push the more central rows ahead of themselves. As a consequence, all cilia are bent, and they all exert their deforming effect on the cuticular plate. In the converse situation, in which the basilar membrane moves toward the scala vestibuli, the relative motion between reticular lamina and tectorial membrane is such that the latter moves toward the stria vascularis. The outermost, tallest, row of cilia is thus bent away from the central axis of the cochlea. In this case, however, the inner rows of hairs are unlikely to follow to the full extent of the excursion. This is the likely case since the hairs are quite independent of one another, and thus adjacent cilia can push but not pull each other. Even if we concede some adherence of adjacent cilia (conceivably due to the mucopolysaccharide molecules that fill the space between the cilia) it is still unlikely that complete symmetry of push and pull movements could be achieved. Thus, stimulation

In defense of linear extrapolation one must mention that attempts to check linearity, albeit over very restricted ranges, by von Békésy (1960) and Johnstone *et al.* (1970) were reported to be successful. In addition, we know that other transducers of considerable physical bulk do seem to operate linearly down to mechanical displacements that are commensurate with the dimensions in question. For example, the condenser microphone does provide linear voltages in proportion to sound pressure down to 0.0002 dyne/cm^2, where the motion of the air molecules, and thus presumably of the microphone diaphragm, is of the order of 10^{-9} cm, or 0.1 Å (Miller *et al.*, 1964). Similarly, when the voltage that activates a loudspeaker is decreased, it can be shown that the displacement of the diaphragm decreases linearly with the driving voltage down to 10^{-10}–10^{-11} cm, or to the very magnitudes that we are interested in. These measurements were made without any extrapolation by the method of laser interferometry (Khanna, 1969). It should also be remembered that the cochlear microphonic potential, which as we shall see

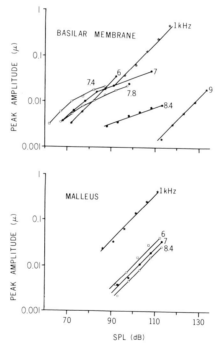

Fig. 4.25. Peak amplitude of the basilar membrane as a function of SPL for several frequencies. Note that the motion of the basilar membrane is linear at 1, 6, and 9 kHz. A nonlinearity appears for 7 kHz at about 70 dB SPL. The nonlinearity becomes more pronounced with an increase in either frequency or SPL. The peak amplitude of the malleus is also a function of SPL. Notice that the malleus vibrated linearly at the SPL's of interest. (From Rhode, 1971, p. 1224.)

is proportional to basilar membrane displacement, is a linear function of sound pressure from about 70 dB SPL to as far down as it is feasible to measure: over at least an 80-dB range. The above points are meant to provide only circumstantial evidence supporting the feasibility of linear extrapolations from von Békésy's measurements.

While the earlier measurements seem to support the notion of linear basilar membrane vibrations, the most recent experiments, those of Rhode (1971), seem to indicate that nonlinearity might influence the system, at least over a limited frequency range. Rhode noted that if his stimulating frequency was so chosen that it was either above or below the best frequency

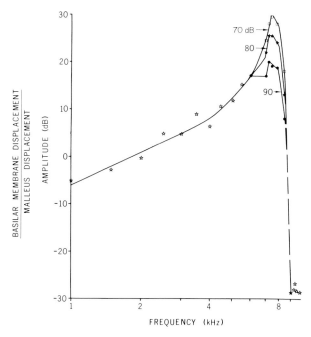

Fig. 4.26. Amplitude of the ratio in decibels of the displacements of the basilar membrane and malleus for three SPL's, 70 (squares), 80 (opaque stars), and 90 dB (circles). Data for displacement of the malleus were obtained at higher intensities and linearly extrapolated to the indicated intensities. Measurements for the basilar membrane had to be extrapolated at several frequencies, including 8.4 kHz. The vibration of the basilar membrane was linear at 1, 6, and 9 kHz, justifying linear extrapolation at these frequencies. The data points for frequencies between 1 and 6 kHz (open stars) were obtained using intensities that varied from 100 dB at 1 kHz to 75 dB at 6 kHz. No test of linearity was run at these frequencies, but the experimental results at 1 and 6 kHz suggest that the basilar membrane vibrates linearly for this range of frequencies at the intensities of interest. Observations from other experiments support this conclusion. The data points for frequencies above 9 kHz (open stars) were determined by using intensities between 115 and 125 dB SPL. (From Rhode, 1971, p. 1223.)

for the point of measurement along the basilar membrane, then the membrane vibratory amplitude was a linear function of the malleus amplitude (and of SPL) for all levels at which he could perform his measurements. In contrast, in the vicinity of the best frequency the membrane vibration exhibited a marked nonlinearity. Figures 4.25 and 4.26 demonstrate these findings. In Fig. 4.25 some input–output functions are shown for basilar membrane and malleus displacements at various frequencies. Note that the functions obtained for frequencies removed from the best frequency (approximately 7000 Hz) are linear; of course, so are all functions that depict middle ear behavior. The curves that are plotted for the best-frequency region exhibit a relatively strong nonlinearity in the direction of saturation at higher driving levels. Another view of the phenomenon is shown in Fig. 4.26, where tuning curves are given in the form of the ratio of basilar membrane and malleus amplitude versus frequency at several sound pressure levels. At the frequencies where the data points are indicated by stars the SPL had no influence on the ratio; in other words, the system was linear. Around the maximum the ratio decreases with increasing sound intensity. Notice that at the lowest sound level used (70 dB SPL) at the best frequency the basilar membrane vibrates with an amplitude that is about 30 dB higher than the amplitude of the malleus. This indicates a considerable gain. At 90 dB SPL the gain is only 20 dB. It is clear that, if the trend were to continue toward lower SPL's, membrane amplitudes at the threshold of audibility would need not be as small as expected on the basis of linear extrapolations of von Békésy's data. If Rhode's results are confirmed, and we remember that they conflict with the observations of von Békésy and Johnstone and his colleagues, then of course it is easier to conceive how basilar membrane movements are translated into hair cell deformation.

2. Brownian Motion as Limiting Factor

As we have seen, if the linear extrapolation of von Békésy's data is used down to threshold levels, the expected displacement of the basilar membrane is very small. The question naturally arises whether this displacement is large enough to be above the thermal noise level, which undoubtedly does create a certain degree of mechanical agitation. This has been a disturbing question for some years. It was originally formulated for the eardrum by Sivian and White (1933), later extended by de Vries (1952), and recently discussed in detail by Harris (1968). We shall present some of Harris' persuasive arguments in a rather sketchy form.

By assuming a 1000-Hz bandwidth, Harris computed that the Brownian motion of air molecules generates a mean pressure fluctuation of 1.27×10^{-5} dyne/cm^2. The usually accepted value of sound pressure corresponding to free-field listening threshold is 18 dB above the pressure level of thermal fluctuations. Thus one can immediately see that Brownian motion of air molecules is certainly *not* the limiting factor of our hearing sensitivity. A more crucial question, however, concerns the energy that is passed by the ossicular chain, by the hydromechanical transducer of the inner ear, and that is distributed to a single hair cell. Clearly this final energy must have a much smaller value than the total that is conducted by the eardrum. Is this energy, absorbed by a single hair cell, above or below the thermal fluctuation of the cell itself? Harris used two methods in computing the relationship between hair cell displacement at the threshold of audibility and that due to Brownian noise. First he assumed that the mechanical coupling among hair cells is very weak. This implies that the cells are loosely suspended and that the displacement of one has little or no effect on its neighbor. Another implication is that, since the average energy of thermal motion of a body is approximately constant, if the mass of the body is small then its displacement and velocity due to the thermal agitation would be large. If the cells are loosely coupled, only the mass of a single cell needs to be taken into account in the calculation. Under such circumstances the signal-to-noise ratio at threshold, that is, the ratio of cell displacement due to the external stimulus to its displacement due to thermal noise, is computed to be -33 dB. This figure implies that the useful displacement would be completely overshadowed by the random fluctuations due to thermal noise. If, however, it is assumed that the hair cells are strongly coupled to one another, one must take the mass of all coherently moving cells and their supporting structures into account in computing thermal fluctuations. Clearly under these circumstances one can expect the amplitudes and velocities that are due to the noise to be considerably reduced. The results bear out the expectations; for the strong coupling case Harris obtained a signal-to-noise ratio of $+22$ dB, which of course is quite favorable. In reality coupling among hair cells, is not completely rigid, but electron microscope studies show that the reticular lamina, which supports the hair-bearing ends of the cells (most likely to be the critical region for stimulation), is a rigid and dense plate that is unlikely to allow much lateral flexibility. Thus while the signal-to-noise ratio of $+22$ dB might be overly optimistic, it is almost certain that even allowing some degree of flexibility of coupling, the ultimate limitation of auditory sensitivity is not thermal motion, even though this limit is closely approached.

V. Laplace Transform and Circuit Models of Cochlear Dynamics

This chapter would be incomplete without a discussion of some very practical modeling efforts aimed at providing computational and measuring convenience. The hydrodynamic model that has been discussed so far is based on our best judgment about the actual physical functioning of the inner ear. This model of course yields a great deal of insight into the system's operation and its dependence on physical parameters such as dimensions and boundary conditions. The results are in the form of partial differential equations and cumbersome partial solutions to these equations. Such results are not ideal for quick computational purposes. Another means of describing the operation of the system is to provide a mathematical structure for computational purposes without any regard to the physics of the system. This method involves the derivation of appropriate descriptive formulas on the basis of curve fitting or matching experimental results. Whenever the only issue of interest is to describe the input–output properties of a system without any need for gleaning insight into the actual "inner working" of the mechanism, the curve fitting method can provide adequate and easy results.

Flanagan (1960) desired just such a mathematical analog of the inner ear and he derived a computational model for its approximation. He studied von Békésy's data of basilar membrane amplitude and phase and first recast these data to make them amenable for curve fitting. The original data on which Flanagan's efforts are based are shown in Figs. 4.8 and 4.10. These curves describe band-pass filters, and to compare them Flanagan normalized them with respect to frequency. His normalized results are presented in Fig. 4.27 as the cross-hatched region. For simplicity he assumed that all the

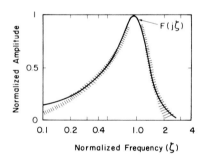

Fig. 4.27. Normalized frequency response of the mathematical model of Flanagan compared with the von Békésy data; spread of 200, 400, 800 Hz. (Adapted from Flanagan, 1960, p. 1177.)

"resonance curves" had the same Q; the lower skirt of the functions was taken to rise at a rate of 6 dB/octave, while the upper skirt was between 20 and 30 dB/octave. Recall that von Békésy's low-frequency phase was shown to be $0°$. Flanagan argued that this is most likely an experimental error, for physical considerations dictate that the dc phase be $90°$ lead. He demonstrated the fit between the experimental curves and three different mathematical functions; we shall present only one of these.

To fit the functions one must consider them to be the graphical representations of a transfer function, namely its magnitude and phase. One complex transfer function that is in an acceptable form is the following:

$$F(s) = c\beta^{4+r} \left(\frac{s}{s+\gamma} \right) \left[\frac{1}{(s+\alpha)^2 + \beta^2} \right]^2 e^{-sT} \tag{4.167}$$

In this expression s is of course the complex frequency that was introduced at the beginning of the last chapter, c is a constant to be adjusted so that the expression yields the proper absolute magnitude, and β^{4+r} is a scale factor used to adjust the variation of amplitude with frequency. Assuming that below 1000 Hz the amplitude maximum rises with frequency at a rate of 5 dB/octave, the value of r can be taken as 0.83. The exponential term e^{-sT} introduces excess phase lag. Without this term the phase of the transfer function would not be sufficient to account for the total phase lag shown by the experimental data. This factor has a physical meaning; it corresponds to a time delay of T seconds. The transfer function itself has a zero at the origin, a real pole at γ, and two pairs of complex poles at $s = \alpha \pm j\beta$. Since constant Q was assumed, it is permissible to relate the real and imaginary parts of the complex poles as $\beta = k\alpha$. For a steady-state condition this transfer function reduces to

$$F(j\omega) = c\beta^{4+r} \frac{j\omega}{\gamma + j\omega} \left[\frac{1}{(\beta^2 + \beta^2/k^2 - \omega^2) + j2\beta\omega/k} \right]^2 e^{-j\omega T} \tag{4.168}$$

The curve fitting process yielded the following parameter values: $\gamma/\beta = 1$, $k = 2$, and $T = 3\pi/4\beta$. Notice that it was necessary to make the delay time T a variable. It is taken as inversely proportional to the resonant frequency β. This general function can be amplitude and frequency normalized to facilitate comparisons with the von Békésy data. This is accomplished by substituting $\zeta = \omega/\beta$ and by plotting $|F(j\zeta)|/|F(j\zeta_{max})|$. Such a plot is given in Fig. 4.27. In the figure the various von Békésy curves are denoted by cross-hatching, and it is clear that the fit of the mathematical model is quite good. This transfer function then represents the ratio and phase between basilar membrane and stapes displacements. It is a linear model, very useful for computational purposes, but it clearly provides no insight into the operation of the cochlea.

To make his computational model more useful, Flanagan (1962) combined it with a transfer function description of the middle ear, to yield a combined middle ear–inner ear transfer function. He chose the simple middle ear description of

$$G(s) = \frac{c_0}{(s+a)\left[(s+a)^2 + b^2\right]} \tag{4.169}$$

with the additional simplifications of $c_0 = a(a^2 + b^2)$ and $b = 2a = 2\pi \cdot 1500$.

When this middle ear model is combined with the previously shown inner ear transfer function, the overall, pressure at the eardrum to displacement of the basilar membrane transfer function is obtained. In Fig. 4.28 the magnitude

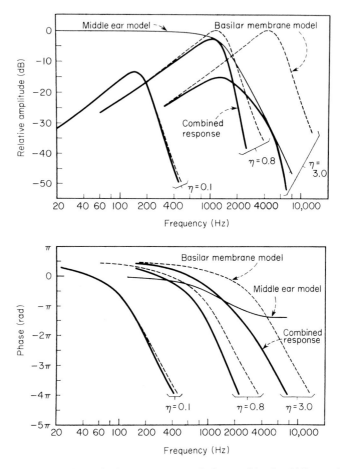

Fig. 4.28. Magnitude and phase responses of the combined middle ear–inner ear model for three cochlear locations whose best frequencies are 150, 1200, and 4500 Hz, corresponding to $\eta = 0.1$, 0.8, and 3.0. (From Flanagan, 1962, p. 975.)

and phase of the combined function are shown. In the plots the parameter $\eta = \beta/b$ expresses the ratio between the best frequency of a given basilar membrane point and the corner frequency of the middle ear response (taken at 1500 Hz). It is quite instructive to note how the low-pass character of the middle ear alters the high-frequency response of basal points on the basilar membrane. A point near the stapes, for example, clearly has a best frequency at which it responds with greater amplitude than any other point on the membrane. The magnitude of response of this point at its best frequency, however, is *not* the largest response that this point can sustain. In fact it vibrates at a greater amplitude at a frequency below its "resonant" point.

Flanagan's computational model has proven to be a very useful research tool. It should be remembered, however, that it is based on basilar membrane tuning characteristics that were described by von Békésy. It is evident from newer data that von Békésy's results underestimate the sharpness of tuning, at least in the basal and central part of the cochlea. As we have noted before there appears to be a systematic growth in the Q of the tuning curves as one moves from apex toward the base. New computational models, using Flanagan's approach, should be derived to match the tuning characteristics of the Johnstone and Rhode measurements; these should take into account the significant increase in Q in the basal region of the cochlea.

Several circuit models of the peripheral auditory system have been constructed by numerous investigators (among them Wansdronk, 1962; Glaesser *et al.*, 1963; Flanagan, 1962). These models usually cascade three blocks, one representing the external, one the middle, and one the inner ear. The modeling of the inner ear is usually based on the recognition that the cochlea is essentially a tapered transmission line. Consequently a model of it can be constructed by cascading an adequate number of circuit segments. Each of these has the same structure but the individual component values are appropriately graduated. Circuit models of this type are very practical means of visualizing motion patterns in the cochlea with various excitation. All the investigator needs is an oscilloscope to measure voltage at a given point (voltage being proportional to displacement), or if the traveling wave is to be visualized a serial sampling arrangement is also required to sequentially display the various points along the simulated transmission line. The circuit model combined with a variety of neural models is of even greater use in testing many neural elements excited with a displacement pattern like that produced by the cochlear partition.

VI. Transient Response

Up to this point our total effort has been directed to the description of the functioning of the cochlear analyzer with harmonic stimuli. While the analysis with sinusoidal inputs has proven to be extremely revealing, it should be kept in mind that this sort of signal is relatively artificial. The inputs that occur in nature are more like a sequence of acoustic transients than a steady-state sinusoid. If for no other reason, it is important to inquire about the transient response properties of the basilar membrane.

In a linear system the frequency response characteristics and transient properties are intimately related. In fact, the transfer function of such a system is identical to the Laplace transform of the system's impulse response. In a nonlinear system, however, a uniquely determined relationship between steady-state and transient behavior is not a necessity. First, let us inquire about the sort of impulse response that can be predicted from the steady-state model assuming that the system is linear. Let us follow this by correlating the impulse response with available experimental data. Finally, let us ask if the assumption of linearity is tenable.

Flanagan (1962) and Siebert (1962) derived impulse response functions for the cochlear partition by taking the inverse Laplace transform of the system transfer function. It is remembered that the latter was obtained by fitting von Békésy's data with an appropriate (not unique and, in Siebert's case, not physically realizable) function of the complex frequency s. The resulting time function (from Flanagan) is demonstrated in Fig. 4.29. Here the

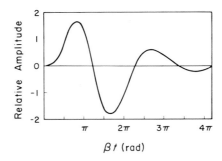

Fig. 4.29. Normalized impulse response of the cochlear partition; β is the best frequency of a given location. (Adapted from Flanagan, 1962, p. 965.)

amplitude scale is relative and the time scale is normalized; as a consequence this response form is general and is adequate to depict the temporal pattern of vibrations at any point along the basilar membrane* when the stapes is given an impulsive excursion. It is also to be noted that the transportation delay to a given point along the membrane is not incorporated in the figure. The response actually begins after a delay that depends on the position. The abscissa time scale is graduated in units of βt radians, where β is the best frequency of the cochlear location whose impulse response is sought. Inspection of Fig. 4.29 indicates that the response is a decaying oscillation with an approximate frequency of β and with relatively rapid (of the order of 20

---

* The model does not take the recently noted increase in Q toward the basal region into account. Consequently actual impulse responses of more basal portions of the basilar membrane should be less damped than those of the apical region.

dB/cycle) decrease in amplitude. The interpretation of this is that, when the basilar membrane is set in vibration with an impulsive stimulus, at any point along the membrane decaying oscillations are sustained having a frequency that is the same as the best frequency of the given point. Thus, for example, a point on the membrane whose best frequency is 1000 Hz would vibrate at this rate, and the total duration of vibrations that would correspond to about 3 cycles would be 3 mseconds. In contrast, the 10,000-Hz point would vibrate at this latter frequency, but for only about 0.3 msecond.

Von Békésy (1943) did attempt some measurements of the impulse response of the cochlear partition. His results were obtained from the apical end of the cochlea and they showed the type of decaying oscillation that we have been discussing above. Von Békésy estimated that the logarithmic decrement of the vibrations was between 1.4 and 1.8. These figures are in agreement with similar values that could be derived from his tuning curves. Aside from these measurements there are no direct determinations of basilar membrane transient response. Some fascinating information can be derived, however, from the temporal pattern of discharges in the 8th nerve in response to click (impulsive) stimuli. The poststimulus time (PST) histograms* of various auditory nerve fibers show that the pattern of firing exhibits some very well defined properties. As we see in Fig. 4.30, where an array of PST histograms from Kiang (1965) are shown, for fibers whose best frequency is below about 5000 Hz the histograms are multimodal, while above this frequency only a single peak can be discriminated. Careful investigation discloses that the latency of the initial peak is inversely proportional to the unit's best frequency, while the interpeak interval is exactly equal to the reciprocal of the best frequency. We thus see that a fiber emanating from the apex of the cochlea (low characteristic frequency) starts responding much later than one that originates in the base (high characteristic frequency). The fact that low-frequency fibers have multipeaked PST histograms in which the successive peaks decrease in size indicates that these fibers respond to a decaying periodic oscillation of the basilar membrane. The period of oscillations (the periodicity in the histogram) is uniquely determined by the characteristic frequency of the fiber, which is the equivalent of saying that it is a function of the location of the fiber origin.

It is clear that the features of the histograms and the computed impulse response are in qualitative agreement in both showing decaying oscillations with a period that is the reciprocal of the best frequency. There are two aspects in which the single-unit data and the computed basilar membrane

---

* A PST histogram provides the number of neural spikes that occur at any given instant after the delivery of a stimulus. Thus in Fig. 4.30 zero time corresponds to the presentation of the stimulus click, the abscissa is the time in milliseconds after this event, and the ordinate is the number of discharges in a given time unit.

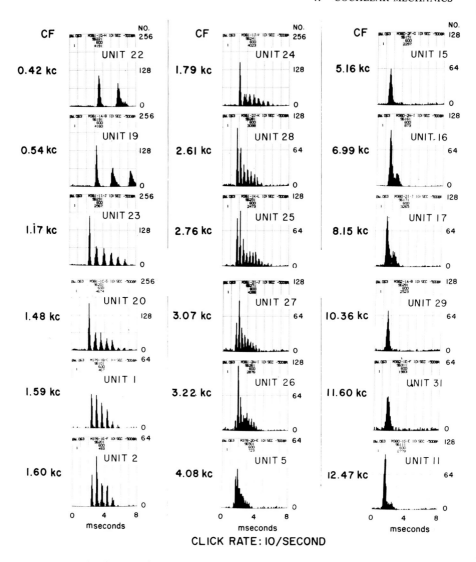

Fig. 4.30. The PST histograms of responses to clicks from 18 units obtained in a single cat. (From Kiang, 1965, p. 28.)

response disagree. First, theoretically there is no need to have an upper-limiting frequency beyond which the oscillations would no longer be periodic; in contrast, beyond approximately 5000 Hz the histograms are unimodal. Second, the decay time of the histograms is significantly longer than what one would expect on the basis of the computed basilar membrane impulse response. The first discrepancy might be due to the limited resolving capability of the computing method that generates the PST histograms. The finite width of the unit interval within which spikes are counted and the statistical jitter in the occurrence of the spikes combine to average out individual peaks (if they exist) in the histogram when these peaks are very closely spaced. The second discrepancy is more serious, it very simply means that the temporal pattern of 8th nerve responses and the tuning characteristics of the basilar membrane as determined from von Békésy's data are not compatible if the system is linear. This incompatibility was noted and emphasized by a number of investigators (Weiss, 1964; de Boer, 1969; Møller, 1970b). It appears that in order to account for the peculiarities of the PST histograms, specifically for their slow decay, either the mechanical tuning of the basilar membrane has to be much sharper than what is indicated by von Békésy's measurements, or the transformation from basilar membrane motion to spike generation in the 8th nerve is a highly nonlinear operation. The more recent measurements of Johnstone and Taylor (1970) and Rhode (1971) tend to indicate that the impasse can be resolved, or at least largely resolved, without the necessity of a nonlinear transformation. The tuning curves obtained by these investigators are sharp enough, so that the impulse response that is predictable from them would have a sufficiently slow decay.

The recent, ingenious experiments of Møller (1970b) prove yet another correlation among the various indices of cochlear function that is directly pertinent to our inquiry. Møller recorded single-unit activity from the rat cochlear nucleus in response to paired clicks with variable interclick intervals. He argued that the response of a linear system to a paired click is the sum of its responses to the individual clicks. The system response (basilar membrane vibration) is assumed to be oscillatory; thus if the second click arrives before the response to the first click dies out, the resulting total response is a function of the arrival of the second stimulus with respect to the first. For example, if the second click is so timed that its response has a positive peak while the response to the first click goes through a negative peak, then the total response is smaller than that to either click alone. Clearly, as the time difference between the two clicks changes one should generate periodic enhancement and reduction in the resulting output. Moreover, the periodicity in this combined response should reflect the periodicity of the individual click response, and its decay rate should be the same. Møller utilized the average firing rate of single units in the cochlear nucleus as the measure of the system output and, as predicted, he noted that this rate shows a decaying oscillation as a function of the interclick interval.

Some of Møller's results are shown in Fig. 4.31. The ordinate is the average number of discharges per click pair, and the abscissa is the time separation between clicks. The two top curves were generated with clicks of equal (solid line) and opposite (dashed line) polarity. The bottom curves merely show the spontaneous activity for reference. The best frequency of this fiber is 5.4 kHz. First we note the periodic decaying oscillation, the interweaving of curves obtained with the two different polarity combinations, the relative slowness of the decay, and significantly that the periodicity is 180 μseconds, corresponding almost exactly to the best frequency, which

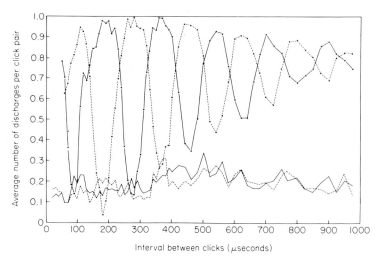

Interval between clicks (μseconds)

Fig. 4.31. Response to paired-click stimulation as a function of the interval between clicks for a unit whose CF was 5.4 kHz. The click pairs were presented in bursts 50 mseconds long with 10 click pairs in each burst, 6/second. The graph shows the mean value of response to each click pair. Dots connected with solid lines represent the response to clicks of equal polarity tallied during the 50-msecond stimulus duration. Dots connected with dashed lines show the response to clicks of opposite polarity. Solid lines and dashed lines in the lower part of the graph show the average discharge rate during the 50 mseconds immediately following each stimulus burst for clicks of equal and opposite polarity, respectively. (From Møller, 1970b, p. 303.)

was determined from the tuning curve of the unit. The determination of the transient properties of a neuron with Møller's two-click method is not confined to low frequencies because of technical limitations as is the evaluation of simple PST histograms. The method is thus capable of resolving the question of whether high-frequency units exhibit decaying oscillations in their activity just as low-frequency units do. The answer is yes, all units show this type of behavior.

Møller obtained both paired-click data and isorate curves (SPL required to elicit a preset number of spikes per signal presentation as a function of frequency, an analog of the tuning curve) from a number of cochlear nucleus units and performed computations to determine how compatible the two types of representation are. He obtained the startling result that the tuning curve that is computed on the basis of the two-click data is considerably narrower than the actually measured curve. In other words, even the relatively sharp neural tuning curves that can be measured with sinusoidal stimuli from cochlear nucleus units are inadequate to account for the temporal, transient characteristics of such units. In fact, a reduction in bandwidth of about twofold was required to bring the steady-state data (tuning curve) in consonance with the transient data. These results indicate that the peripheral auditory analyzer has a narrower effective bandwidth for transient stimuli than for steady-state stimuli. Interestingly these results agree with some of Møller's (1970a) other findings, that the bandwidth is narrower when obtained with a wide-band noise stimulus than when determined with pure tones, and also with the paired-click experiments of Goblick and Pfeiffer (1969), which demonstrated the presence of a distinct nonlinearity. Thus there appears to be strong evidence for nonlinear performance in the cochlea and possibly in the 8th nerve network.

CHAPTER 5

Cochlear Potentials

I. Classification of Potentials

In this chapter the electrical events that are measurable from the cochlea are discussed. Among the cochlear potentials two main categories are distinguished: direct (dc) and alternating (ac) potentials. Three dc voltages have been identified; these are the positive endocochlear potential (EP) discovered by von Békésy (1952), the negative potential within the organ of Corti, again first identified by von Békésy (1952), and the summating potential (SP), which was first described by Davis and colleagues (1950). The ac potential, commonly known as cochlear microphonic (CM), was identified by Wever and Bray (1930). Two of these potentials, the SP and the CM, are stimulus related, while the positive and negative dc resting potentials are present as the consequence of basic metabolic processes. It is commonly assumed that these resting potentials supply at least part of the electrical energy that is manifested in the stimulus-elicited voltages: SP and CM. It is also a fairly common assumption that the CM and SP are receptor potentials of the auditory sense organ (Davis, 1961a) or, stated differently, these potentials are assumed to be the first electrical events in the sound stimulus–auditory perception chain. With this framework in mind the detailed discussion of the potentials can now begin.

II. Resting Potentials

A. ENDOCOCHLEAR POTENTIAL (EP)

In 1950 von Békésy noted that, when measured in reference to a point on the cochlear bone, small dc potentials could be recorded from the perilymph in either cochlear scala. These potentials did not exceed 3 mV and they had a relatively complicated distribution pattern. Von Békésy was of the opinion that the resting potential originated from within the cochlear partition, but he did not prove this correct contention until 1952. Von Békésy's motivation in questioning whether dc potentials were present in the cochlea was that such potentials clearly demonstrate a continuous consumption of energy. If such a metabolic (chemical) energy source is available then the acoustic stimulus is not required to supply whatever energy is necessary for generating stimulus-related electrical events in the cochlea. Instead, the acoustic stimulus can serve to merely trigger the release or conversion of the local energy.

After developing techniques for penetrating Reissner's membrane and the organ of Corti with microelectrodes without causing undue damage to these structures, von Békésy (1952) succeeded in describing the detailed dc potential pattern within the cochlea. By presumably equalizing electrode–fluid contact potentials in scala vestibuli, von Békésy designated the resting potential there as zero. Inside Reissner's membrane a negativity amounting to about 20 mV was noted, while inside the scala media a high positive potential, about 50–80 mV (which became known as the EP later), was measured. Inside the organ of Corti −40 mV was recorded, while the scala tympani was slightly negative, about −2 mV. It should be immediately noted, lest confusion arise, that present-day investigators customarily refer their potentials to the scala tympani, which is then assumed to be at zero potential. Consequently in scala vestibuli one would measure a slight positive potential. Contemporary measurements indicate that the normal value of EP is higher than that obtained by von Békésy. In 51 cat cochleae Peake *et al.* (1969) found that 88 % had EP values between 90 and 115 mV, the average being approximately 100 mV. The same authors noted that the potential difference between scalae vestibuli and tympani hovers around zero value; 90 % of 38 measurements were within ± 10 mV with an average of 0 mV.

After von Békésy's initial observations, the EP underwent extensive scrutiny. Special efforts were made to find the source of this high positive potential, to discern its role in the hearing process, and of course to investigate several of its properties.

One of the first important observations about EP pertained to its independence from the unique chemical composition of the endolymph [high concentration of potassium (K) and low concentration of sodium (Na), not unlike intracellular fluid]. Tasaki *et al.* (1954) effectively replaced perilymph (high sodium concentration) with KCl solution. This manipulation largely abolished the cochlear microphonic potential but it did not affect the EP recorded from scala media. If EP depended on the concentration gradient of K^+ ions between the inside and outside of scala media then it should have been diminished when such a gradient was abolished by the replacement of perilymph. Thus it appeared that, while the chemical composition of the content of the endolymphatic space is fairly unique, this composition is probably not responsible for the production of endocochlear potential. This viewpoint was further substantiated in subsequent experiments by Smith and colleagues (1958), who compared dc potentials in the cochlear duct and in the utricle and found the former to be about +65 mV, the latter only +4 mV in spite of the similar chemical composition of the fluid media at these locations. These observations were further confirmed by a detailed study on dc potentials throughout the labyrinth by Eldredge and co-workers (1961). It is then clear that, while endolymph and EP coexist within the cochlear duct, the latter is not a direct consequence of the former.

The source of the EP was established by Tasaki and Spiropoulos (1959), who drained the endolymph from the cochlear duct and then explored the boundaries of the duct with a microelectrode. They succeeded in recording the usual high positive potential from the surface of the stria vascularis, but at no other point within the scala media did they find a similar polarization. Additional support for the stria as the site of origin of EP was garnered by an experimental series of Davis et al. (1958b) in which they surgically obstructed the cochlear vein, thus creating atrophy and necrosis of cells in the stria vascularis. In those cases where subsequent histological examination confirmed that venous obstruction had damaged the stria vascularis, the EP was shown to be severely depressed, from the normal +77 mV to about +15 mV. The companion experiment of Davis et al., in which they accomplished hair cell degeneration (by streptomycin poisoning) without affecting the stria, showed that no detriment in EP is to be expected as long as the stria is intact, even though the hair cells might be destroyed. Similarly, Tasaki and Spiropoulos (1959) demonstrated that in waltzing guinea pigs (who have no hair cells) the EP is normal; thus the hair cells could not in any way be responsible for the production of the positive polarization of the cochlear duct.

Let us now discuss the effect of sound on the EP in somewhat more detail. When von Békésy (1950) discovered that a dc potential exists in the cochlea, he also noted that this potential can be modified by introducing sound stimuli. Von Békésy recorded his potentials from the round window or in its vicinity, from the perilymph of scala tympani. Since he found that upon presenting a sound stimulus the resting potential decreased at these locations, he designated this change in polarization as "dc fall." He noted, however, that at other recording sites the resting potential could also increase due to sound. The dc fall was sustained as long as the sound stimulus lasted, although in anoxic animals or in response to extremely loud sounds the dc fall increased for a while before starting to decline.*

Misrahy *et al.* (1958a) noted a decrease in dc potential upon presentation of a loud sound. When the change in resting potential in response to sound stimulation is recorded from the perilymph, the time course of the change corresponds to that of the stimulus. In other words, when sound is presented, a dc shift is immediately seen and the shift is maintained at a constant level as long as the stimulus is on. In contrast, if the recording is made from the endolymph then in response to a steady tone a gradual change in the dc level is seen (Johnstone, 1968). If the change in EP is graphed as the function of the logarithm of stimulus duration then a straight line obtains (if one discounts the first 10 or so milliseconds, during which the change is more abrupt). The rate of diminution in EP is approximately 2–4 mV/decade-time. Because of the difficulties in prolonged dc recording the logarithmic relationship was established for about 5 decades of time only (about 20 minutes). Johnstone's data apparently corroborate the findings of Honrubia and Ward (1966), who noted that when a recording was made from the scala media the magnitude of dc shifts in response to sound stimuli depended directly on the duration of the tone presentation. It is appropriate to alert the reader to a state of general confusion in the literature concerning the relationship between what we have designated as change in EP in response to sound and what is generally known as summating potential (SP). At this stage there is no reason to assume that the two phenomena are different. The effects of various chemical agents and of anoxia on this resting potential will be discussed in Section VI.

The EP is clearly not merely a diffusion potential but is maintained by active secretory processes. The clearest indication of this is the course of EP during anoxia. As we shall see, the fact that the EP disappears almost instantaneously after the onset of oxygen deprivation indicates that active membrane processes are necessary for its maintenance. As soon as these processes are inhibited by anoxia, the potential of the endolymphatic space starts to move toward the K^+ diffusion potential. This potential is negative (not too dissimilar from the familiar intracellular negativity) and it is maintained by K^+ diffusion down its concentration gradient across the basilar and Reissner's membrane. In the normally functioning cochlea the actual EP is the result of a balance between the positive secretory potential (generated in the stria vascularis) and the negative diffusion potential (due to the K^+

_____

* It is surely realized that von Békésy's "dc fall" and Davis' "summating potential" are the same entity.

gradient). If a manipulation of the state of the cochlea affects either mechanism then the EP can change in either direction, toward more positive or toward more negative. The latter is seen in anoxic cochleae, the former in situations when the K^+ gradient between endolymph and perilymph is reduced. Such a change occurs for example when the K^+ concentration of the perilymph is artificially raised. In this case the EP does actually increase (Konishi and Kelsey, 1968a).

The ionic composition of the endolymph is apparently maintained by active transport processes that are intimately tied to the cells of the stria vascularis. These processes are highly oxygen dependent and they maintain the normal sodium, potassium, and chloride concentrations of the endolymph (Bosher and Warren, 1968). It is apparent that both the characteristic ionic content and the characteristic positive potential of the endolymphatic space are the results of a specific metabolic activity within the stria vascularis. The question naturally arises as to the primary function of the stria. Is it the maintenance of the chemical balance with the generation of the EP as an epiphenomenon, or is it the other way around? There does not appear to be an unequivocal answer to this inquiry, even though it appears more likely that the unusual chemical concentration of the endolymph is of primary importance.

Some interesting experiments of Bosher and Warren (1971) shed some light on the development of these two phenomena: ionic content and EP. These authors studied the changes in EP and in endolymphatic ionic concentrations in newborn rats. They noted that all ionic concentrations had attained near-normal levels from the earliest time after birth, but in contrast the EP was very low up to the 11th day after birth. Between the 12th and 15th day the EP increased at a marked rate, growing by about 50 mV in a 48-hour period. Histological examination revealed that all structures in the cochlea, including the cells of the stria vascularis and the organ of Corti, were fully developed by the time the rapid increase in EP commenced, with the exception of the cells of Claudius. The latter cells attained their final development in the very period during which the EP underwent its rapid increase. It would thus appear that endolymphatic ionic concentration and EP are independent phenomena since they develop in a serial instead of a concurrent manner. A more likely explanation is that suggested by Bosher and Warren, that the source of the EP develops as the cells in the stria mature. The source is responsible for both EP and ionic content, and thus both characteristic phenomena appear simultaneously. It must not be forgotten that what one measures as EP is only a voltage drop across the equivalent cochlear resistances and not the actual source voltage. Thus one can have a full-blown source voltage but if the load resistance is low the measured voltage drop will also be low. It appears then that during early development the resistance pattern of the cochlea changes, conceivably as a consequence of the maturation of Claudius' cells.

B. INTRACELLULAR NEGATIVITY WITHIN THE ORGAN OF CORTI

When von Békésy penetrated the organ of Corti with fluid microelectrodes (1952), he noted within the organ a negative potential amounting to 40 mV with respect to the scala tympani. He assumed that this potential arose from the cells of Hensen and Claudius. Tasaki *et al.* (1954) confirmed the existence of a large negative potential (about 50 mV) in the cellular layer above the basilar membrane. They considered this potential to be cellular in origin; in other words, the negativity measured was presumed to correspond to the intracellular resting potential common in all living cells. Later measurements showed that the negative potential can be of the order of 70–100 mV. Its *intra*cellular nature has been accepted (Davis, 1960) by most investigators. However, over the years a second school of thought has developed concerning this negative potential. According to this other view, the negativity is *inter*-cellular, indigenous to the fluid spaces within the organ of Corti.

The first observation to conflict with the intracellular hypothesis was that of Tasaki and Spiropoulos (1959). They noted that the negative potential is clearly present even when recording is made with pipettes as large as 15 μ tip diameter, which could not have penetrated the cells of the organ of Corti. Tasaki and Spiropoulos suggested that the fluid surrounding the hair cells is negatively polarized. This viewpoint was adopted and advanced by Butler *et al.* (1962) and Butler (1965). They suggested that this potential might properly be called "cortilymphatic potential," since it is recorded from the region that is presumably filled with a fluid which Engström (1960) termed cortilymph. Cortilymph was assumed to be different from both endolymph and perilymph. Endolymph must be ruled out as the fluid surrounding the bottom of the hair cells and the nonmyelinated dendrites of the 8th nerve, for its chemical composition is like that of intracellular fluid. Nerve conduction could not be maintained in such a bathing medium. Pure perilymph is unlikely to surround the hair cells, for Lawrence and Clapper (1961) showed in histological sections that the fluid spaces inside the organ of Corti stained unlike perilymph.

The implications of a negative extracellular polarization of the fluid space surrounding the hair cells are somewhat disturbing. This potential can apparently be recorded for sustained periods *only* with large-diameter electrodes. Fine pipettes record negativity (presumably intracellular) but can maintain it for only very brief periods (Konishi and Yasuno, 1963; Dallos, 1968; Peake *et al.*, 1969). This indicates that fine electrodes pick up the intracellular potential but then presumably damage the cell so that its polarization is destroyed. In order to maintain the negative potential one must resort to recording with large electrodes, which cannot penetrate cells. It is interesting that with 2-μ-tip electrodes, which is an intermediate size, Lawrence (1967) was able to hold the organ of Corti negativity for approximately 2 minutes. It seems then that the duration of maintainability of the negative potential is directly proportional to the size of the recording electrode.

If the potential is truly extracellular in origin, it is difficult to explain why it cannot be held for long durations with fine electrodes. On the other hand, the large electrodes cannot record intracellularly. There appears to be a contradiction here; however, it need not be so. When a fine electrode enters a cell it records the common intracellular negativity but it injures the cell during penetration. If the injury is severe the cell dies within a brief time. With fine electrodes it is also possible to lose contact with a cell and thus to observe an apparent cessation of potential pickup. In contrast when a large electrode is pushed into a layer of cells it injures several of these and records the injury potential in the process. The injury potential is maintained for considerable time intervals. These considerations indicate that it is likely that all negative potentials within the organ of Corti are of cellular origin; with small electrodes one records the normal intracellular polarization, and with large electrodes one records the injury potential.

A second objection to the assumption that the negative potential is extracellular can be raised on theoretical grounds. The hair cells and the dendrites of the 8th nerve are surrounded by the fluid (cortilymph) that is supposedly negatively polarized. The inside of cells and of dendrites is negative with respect to interstitial fluid. This negativity is maintained by selective ion transport across the semipermeable cell membranes. The usual intracellular negativity is of the same order of magnitude, 70–100 mV, as the presumed extracellular organ of Corti potential. Thus if the intercellular spaces are truly negatively polarized, the potential difference implies a permanent depolarization of the cell, or dendrite, which would result in the inability of these structures to sustain *active* membrane processes. While spikes have never been demonstrated in hair cells or within the organ of Corti, their presence in the dendritic processes cannot be ruled out. Even if active propagation within the organ is not the mode of communication, it is highly improbable that all cells, dendrites, and telodendria would function therein in a state of permanent depolarization.

In a systematic study, Lawrence (1967) measured the various resting potentials within the organ of Corti. He used controlled penetrations from both the tympanic and vestibular sides, and at various points across the basilar membrane. His electrode consisted of 2-μ glass pipettes filled with various electrolytes. Lawrence confirmed the presence of both the negative resting potential and the positive endocochlear potential. It is interesting to note that he could not maintain the negative potential within the organ of Corti for significant durations. As soon as the forward thrust of the electrode stopped, the negative potential began to drop and it tended to disappear within a minute. When the electrode was filled with 0.5 M Na$_2$SO$_4$, the potential dropped, but it did not disappear completely. Negative potential in any significant amount was recorded only during forward motion of the electrode. Upon withdrawal, the negativity was either completely absent or greatly diminished. Lawrence believes that the basilar membrane controls the selective ion transport that creates the negative potential within the organ of Corti; he thus subscribes to the hypothesis that the negative potential is *inter*cellular. However, some of Lawrence's own findings, more specifically the fact that the negativity is mostly absent during the withdrawal of the electrode, substantiate the belief that we are dealing with an injury potential. Such a potential would quite naturally be more prominent when the electrode exerted considerable pressure on the cells than during its motion out of the medium.

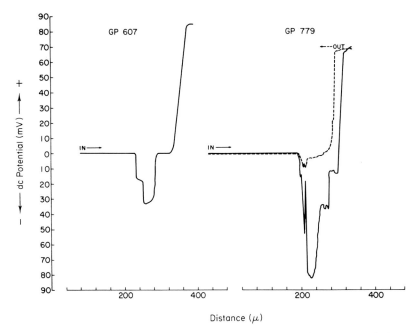

Fig. 5.1. The dc electrical potential change as the electrode is advanced through Deiters' cells. There is, first, the negative potential and then a gradual change and rise to zero potential, until the positive potential of the endolymph is reached. The double plateau of GP 779 may indicate the penetration of hair cells. At the moment of rise from zero to positive dc, the ac potential reverses 180° (not shown). Electrodes: GP 607, 3 M KCl; GP 779, 0.5 M Na$_2$SO$_4$. (From Lawrence, 1967, p. 299.)

One finding of Lawrence is very provocative and should be discussed in more detail. He noted that, when the electrode penetrated the organ of Corti at a point where it did not encounter the tectorial membrane during its travel, an extremely abrupt change from high negativity (organ of Corti) to high positivity (scala media) took place. In contrast, during penetrations passing through the tectorial membrane, instead of an abrupt sign change, the potential returned to zero and stayed there for the duration while the electrode presumably dwelled within the tectorial membrane. Figure 5.1 shows the variation of dc voltage in two such penetrations. These results are provocative, for they suggest that the boundary of EP on the organ of Corti side is not the reticular lamina but the tectorial membrane. Prior to Lawrence's experiments it was universally accepted, on the basis of the experiments of von Békésy (1952) and Tasaki et al. (1954), that the border line of the region where the endocochlear potential is measurable coincides with the reticular lamina. As we shall discuss in the following section, concomitant with the abrupt change in dc potential the CM reverses phase during penetration of the organ of Corti. This phase reversal led Tasaki et al. (1954) to suggest that the source of origin of the CM is in the region of the reticular lamina, that is, at the hair-bearing pole of the hair cells. Lawrence's findings would suggest that the CM itself might not originate in hair cells but in the tectorial membrane. We shall discuss this issue later in more detail, but here we shall confine ourselves to some observations of Lawrence (1965, 1967) and to some results of Davis (1965) and of Peake et al. (1969).

Davis observed that the *structure* of the tectorial membrane makes it an unlikely candidate for sustaining a high potential difference across it, or across its surface. He noted that the tectorial membrane is not cellular, is 93 % protein material, and is anisotropic (Iurato, 1962). It does not possess a surface membrane that could sustain either a potential or a concentration gradient. On this basis the tectorial membrane appears electrically "transparent." Peake et al. (1969) repeated Lawrence's (1967) experiments in attempting to map the dc electrical profile of the cochlea. Their main effort centered on correlating anatomical and electrical measurements, and they concluded that in general "It is not possible . . . to arrange the dc profile and the anatomical section to give a reasonable correspondence of distances" (p. 297). To explain, the recording electrode, when advancing, pushes the delicate structures within the cochlea over considerable distances before penetrating them. Consequently a knowledge of the depth of electrode insertion does not always reveal the exact anatomical location of the electrode tip. In Fig. 5.2 an example of this lack of correspondence is shown, the recorded electrical profile (potential versus measured electrode position) and the actual anatomical profile are superimposed. Note that the positive EP was maintained over a distance that is about twice as long as the width of the

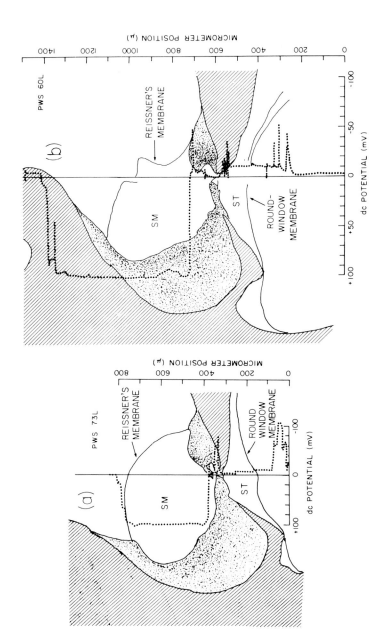

Fig. 5.2. Two dc profiles (dotted) superimposed on the outline of photomicrographs containing a clear indication of the electrode track through the tunnel. No matter how the dc profile is moved up and down with respect to the histological section, it is difficult to associate the changes in potential with the structures. (From Sohmer *et al.*, 1971, p. 582.)

scala media at the level of penetration. The reason undoubtedly is that the electrode distended Reissner's membrane over such a large distance that it did not leave the positive region during its travel. The implication of these findings is simply that it is difficult to assign a particular anatomical location to electrical potentials as obtained during microelectrode penetrations of the cochlea. Peake *et al.* (1969), Bosher (1970), and Schwartzkopff (1970) further comment that they were not able to obtain a zero-potential region between the organ of Corti negativity and the scala media positivity during microelectrode penetrations. It is said that during some of these penetrations the electrode had undoubtedly passed through the tectorial membrane. It is probably more realistic at this time to assume that the tectorial membrane is electrically transparent.

III. Stimulus-Related Potentials

A. COCHLEAR MICROPHONIC (CM)

1. Properties

Wever and Bray (1930), while studying the electrical potentials recorded from the auditory nerve of cats, observed the curious phenomenon that if these amplified potentials were led to a loudspeaker then words spoken into the cat's ear could easily be recognized. Wever and Bray thought that they were dealing with the responses of the nerve itself. However, Adrian (1931) objected to this notion and suggested that the electrical changes were generated in the cochlea and were passively conducted by the nerve to the recording site. Adrian suggested that the potentials are due to some kind of *microphonic* (hence the name) action within the inner ear. He also noted that the round window proved to be an optimal extracochlear recording site. Saul and Davis (1932) supported Adrian's contention, as did Hallpike and Rawdon-Smith (1934). The views of Saul and Davis (1932) and Davis *et al.* (1934) were shown to be correct, and the CM came to be known as the electrical response of the cochlea. The latter writers proposed specifically that the CM arises from the hair cells of the cochlea in a process of mechanical deformation. Other authors suspected that the genesis of the CM might be in the vibration of a polarized membrane within the cochlea (Hallpike and Rawdon-Smith, 1934). It was thought possible that either the tectorial or Reissner's membrane might be appropriately polarized. It is fascinating, to me at least, that these arguments concerning the source of CM are still not settled, more than 35 years after they were first enunciated. While Davis' hair cell hypothesis has been accepted by most, a number of other alternatives have been suggested recently. We shall attempt an evaluation of these hypotheses later in this chapter.

a. Spatial Pattern. The most distinctive feature of the CM is that its waveform replicates (to a degree) the moment-to-moment pressure variation of the stimulating sound. This replication is perfect if the stimulus is a pure tone of moderate or low intensity. Complex sound pressure changes are not reproduced with an unaltered waveform because of the frequency-dependent amplitude and phase characteristics of the middle ear–inner ear system. In other words, individual frequency components in the stimulus suffer varying degrees of attentuation and relative phase shift, and consequently the composite CM waveform differs from the shape of the complex pressure wave. At high intensities, because of the presence of amplitude distortion (nonlinear effects), the generated harmonic components also alter the shape of the CM waveform, even if the stimulus is only a single pure tone. In the intensity range where nonlinear distortion is not significant, it is best to describe the CM waveform as one that mimics the vibratory pattern of the cochlear partition. This description of course takes the frequency-dependent amplitude and phase effects into consideration. To explain, it is assumed that at a given location along the cochlear partition a CM voltage is a fair replica of the displacement–time pattern of that point of the partition. The magnitude and phase of the CM are thought to vary along the cochlear partition in accordance with the traveling wave.

Tasaki *et al.* (1952), using the then recently developed differential-electrode technique (Tasaki and Fernández, 1952), presented extensive data on both amplitude and phase variation of the CM along the length of the cochlea. Tasaki *et al.* measured the response at four locations along the guinea pig cochlea and plotted phase and amplitude distribution curves. Their data are most illuminating, and based on them the direct correspondence between microphonic distribution and cochlear motion pattern was established beyond any doubt, even though due to the choice of experimental procedure the data are somewhat difficult to interpret. Tasaki *et al.* chose the potentials obtained from a set of differential electrodes inserted near the round window as the reference for their measurement of CM in the first turn, while for all measurements of CM in turns 2, 3, and 4 the first-turn CM served as reference. Thus they obtained CM potential curves from the higher turns by keeping the CM output of the first turn invariant and adjusting the sound pressure. Similarly, phase shifts of CM in the higher turns were measured in reference to the phase of the first-turn CM. Their amplitude plots seem to imply that below a certain frequency all turns respond with a flat characteristic; beyond that frequency there is a precipitous drop in CM. Von Békésy's measurements of the traveling wave envelope do not suggest such a "low-pass" characteristic; instead, clear maxima were seen. Stating it differently, at any point along the cochlea there is a frequency for which the vibratory amplitude is maximum. For either lower or higher frequencies the magnitude of vibration is less at that point. One thus expects to see a similar best frequency of the CM for a given electrode location. The reason that the Tasaki *et al.* data do not behave this way is simply due to their equalization process whereby the electrical output of the first turn was kept constant instead of either the sound pressure level of the eardrum or the amplitude of vibration of the stapes. Zwislocki (cf. Tasaki, 1957) first noted this reason for the apparent disharmony between the first available CM distribution data and von Békésy's observations.

The same objections that apply to the amplitude data of Tasaki *et al.* of course also apply to their phase data. In addition to measuring phase, these authors carefully computed the travel time of the disturbances as manifested by the appearance of CM at various points along the cochlea. The striking observations that emerged from the data are, first, that the travel time is frequency dependent and, second, that in the higher turns there is an apparent extremum. The finding that travel time is not constant with frequency is a potentially very significant observation. The reader will recall from Chapter 4 that the theoretical treatment of cochlear mechanics revealed that phase velocity and consequently travel time to a given point in the cochlea are independent of frequency. It will also be remembered that this result was a direct consequence of the original assumption that the so-called "shallow-water treatment" of cochlear dynamics is adequate; i.e., a one-dimensional analysis is sufficient. Remember that, in shallow water, $c = (gh)^{1/2}$; i.e., the velocity is independent of wavelength. If the experimental data indicating the contrary as far as the CM is concerned are correct, then a one-dimensional treatment of cochlear mechanics is neither adequate nor appropriate. It appears now on the basis of newer information (Tonndorf, 1970a; Nordmark *et al.*, 1969; Dallos and Cheatham, 1971) that when CM measurements are kept within limits of their legitimate use they indicate that the travel time *is* independent of frequency.

To explain, we must again consider some properties of the differential-electrode recording (with which the data in question were generated). The fundamental assumption of the method is that differential electrodes see local sources in opposite phase and remote sources in-phase. The phase measurement obtained with differential electrodes can be legitimate only if the output of the local source is considerably in excess of that of the remote source. If the remote source dominates the electrical signal at a given electrode location, the measured phase reflects it instead of the local situation. Consequently phase measurements with differential electrodes (and of course with single electrodes even more so) should be restricted to frequencies *below* the cutoff frequency of a given electrode pair. The cutoff frequency can best be estimated from the relative phase shift between the two electrodes of the pair. Above the cutoff there is no phase difference between them, but in the region of the

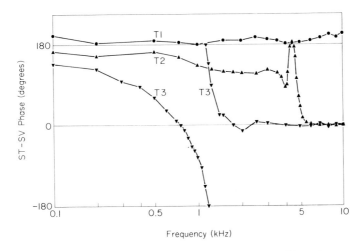

Fig. 5.3. The CM phase difference between potentials measured in scalae tympani and vestibuli as the function of stimulus frequency at a constant 70 dB SPL. Data from three individual guinea pigs are shown; the electrodes are located in turns 1, 2, and 3, respectively. Positive phase indicates lead. (From Dallos *et al.*, 1971, p. 1145.)

cutoff the phase between them changes radically, indicating the interaction of local and remote components. In Fig. 5.3 such phase plots are shown for electrode pairs in the first three turns. They indicate that, in turn 1, measurements are certainly legitimate below 10 kHz, in turn 2 below 4 kHz, and in turn 3 probably below 500 Hz. We have no data for the fourth turn, but since the Tasaki *et al.* recording was not a true differential recording from that turn, their fourth-turn results should probably not be considered too quantitatively, due to the large amount of remote response. In this light their time lag data no longer look so forbidding. If one replots those points that can be relied on for quantitative inferences then, in spite of a paucity of usable points, the data seem to support, or at least not contradict, the assumption that waves of different frequencies travel in the cochlea with the same velocity and thus the travel time is independent of frequency.

When the CM phase as referred to that of the sound in front of the eardrum is carefully measured for a wide range of frequencies and then the travel time as reflected by the CM is computed from the relation $T = \phi/2\pi f$, plots in the form shown in Fig. 5.4 can be obtained. Here the ordinate is travel time to the location of the recording electrode pair (in second turn approximately 10 mm and in third turn approximately 14 mm) and the abscissa is the test frequency. It is quite clear that the travel time is quite invariant with frequency at either recording site up to the cutoff frequency, beyond which the dominance of remote CM invalidates the computed time values.

Apparently Tonndorf (1958b) was the first to publish CM distribution

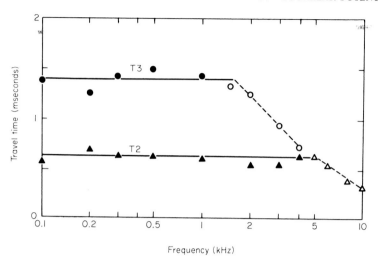

Fig. 5.4. "Travel time" of CM as the function of frequency from two electrode locations (turn 2 and turn 3). The time information is computed from phase data on the basis of $T = \phi/2\pi f$. (From Dallos and Cheatham, 1971, p. 1142.)

functions, recorded with differential electrodes from guinea pig cochleae, that were obtained with methods that make them more amenable for comparison with the traveling wave amplitude pattern. Tonndorf recorded CM response from several cochlear turns, for a wide range of frequencies, while keeping the sound pressure level roughly constant. Under these conditions the CM magnitude at any given recording location was shown to vary with frequency, as we would anticipate on the basis of von Békésy's (1951) observations. Similar data had been produced, but at lesser intensities (which is more favorable since the response is more likely to be linear), by Laszlo (1968), who presented normalized CM amplitude functions for three electrode locations.

Extensive data were collected on CM spatial patterns by Honrubia and Ward (1968), who recorded with KCl-filled pipettes from the scala media of guinea pigs. These authors inserted their recording electrodes into the scala media through small fenestras made on the bone over the stria vascularis. Recordings were made from all four turns of the cochlea. In Fig. 5.5 four plots are shown depicting the longitudinal distribution of CM for four frequencies over a wide range of intensities. A number of important observations can be made on the basis of these very clean data. First, there is a clear spatial preference for efficiently producing a particular frequency CM from one location to another. In accordance with von Békésy's observations the maximum response moves toward the base with the increase in stimulus frequency. This can be seen particularly clearly at low stimulus intensities.

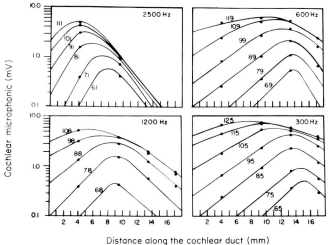

Fig. 5.5. Longitudinal distribution of the CM recorded inside the scala media. Responses were obtained for four different frequencies, same guinea pig. The parameters are the SPL's. (From Honrubia and Ward, 1968, p. 953.)

Again in conformity with the shape of the traveling wave envelope the proximal side of the distribution curves is much shallower than the distal side. The slopes become steeper with increasing frequency, the change is about 2 : 1 between 3000 and 300 Hz. The authors noted that with increasing intensity the point of maximal CM shifted toward the base quite radically; the overall shift within the SPL's studied was some 4 mm. This phenomenon will be discussed in somewhat more detail later in this section. A good quantitative relationship between the location of maximum sensitivity and the location of maximum voltage is given in Fig. 5.6. The point of maximum sensiti-

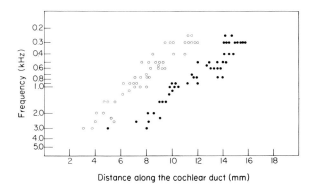

Fig. 5.6. Location of the points of maximum sensitivity (●) and maximum voltage (○) of the CM along the cochlear duct. (From Honrubia and Ward, 1968, p. 954.)

vity of course corresponds to the electrode location where the CM could be detected with the least SPL. It is clear that, irrespective of the frequency, the maximum CM is produced approximately 4 mm more basally than where the CM first appeared.

In Figs. 2.9 and 2.10 we presented some of our data showing CM iso-potential curves that can also be used to assess the sensitivity of two cochlear locations. In these plots the low-frequency sensitivity improves at a rate of 20 dB/decade up to a frequency at which the sensitivity of the electrode location is maximal. This *apparent* best frequency is approximately 500 Hz for turn 3, 750 Hz for turn 2, and 1000 Hz for turn 1. Below the frequency of the shallow minimum the sensitivity is better for electrode locations that are more remote from the stapes. Probably more characteristic of a given electrode pair than the point of best sensitivity is the frequency at which the sensitivity begins to decrease in a quite radical manner. These frequencies are 1000 Hz for turn 3 and 4000 Hz for turn 2. Beyond these cutoff frequencies the sensitivity of the differential electrodes decreases at an approximate rate of 100 dB/decade. It is apparent that when one compares the mechanical tuning curves discussed in Chapter 4 and the CM sensitivity curves studied here that discrepancies exist, especially in the location of the best frequency. One can estimate that at the first-turn electrode location for the guinea pig the maximal mechanical vibration occurs at about 9000 Hz, the comparable figures for turns 2 and 3 being 1750 and 500 Hz, respectively. The agreement is excellent for turn 3, but the other CM sensitivity functions peak at too low frequencies. The discrepancy is particularly striking for the basal-turn results. The primary reason for the early appearance of the CM sensitivity peak is that the results incorporate the filter effects of both middle ear and cochlea. In guinea pig the middle ear transfer function decreases at an approximate rate of 6 dB/octave above 500–1000 Hz. If one corrects plots such as those in Fig. 2.10 for the middle ear effect then the curves do show shallow extrema in the vicinity of 2000 and 9000 Hz for turns 2 and 1, respectively; of course these values are in good agreement with the corresponding mechanical tuning characteristics.

In summarizing the various pieces of evidence concerning the longitudinal distribution of the CM we note that these spatial patterns are at least in qualitative agreement with the traveling wave envelope and phase patterns. The microphonic tuning curves, irrespective of recording method (i.e., differential or scala media), are *not* narrower than the mechanical tuning curves. Thus, at least as reflected in the gross microphonic potential, there is no sharpening of spatial patterns between mechanical motion and the first electrical sign of this motion, i.e., the CM. The basal shift in the CM with increasing intensity is much more pronounced than what might occur in the mechanical process and is most likely a simple consequence (as we shall attempt to demonstrate later) of the nonlinearity of the CM input–output functions.

While discussing the distribution of CM along the length of the cochlea, it is important to allude to a seeming controversy over this distribution. One school of thought (Wever and Lawrence, 1954) is that all tones, regardless of their frequency, activate all parts of the cochlea. This activation is stronger or weaker at a given point depending on stimulus frequency, but all frequencies create a spread of activity over the entire length of the cochlea. The corollary of this contention is that all frequencies generate CM from all segments of the cochlea. Again the magnitude is dependent on frequency, but there is no "silent" region for any frequency. Wever and Lawrence base their arguments on results obtained in studies of sound damage to guinea pig ears. Two observations are pertinent.

First, when the ear is stimulated with intense pure tones, the damage sustained is not limited to the frequency band around the injurious tone but in general spreads to all frequencies. This was shown (Smith and Wever, 1949) by injuring the ear with tones of 300, 1000, 5000, and 10,000 Hz at an intensity of about 130 dB SPL. The three lower tones produced relatively flat diminution of CM as measured on the round window by about 25 dB between 100 and 10,000 Hz. The highest damaging tone alone created a slightly frequency-dependent CM loss, sloping from about 5 dB at 100 Hz to about 20 dB at 10,000 Hz. Histological studies on these animals indicated fairly wide patches of damage, localized roughly in the region of the basilar membrane that is maximally responsive to the frequency of the damaging tone. Thus the first experiment indicates that no matter what damaging frequency is used, all frequency CM's suffer.

The second observation of Wever and Lawrence is based on the unpublished experiments of Alexander and Githler (1954). Here damage was produced by a 300-Hz tone, which damaged all hair cells except for a few in narrow regions at the two extreme ends of the cochlea. In spite of the widespread annihilation of the hair cells, round-window CM could be obtained at all frequencies between 200 and 10,000 Hz with a flat loss of about 55 dB. This second experiment would indicate that even a very limited region of the cochlea can respond to all tones.

In contrast to the above arguments are the observations of Tasaki and Fernández (1952), Tasaki *et al.* (1952), and Davis (1957). These investigators contend, as we have seen, that the CM distribution as well as the form of vibratory pattern are markedly asymmetrical. Accordingly, the basalmost portion of the cochlea responds to all tones, mechanically and in producing CM. However, the apical region does not vibrate at all at high frequencies, and no high-frequency CM comes from this segment. We have already reviewed some of the evidence that supports this viewpoint, namely, the

CM distribution functions recorded from various turns of the cochlea by Tasaki and colleagues. Further evidence comes from the work of Tasaki and Fernández (1952), who recorded CM activity with differential electrodes from various turns of the guinea pig cochlea while the CM response was selectively suppressed in certain cochlear regions. Two methods of suppression were used. One of these methods entailed the introduction of KCl solution into the perilymphatic space either in the basal turn or at the apex. The other method consisted of passing dc current through the cochlear partition in the basal turn. Both experimental methods yielded similar results: It was possible to suppress the CM activity in either the basal turn or at the apex without substantially affecting the electrical response from the other recording site. These results argue for the independence of CM-generating sites from one another. Furthermore, since low-frequency CM could be recorded from the basal turn without alteration when the response of the apex was severely diminished, it became clear that the first turn does generate CM at all frequencies. However, it was also shown that under no circumstances could significant CM be recorded from the third or fourth turn in response to high-frequency stimuli.

The observations of Misrahy et al. (1958) are also highly pertinent here. They recorded CM from the scala media of the first turn of guinea pig cochleae with micropipettes. During recording they progressively destroyed the cochlea by amputating successive turns from the fourth turn down. It was striking that the removal of the higher turns did not have a significant effect on the CM from the basal turn. The implication is clear: From the basal turn, one records activity that is generated therein, and the higher turns have very little influence over this response.

We are now in a position to reconcile the apparent controversy between the Wever–Lawrence and the Tasaki–Davis schools. The major difference is of course due to the recording technique. While Wever and associates use round-window electrodes routinely, Davis and colleagues base their results on differential recording. The fact that Wever and Lawrence obtained relatively flat losses in CM irrespective of the frequency of the damaging tone indicates that the output of the basal turn (which is registered primarily by the round-window electrode) was uniformly reduced at all frequencies. Similarly the case cited in which most of the hair cells were gone, with the exception of a few at the extreme ends of the cochlea, and in which a flat loss was obtained, again points to the fact that it is the condition of the basal turn which determines the CM output from the round window at all frequencies. It should be mentioned for the sake of clarity that the basal turn would control the round-window response *only if* it were healthy or at least less damaged than the higher cochlear turns. To explain, if the basal-turn response were suppressed (by damage, polarization, or other means) then at low frequencies the remote response from the higher turns would dominate the recording. For example, the sensitivity difference at 500 Hz between turns 1 and 3 is approximately 15 dB, while the rate of attenuation for single-electrode recording is approximately 2 dB/mm. Since the best location for 500 Hz from the round window is approximately 14 mm, the attenuation for potentials originating there is about 28 dB. Consequently if both the first and third turns are functioning properly, the contribution of the third-turn response to the round-window recording is about 13 dB less than the contribution of the basal turn. If the basal-turn potential is suppressed by more than 13 dB, the remote response controls the recording.

Lest it be assumed that the differential-electrode recording technique can insure the complete elimination of remote response components, attention is called to the usual pattern of third-turn microphonics at high frequencies. When inspecting CM isopotential curves obtained from the third turn (e.g., Fig. 2.9) one notes that beyond the most sensitive region the curve rises at an approximate rate of 100 dB/decade, but the rate of rise decreases significantly beyond 4000–5000 Hz. Thus measurable microphonic potential can always be produced at high frequencies even though the differential-electrode method is used. This microphonic can be either local activity or uncanceled remote CM. In the past, we have tacitly assumed that the presence of microphonics at high frequencies is a consequence of imperfect electrode placement, manifested by excessive pickup of remote microphonic. This contention, however, needed experimental verification. The method of localized alteration of the electrical properties of the cochlear partition by dc polarizing currents (Tasaki and Fernández, 1952) appeared to be a promising way to determine if the aforementioned high-frequency activity in the third turn is truly locally generated or merely a conducted remote response. The following argument is offered.[*] If the CM in the basal and second turns is suppressed, then the third-turn response can either diminish or stay unchanged at high frequencies depending on the origin of this third-turn response. If the response is actually generated in the basal or second turns and is merely a remote response in the third turn, then its depression in the first and second turns should result in a like change in the third turn. Conversely, if the high-frequency response recorded in the third turn does originate in that region, then the alteration of the microphonic in the lower turns should not affect it.

To produce electrical polarization of the two lower turns, we placed, in addition to the recording electrodes, pairs of stimulating electrodes in some of our animals. These electrodes were glass pipettes with approximate tip diameters of 20 μ, filled with Ringer solutions. These pipettes were connected to the dc current source with Ag–AgCl wires. When the microphonic was

[*] From Dallos (1969a).

to be reduced in both the first and second turns, the current was passed between scala vestibuli of the second turn and scala tympani of the first turn.

Some results of the polarization experiments are shown in Fig. 5.7. In this figure, the change in CM due to 100-μA polarizing current is shown in both first and third turns. The second-turn scala vestibuli electrode is negative in this case. Recording was made with the differential-electrode method from both turns. The 100% response corresponds to a CM of 3 μV. The effect of polarization on the basal-turn response is only slightly frequency dependent; the CM decreases from about 85% at 300 Hz to 65% at 10,000 Hz. Below 2000 Hz, no change in the third-turn response is detectable but, above that frequency, the CM drops rapidly and, above 4000 Hz, the decrease in the third-turn response due to polarization is very similar to what is seen in the basal turn.

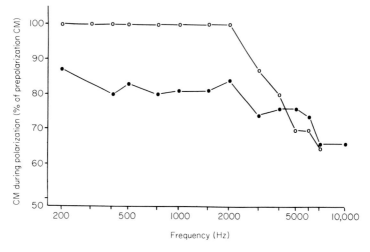

Fig. 5.7. The CM during polarization with 100-μA dc current expressed as the percentage of the no-current value. Polarizing electrodes are in scala vestibuli of turn 2 (negative) and scala tympani of turn 1 (positive). The 100% CM level corresponds to 3 μV. First turn, ●; third turn, ○. (From Dallos, 1969a, p. 1005.)

The first important conclusion that can be drawn from the plots of Fig. 5.7 is that the polarizing current did not spread to the third turn to any appreciable degree. If the current had spread toward the higher turns, then a decrease of the low-frequency response from the third turn would have been expected. Thus, one can operate on the premise that, under the experimental circumstances considered, the polarization did not affect the local response in the third turn. Up to 2000 Hz, the local third-turn CM appears to be so much greater than any remote CM that the diminution of the latter due to polarization has no measurable effect on the former. Above 2000 Hz, the remote CM becomes comparable in magnitude to the local CM, and thus a decrease in the remote response does affect the composite potential. This is seen by the decline of the third-turn response. Around 4000 Hz, the remote CM becomes much larger than the local CM of the third turn, and as a consequence the potential recorded from the third-turn site declines in proportion to the diminution of the remote response.

These considerations seem to indicate that at high frequencies the local contribution to the CM recorded from the third turn is quite negligible. Stated differently, the rate of decrease of the local CM in the third turn is almost certainly higher than the response above 5000 Hz in Fig. 2.9 would indicate. This is because, apparently at high frequencies, remote CM becomes large compared to local CM, and thus the high-frequency portion of the third-turn isopotential curves reflects this conducted remote response as opposed to locally generated microphonics. It is then proper to conclude that high-frequency activity in the apical region of the cochlea is either nonexistent or truly inconsequential. The difference in sensitivity of the third-turn electrode location from its best frequency to 10,000 Hz is about 90 dB. This difference considerably underestimates the change in sensitivity for the local response.

One final comment concerns the ability of the cochlea, as manifested in CM, to function as an envelope detector. It is well known that human beings can perceive a pitch corresponding to the periodicity of interruptions in a noise signal or high-frequency sinusoid. The question naturally arises whether one can detect a CM in the cochlea that would correspond to the interruption frequency. In other words, let us assume that we interrupt or modulate a high-frequency (say, 8000-Hz) sinusoid at a low rate (say, 400 Hz). Can a 400-Hz CM be detected from the apex of the cochlea? There has been some controversy over this question in the literature (Deatherage *et al.*, 1957; Leibbrandt, 1966; Glattke, 1968) but the answer is relatively simple. No locally generated CM corresponding to the repetition frequency can be measured from the apex, at least not up to very high sound levels where nonlinear distortion confounds the picture. Some response can apparently be seen when recording with single electrodes, but if the proper differential-electrode technique is used this remote response (which appears to be a sum of SP and AP) is eliminated.

b. Input–Output Relations. The relationship between CM magnitude and sound intensity has become a familiar one. In Fig. 5.8 a typical, so-called input–output function is shown. Customarily such functions are plotted on double logarithmic coordinates. In such a coordinate system power functions plot out as straight lines, with the slope of the line corresponding to the exponent. The typical CM input–output function consists of three distinct

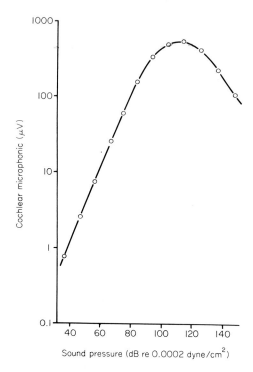

Fig. 5.8. Input–output relationship in cochlear turn 1. The curve represents the electrical response (CM) from a given cochlear turn as a function of the input sound pressure level.

segments. The first segment is represented by a straight line with unity slope.* In this region the CM is directly proportional to the strength of the stimulating sound. The relationship is linear and simple. This region extends from the lower limit of measurement up to a frequency-dependent intensity where departure from linearity is accompanied by the appearance of harmonic distortion components. Cochlear microphonic response has no demonstrable threshold. The linear segment has been measured down to 0.005 μV (Wever, 1966), and there is no reason to assume that, with further improvements in instrumentation, this value could not be lowered. Clearly the lower measurable

---

* It is possible to record input–output functions with straight-line segments whose slope is different from unity. Careful scrutiny of such functions almost invariably discloses that as a consequence of the measuring technique the experimenter did not record pure CM potentials. Contaminants that can significantly change the slope are noise and whole-nerve action potentials. The presence of noise results in slopes shallower than 1, while a significant amount of AP can interact with CM to either decrease or increase the slope. The AP is a contaminant of course at low frequencies only. In our experience the most significant interactions between CM and AP occur between 750 and 1500 Hz.

limit depends only on the interaction of system noise, biological noise, and instrumentation technique.

The apparent point of departure from linearity depends on frequency, cochlear location, and measuring technique. When measuring from the round-window membrane, Wever (1949) noted that the departure from linearity of the guinea pig CM is at a fairly uniform level of about 350 μV up to 1000 Hz. At higher frequencies linear responses are confined to gradually lesser and lesser CM values, until at 15,000 Hz the CM becomes nonlinear at 40 μV. Tasaki *et al.* (1952) compared input–output functions obtained from the first, second, and third turns at a number of frequencies. They stated that the limit of linearity is reached in any turn at progressively lower CM levels as frequency increases. Tasaki *et al.* also remarked that the limit of linearity is attained at lower frequencies in turn 3 than in turn 2 for comparable stimulus levels. While they did not state this, similar conclusions can be drawn from their data on the relationship between the turn 1 and turn 2 responses. In general the Tasaki *et al.* data clearly suggest that for *any* given frequency the widest range of linear response can be obtained from the basal turn, followed by the higher turns in order. The general tendency is clearly indicated by a set of input–output functions shown in Fig. 5.9. These functions were obtained from the Tasaki *et al.* article. It is quite instructive to study these functions in some detail. First note that the horizontal position of the function reflects the *sensitivity* of a given electrode location to a certain frequency. Accordingly at low frequencies the third-turn responses are greater for a given sound level than the first-turn responses. In other terms, the third-turn function is farther to the left. As frequency increases, the relative positions of the functions change and at higher frequencies the first-turn function shows greater sensitivity. If we examine the point of departure from linearity in the first-turn functions, we note a remarkable uniformity, at least for the six frequencies examined. The point in question occurs between 90 and 100 dB SPL, corresponding to a CM of roughly 1 mV. Note that this is in good agreement with the round-window data of Wever. The point of nonlinearity of the third-turn response, however, occurs at lesser and lesser CM and at lower and lower SPL as the stimulus frequency increases.

The second region of typical input–output functions is between the departure from linearity and the maximum of the function. This region is characterized by an increasing amount of harmonic distortion occurring in the CM. In this region if the rms values of the fundamental and all of its harmonics are added, the resultant function is said to rise as a straight line (Wever and Lawrence, 1954). This indicates that this second region is characterized by the conversion of energy to upper partials, and thus this is a region of simple saturation. As intensity increases, the total CM curve (fundamental

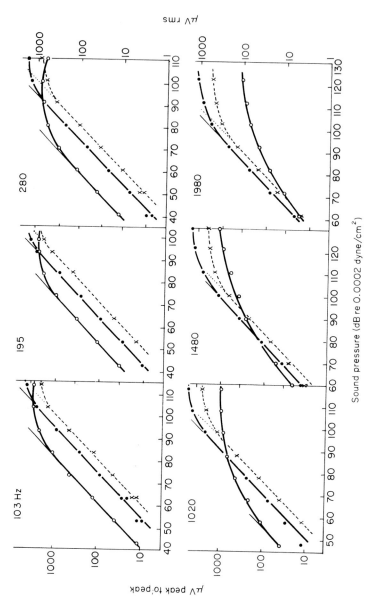

Fig. 5.9. Voltages (peak to peak) of the cochlear microphonic from turn 1 and turn 3 as a function of sound pressure level. Heavy line, turn 3 (differential electrodes); lighter line, turn 1 (differential electrodes); broken line, turn 1 (scala tympani) referred to neck. The last is practically the equivalent of the classical round-window–neck combination. The measurements were from oscillograms. (From Tasaki *et al.*, 1952, p. 506.)

plus all harmonics combined) also ceases to rise linearly, which signifies that there is actual diminution in the CM energy. This is the region of overloading.

The maximum point on the CM input–output function behaves quite the same as the point of nonlinearity does. With round-window recording the CM maximum is relatively constant to 750 Hz, beyond which it decreases exponentially with increasing frequency. From the Tasaki *et al.* plots of Fig. 5.9 we note that the maxima of the first-turn plots are remarkably constant up to about 2000 Hz. Presumably at higher frequencies these maxima would decline in accordance with Wever's round-window data. Observing the third-turn plots of Fig. 5.9, we see a fairly clear-cut reduction in the maximum CM with increasing frequency. More data on the dependence of CM maximum on recording location and frequency were collected by Tonndorf (1958b). From his plots it seems that the maximum CM at low frequencies is greatest in turn 3 and smallest in turn 1. This tendency does not agree with the Tasaki *et al.* data or with our own experience. It appears from Fig. 5.9 that no matter what the frequency is, the maximum CM is always greatest in the basal turn.

While the maximum CM that can be recorded from the perilymphatic scalae is of the order of 1 mV rms, the corresponding maxima when recorded from scala media are much greater. From the data of Honrubia and Ward (1968) we can deduce that from the basal turn at low frequencies one can record CM as large as 8 mV. The maxima as recorded from scala media behave as we have seen above: the higher the frequency the lower the maximum from any given recording site, and in general the further away from the base the lower the maximum for any given frequency. There are some exceptions to this last contention in the Honrubia–Ward data; particularly at the lowest frequencies, the higher turns appear to produce larger potentials than the base. The differences, however, are not sufficiently impressive to discard the above-formulated generalization that the basal turn can produce maximal CM under any condition. Note, however, that this observation is not contrary to the traditional place principle. The *sensitivity* of the third turn is considerably greater for, say, 1020 Hz than that of the base. This is clearly seen in the appropriate plot of Fig. 5.9. At low sound levels the third turn produces considerably greater CM than does the base. But the linear region in the base is more extensive, and thus, while the third-turn response saturates, the basal-turn response continues to grow. Thus the CM produced in turn 1 overtakes the CM originating in turn 3 in magnitude as the intensity of the stimulus increases. This clearly means that the distribution pattern of the CM changes with intensity. This change was demonstrated with particular clarity and was emphasized by Honrubia and Ward (1968).

To underscore and explain this phenomenon two schematic constructions are shown in Fig. 5.10. In each we assume several hypothetical displacement

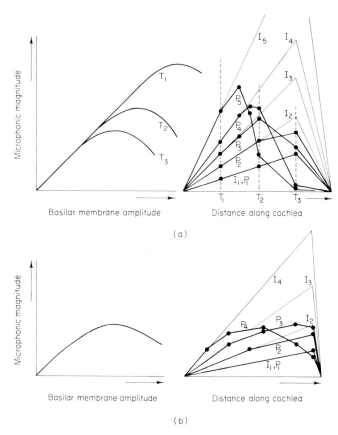

Fig. 5.10. Schematic construction demonstrating an apparent basal shift of CM activity with increasing intensity without any spatial shift of the underlying traveling wave pattern. The construction of hypothetical CM spatial patterns (heavy lines denoted by $P_1, \ldots, P_5$) proceeds as follows. The traveling wave spatial patterns are assumed to be triangular for simplicity. Their magnitude increases with intensity without a change in the location of the maximum (thin lines denoted by $I_1, \ldots, I_5$). At a given point along the cochlea and at a given intensity the ordinate of the appropriate I function is measured. This measurement is used as the abscissa in the hypothetical microphonic input–output function (given in the left side of each panel) to obtain the corresponding CM value, which is then inserted in the spatial plot to form a point on the appropriate P function. In panel (a) in accordance with experimental data it is assumed that at any given location the CM input–output function is different. Specifically, greater linear range is assumed to correspond to functions at more basal locations. Three functions, T_1, T_2, and T_3, are shown to correspond to the three points T_1, T_2, and T_3. For the sake of clarity points are obtained for intermediate points (and functions) between T_1 and T_2 but the corresponding input–output functions are not plotted. In panel (b) a similar construction is shown, but here matters are simplified by assuming that all locations have the same CM input–output function. Even with this assumption a clear (albeit less pronounced) basal shift of the CM is demonstrated.

patterns (triangular for simplicity) for a few stimulus intensity levels of a given frequency stimulus. These displacement patterns are drawn with thin lines. Note that we assume that with increasing intensity the location of the vibratory maximum does *not* change. There are three locations where we wish to find the CM magnitude, and the CM input–output functions that apply to these locations at our frequency are shown at the left of the figure. Note that in panel (a), in conformity with our experimental observations, the input–output functions are shown to become nonlinear at lesser and lesser intensities from the higher-turn locations. We now simply measure the displacement magnitudes at any point (T_1, T_2, or T_3) and obtain the corresponding CM magnitude from our hypothetical input–output functions (T_1, T_2, or T_3); the resultant points are shown connected with heavy lines. In panel (b) a similar construction is shown but here we did assume that *any* cochlear location has an identical input–output function. Now let us reiterate. The thin lines are hypothetical envelope patterns for basilar membrane motion at various intensity levels. The heavy lines are corresponding CM distribution patterns. While these constructions are admittedly quite crude they are also simple and illuminating. They show that to infer from CM distribution patterns to basilar membrane motion patterns is a somewhat risky business, especially at high intensity levels. We thus see that as one consequence of the nonlinearity of the input–output functions, and particularly of the lowering of the level of nonlinearity in the higher cochlear turns, the peak CM response at any frequency tends to migrate toward the base as intensity increases. As our construction shows this phenomenon can occur *without* a concomitant migration of the peak basilar membrane displacement.

The following comments concerning the CM input–output functions are related to the final, declining stage of these characteristic curves. Invariably if intensity is raised to sufficiently high levels, the CM functions go beyond their maximum and begin to decrease. This phenomenon indicates that a process in excess of a simple saturating type of nonlinearity is in effect at very high sound levels. As a consequence of the operation of this process the total electrical output from the cochlea actually decreases. This point is worth emphasizing for it is not only the fundamental frequency component of the response that declines in this region, but also the total rms response. Thus the decline is not associated with a conversion of energy from the fundamental frequency to harmonic components. This latter type of process probably operates to some degree below the maximum of the input–output function (Wever and Lawrence, 1954) but cannot account for the observed behavior beyond the maximum. The process that results in the decline of the microphonic magnitude is somewhat of a mystery. Several explanations have been proposed, but no hard evidence exists.

Wever (1949) integrated this phase of the function into his theory of CM generation, according to which deformation of the hair cell membrane results in the alteration of the surface charge of these membranes and thus of the external potential field (see more details later in this chapter). The original charge of the membrane is maintained in this scheme by a polarization of the cell's interior with respect to the external medium. It is assumed that this resting polarization is reduced when very intense stimuli are forced upon the cell, and as the consequence of the reduction of the base polarization the variable, stimulus-related response component would also be reduced. According to this scheme there are three regions of operation, corresponding to the three phases of the input–output function. The first is linear operation. The second is where the variation in surface charge generates potential changes that are commensurate with the base polarization and consequently create nonlinear effects such as clipping; this would be the region where energy is transposed from the fundamental to harmonic frequencies. Finally, in the third phase the base polarization would be reduced due to overstimulation and here the total response would decline.

Whitfield and Ross (1965) extended their phase-cancellation scheme (details below) to propose a mechanism for the high-level decline of the CM input–output function. They simply assumed that at high levels those generators that are on the segment of the membrane that is undergoing the largest excursion will limit their output due to nonlinearity. In contrast other generators, out of phase with the maximally stimulated ones, would still increase their outputs. As a consequence the total potential would actually decrease. Laszlo (1968), in his computer simulation of the modified Whitfield–Ross scheme, examined this proposition and found that it does not work. The only way he could obtain a decreasing gross CM characteristic was to assume that the individual generators themselves had a decreasing high-level portion in their respective input–output functions. It is probably safe to say that this issue is far from being settled. It is one of those situations, common in auditory physiology, in which more solid experimental evidence is needed to augment theoretical considerations. The declining phase of the input–output characteristic has more than theoretical importance since stimulation in this region invariably results in at least temporary, and often permanent, impairment of hair cell function. The mechanism of hair cell damage due to overstimulation is clearly manifested in the outward sign of declining CM output. Consequently the understanding of the latter would provide clues to the understanding, and possible prevention, of the former.

c. Meaning of Gross Cochlear Microphonic. Armed with the understanding of the basic properties of the CM as recorded from various cochlear locations, we are now in the position to inquire how this potential is related to the outputs of its individual generators. While there are several theories to the contrary, it is fairly widely accepted that it is the cochlear hair cell that generates the CM. For any stimulus there are hundreds or thousands of hair cells undergoing stimulation, and they all presumably produce some CM. The question now is, how are the outputs of these multitudes of sources combined to produce the CM response that is recorded by our electrodes or, the converse, how can we infer the output of an individual source from the overall recorded CM? This is a very real and serious issue because on the answer depends the value of much of the CM literature. In Chapter 2 we devoted considerable space to discussions on the relative merits and limitations of the various CM recording methods. We saw that round-window recording and any single intracochlear electrode recording emphasize the CM contributions of proximal generators, but also respond to remote sources. This type of recording is not selective enough to provide good indication of localized events and yet not general enough to indicate the overall state of CM production of all cochlear generators. We note that the differential-electrode technique improves the selectivity of the recording to a great extent, and thus by sampling the response with several pairs of spatially separated differential electrodes one can obtain a fair representation of relatively localized events and also the overall trends. It appears that recording from the scala media provides a somewhat lesser degree of selectivity than does the differential-electrode technique. Even though the latter methods are stated to be selective, we must keep in mind the very real limitations on the spatial resolving power that they can provide. Even optimistic estimates do not claim that one could record selectively from less than about 1.5–2 mm of the cochlea. Over such a distance there might be about 600 hair cells whose output potential would strongly contribute to the CM recording from that region. We can rephrase our inquiry then and ask, how do the outputs of these cells summate to produce the measured CM? Is there any resemblance between what we measure (the CM) and the outputs of the individual cells in, for example, magnitude or waveform?

Whitfield and Ross (1965) were the first to attempt to treat this issue in a semiquantitative manner. They noted that for a given stimulus the generators are excited in proportion with the traveling wave activity at their respective location. Consider two hair cells, A and B. The output of hair cell A is a potential of magnitude and phase that corresponds to the magnitude and phase of membrane displacement at cell A, while the output of B is related to the magnitude and phase of displacement of cell B. Clearly both magnitude and phase of the outputs of these two cells are different at any instant; they contribute vectorially to the overall potential that can be recorded. Of course so do all the other cells within the pickup range of the recording electrode. Consequently the measured potential is the vectorial sum of the outputs of several hundred generators. In fact, theoretically every single excited cell in the cochlea contributes to the recorded potential, each with different magnitude and phase. Of course, distant cells contribute relatively little and their effect can be safely neglected in a normal preparation. It is clear that the recorded CM does not really correspond to the output of *any* cell in magnitude, phase, or waveform. Instead, it is a weighted vectorial sum of the outputs of a very large number of cells. One consequence of this is that the lower the frequency, the better the recorded CM represents the outputs of individual generators and the better the representation on the proximal as opposed to the distal side of the traveling wave.

To see the validity of these contentions let us consider the spatial extent and phase characteristics of traveling waves for low and high-frequency stimuli. We know that high-frequency traveling waves are much more limited in their overall active region than are low-frequency traveling waves. Consequently the gradient of phase changes is greater at high frequencies. To see this quantitatively one can consult Fig. 4.5. Consequently, an electrode located for example in the basal turn would see much more rapid phase changes from generator to generator within its pickup area for a high-frequency as opposed to a low-frequency stimulus. In Fig. 5.11 this situation is illustrated by two hypothetical phase distribution functions for a low (a) and a high

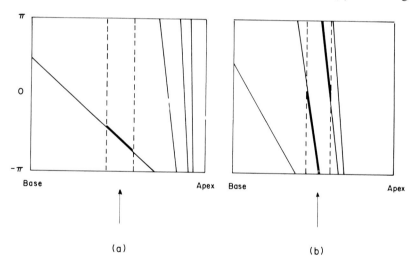

Fig. 5.11. Schematic representation of the hair cell excitation phase (and CM phase) along the length of the cochlea at a low-frequency input (a) and at a high-frequency input (b). In both cases the recording electrode is located at the same point (arrow). The effective pickup area of the electrode is denoted by the dashed lines. Note that in case (a) the phase change within the pickup region is moderate, in other words virtually all significant CM sources are in phase, but in case (b) there is a very rapid phase shift within the pickup zone.

frequency (b). The location of the recording electrode [same for both case (a) and (b)] is designated with an arrow, and the region from which this electrode is assumed to pick up potentials is between the dashed lines. Now observe that the phase of the generators that produce the CM changes very rapidly within the pickup area in panel (b) but quite gradually in (a). This means that the electrode in (b) "sees" a set of generators with quite inhomogeneous phase distribution, while the phases in panel (a) are highly similar. Clearly, if all other conditions are equal, the resultant signal picked up by the electrode in case (b) will be much smaller than that recorded in (a). This is because many of the generators in case (b) would find themselves in phase opposition with others, and thus the contributions of these generators would tend to cancel one another in destructive interference. In case (a), at a lower frequency, the phases of the various generators within the active area are quite homogeneous, and consequently there is very little cancellation among them. It is clear that we can extend our argument and consider what would happen in case (a) if we moved the recording electrode toward the apex. In this case, even though the frequency is low, the recording electrode would be in that region of the traveling wave where the phase changes rapidly, and of course phase cancellations would occur here also.

It appears that CM recording tends to reflect faithfully the average magnitude and phase of the generators within the effective pickup area of the electrodes if these electrodes are situated on the proximal side of the traveling wave envelope. This means that for any given recording site there is a progressive bias against high frequencies. For example, in the basal turn this bias would become significant above 8000–10,000 Hz, and in the third turn above 750–1000 Hz. Whitfield and Ross expanded these arguments to explain why the summating potential response to a high-frequency tone can be greater than the CM response and also why "clean" CM waveforms should be seen in the presence of a large amount of harmonic distortion. Clearly the phase cancellation effects do not apply to the dc potential (SP) and thus their arguments concerning it are sound. As we shall show in the next chapter, however, cochlear harmonics do not have their own traveling wave pattern (except at very high intensities), and consequently the phase cancellation argument that would penalize harmonics more than fundamental components is not valid.

Kohllöffel (1971) expanded and further quantified the arguments of Whitfield and Ross (1965). He worked with the hypothesis that the activity recorded by any cochlear electrode is a weighted average of the outputs of all hair cells. If the distance from the stapes is denoted by x and the output of the hair cell at point x is denoted by $H(x)$, then an electrode at $x = x_0$ would record a potential,

$$CM(x_0) = \int H(x)W(x_0 - x)dx \qquad (5.1)$$

where $W(x_0 - x)$ is a weighting function showing the attenuation for a potential that is generated at x and recorded at x_0. The integration has to be carried out over the entire length of the cochlea. One recognizes that the above formula is the convolution integral. Kohllöffel noted, as did Whitfield and Ross, that high frequencies are expected to be more severely influenced by this "spatial filtering" than low frequencies. He noted in fact that, as a direct consequence of the varying phase and amplitude contributions of the members of the generator array, amplitude minima and abrupt phase shifts should be observable in the gross recording. To substantiate this he placed an array of 12 electrodes, spaced 150 μ apart, in the scala tympani of the basal turn of the guinea pig cochlea and recorded CM responses from the array at several frequencies at constant SPL. Some of his results are shown in Fig. 5.12, for both CM amplitude and phase (re an unspecified reference). The important features that can be gleaned from these data are that there indeed can be seen amplitude minima (note the 13.5-kHz or the 13.75-kHz plots) and abrupt phase shifts from lag to lead (note the 13.5-kHz plot). This demonstration clearly underscores what we have stated above: One can infer from gross CM recording to the individual hair cell (or small group of cells) output *only* for stimulus conditions that generate a traveling wave whose peak is distal from the electrode location. It is clear that Kohllöffel's experimental conditions (purposely) did not meet this criterion in that the amplitude and phase pattern of his high-frequency traveling waves changed considerably over the extent of his electrode array, and thus the phase cancellation effects operated powerfully.

While we are discussing the limitations and interpretation of gross CM recording it is appropriate to consider some possible shortcomings of the differential-electrode recording that are implied in the results of Weiss *et al.* (1969, 1971). These authors recorded CM with microelectrodes from cat cochleae from all three scalae of the basal turn while penetrating through the round-window membrane and through the basilar and Reissner's membrane, depending on which scala they wished to record from. They were interested in relative changes in CM phase and magnitude from one scala to another at any given stimulus intensity and frequency. We shall discuss their results with the aid of Figs. 5.13 and 5.14. In the former figure the ratio of CM magnitude in scala media (SM) and scala tympani (ST) is given as the function of frequency for eight animals. In the latter figure the phase shift between scala media and tympani CM is shown, again as the function of frequency at a constant SPL and for five animals.

In the magnitude plot one can discriminate three zones. Below 1000 Hz the difference generally decreases with increasing frequency, between 1000 and 2000 Hz there is a distinct maximum, and above 2000 Hz the results are scattered and their interpretation is difficult. One can say that at least below

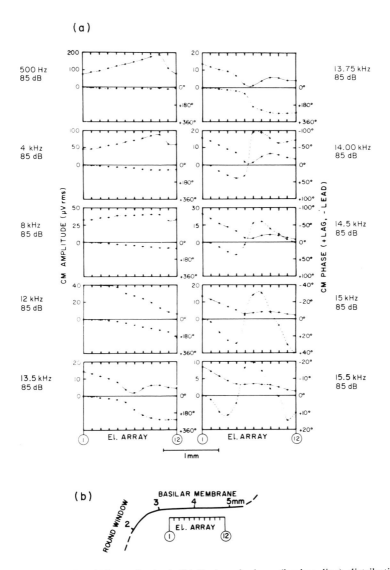

Fig. 5.12. (a) The CM amplitude (solid line) and phase (broken line) distribution along the electrode array at different frequencies. At 13.5 kHz the phase changes from lag to lead within the array. (The phase angles in this figure are referred to the most basal electrode of the array.) (b) The position of the electrode array in the basal ST is shown in relation to the longitudinal dimension of the basilar membrane. (From Kohllöffel, 1971, p. 29.)

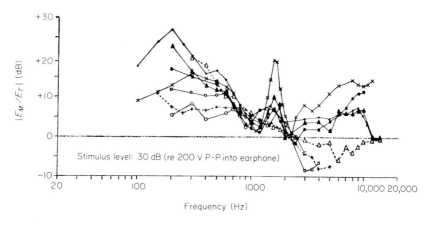

Fig. 5.13. Ratio of magnitudes of cochlear potentials across the organ of Corti (E_M/E_T) versus frequency for eight cochleae. (From Weiss *et al.*, 1971, p. 593.)

2000 Hz the SM potential is in excess of the ST potential by differing amounts up to 25 dB. Weiss *et al.* also provide similar CM magnitude plots for scala media (SM) versus scala vestibuli (SV). These plots are relatively uniform and indicate that the SM potential exceeds the SV potential by less than 5 dB over most of the frequency range. The conclusion then is that large differences in magnitude can be expected between SV and ST microphonic. In two animals the authors eliminated the contribution of whole-nerve action potentials by cutting the auditory nerve prior to the experiments. The results for these two animals are not radically different except between 1000 and 2000 Hz, where no maximum was seen for these animals in the SM versus ST magnitude plot. These results would seem to indicate that aside from the already discussed contribution of the AP (see Fig. 2.6) there are additional asymmetries between recordings from the scalae vestibuli and tympani of a given turn. The phase plots of Fig. 5.14 further amplify this contention. We note there that aside from the large variability from one animal to another, the general trend is that phase difference between SM and ST is negligible at very low frequencies and it tends toward 180° at higher frequencies. The authors also indicate that the phase difference between SM and SV is negligible. Thus it seems that the traditionally accepted relationship between the magnitude and phase of the CM in scalae vestibuli and tympani might need to be revised. It is remembered that the tacit assumption is generally made that on the two sides of the cochlear partition the electrodes see the source with the same (or approximately the same) magnitude and in opposite phase. Here these expectations are not borne out.

In our laboratory some comparison experiments have been made with partially different results. Instead of using a single microelectrode and sepa-

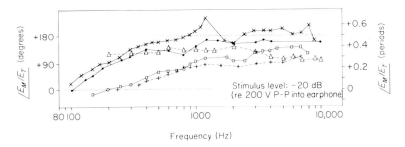

Fig. 5.14. Phase difference of cochlear potentials (scala media minus scala tympani) versus frequency. Solid lines correspond to data obtained from normal cochleae. Dashed lines correspond to data obtained from animals whose auditory nerve have been severed. (From Weiss *et al.*, 1971, p. 594.)

rate measurements from all three scalae during the course of a penetration, we placed the customary gross electrodes in the scalae tympani and vestibuli of the cat first cochlear turn. Our phase measurements were made directly between these two electrodes: some results are shown in Fig. 5.15. It is clear that, while the phase difference between the two electrodes is not exactly 180°, it is very close to 180° between 100 and 10,000 Hz; the departures appear to be negligible, except in the vicinity of 1000 Hz.

We expanded this line of investigation somewhat and made similar magnitude and phase measurements in the first three turns of guinea pig cochleae. These measurements are sufficiently illuminating to make them

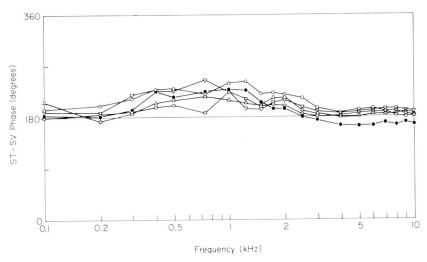

Fig. 5.15. The ST—SV microphonic phase for five cats with electrodes in the first turn of the cochlea. Stimulus level: 70 dB SPL. (From Dallos *et al.*, 1971, p. 1151.)

worthy of discussion in some detail here. In Fig. 5.3 comparison was presented between the phase plots of three different animals, one each for turn 1, 2, and 3. These three were completely representative animals. The plots of Fig. 5.3 were all obtained at a constant 70 dB SPL. In this figure, as in our results for cat, one sees no significant departures from 180° in the turn 1 phase over most of the frequency range of interest, i.e., from 100 to 10,000 Hz. Note that in the higher turns the phase difference approximates 180° at low frequencies, but at higher frequencies radical phase changes take place. In the second turn, between 4000 and 5000 Hz the phase difference undergoes a radical shift, and above 5000 it settles to zero. In the third turn the radical phase change takes place between 1000 and 1500 Hz, and above 2000 Hz the phase difference is zero. What is the meaning of these results? At frequencies that create substantial responses in the region of the electrodes the locally generated CM dominates the recorded potential. This local CM is generated largely " between " the electrodes and is consequently seen with approximately 180° phase difference. This situation applies at least up to 8000 Hz in turn 1 (one can see the beginning of a rise in phase between 8000 and 10,000 Hz), up to 2000–3000 Hz in turn 2, and approximately 500 Hz in turn 3. At high frequencies, above 2000 in turn 3, above 5000 in turn 2, and probably above 17,000 Hz in turn 1, the contribution of remote CM sources to the overall potential exceeds the contribution of the local source, and both electrodes tend to see the remote source in the same phase. Consequently at high frequencies the $SV - ST$ phase difference is zero. In the transition zone the phase changes rapidly and radically as the balance of dominance shifts from local to remote CM.

The reason that in a coiled cochlea we observe these bizarre phase effects is that there is considerable cross talk between adjacent turns, particularly between higher turns. Thus for example at 2000 Hz there is very little local activity in turn 3 but a great deal of activity in turn 2. The electrical insulation between turns 2 and 3 is poor, and consequently both third-turn electrodes see the second-turn remote source in approximately the same phase. Another manifestation of cross talk between turns can be discerned from the low-frequency behavior of second-turn responses. We have measured the SV versus ST phase in the second turn for ten guinea pigs. Six of these showed the type of low-frequency phase difference that was illustrated in the second-turn plot of Fig. 5.3; that is, in these animals the phase between SV and ST was approximately 180°. The phase difference in the other four animals was approximately zero. Thus a dichotomy in phase difference is clearly seen, and the question is, what causes such behavior? To answer this we investigated the low-frequency magnitude differences between the second-turn SV and ST microphonic. It was noted that in cases where the phase was close to 180° the SV and ST electrodes showed only moderate sensitivity differences; going hand in hand with the zero difference, however, was a marked inequality between SV and ST potentials. The scala vestibuli electrode invariably registers potentials in excess of the scala tympani electrode. In the latter group, however, the differences were of the order of 20 dB. It should quickly be noted that all preparations satisfied our placement criteria (cf. Chapter 2, Section II,A,1,c); in other words, at high frequencies the electrodes did record the same CM.

The meaning of the above observations seems clear. At very low frequencies the third turn produces considerably more CM than the second. In cases where the insulation between turns 2 and 3 is poor the second-turn SV electrode picks up more CM from the third turn than from its own location. Thus neither the magnitude nor the phase difference between the SV and ST electrodes reflects the behavior of the local CM component. In those cases, however, where the electrical insulation between turns 2 and 3 is better, or probably the electrode placement is superior, the local component is reflected in the similarity of the magnitude and near-180° relation in phase between ST and SV recordings.

The influence of CM conducted from adjacent turns on single-electrode recording forces interesting and very consistent patterns on the CM versus frequency functions. In Fig. 5.16 three examples of such patterns are shown. The three panels of the figure contain median CM isopotential contours for ST and SV electrodes from the first three turns of guinea pig cochleae. The one consistent finding that is most conspicuous in these graphs is that the SV electrode is always more sensitive than the ST electrode at the lowest frequencies. The sensitivity difference is a relatively modest 4 dB for the first-turn electrode pair, but it is a very significant value (up to 15 dB) in the second turn. The low-frequency advantage of the SV electrode prevails up to a frequency that appears to be quite consistently observed from turn to turn. This crossover frequency at which the two electrodes become equally sensitive is approximately 275 Hz in turn 3, 1000 Hz in turn 2, and 2000 Hz in turn 1. The low-frequency region within which the SV electrode is more sensitive is usually followed by a frequency band in which the two electrodes record equal amounts of electricity. This band extends all the way to approximately 13,000 Hz in turn 1, to 2500 Hz in turn 2, and it is nonexistent in turn 3. To explain, in the lower turns the two electrodes are equally sensitive between the crossover frequency and the aforementioned higher frequency limit. Beyond this higher frequency they diverge again. The third-turn electrodes, however, diverge immediately beyond their low-frequency crossover of 275 Hz and do not show a band of frequencies in which equal sensitivity prevails. Above the region of equality the scala tympani electrode becomes more sensitive and stays so for a narrow frequency region. Thus in the third turn the ST electrode regularly exhibits greater sensitivity than its pair between

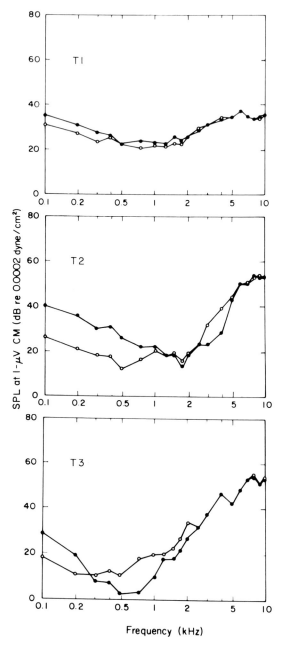

Fig. 5.16. Median isopotential curves for scala vestibuli (open circles) and scala tympani (closed circles) from the first three turns of the guinea pig cochlea. Number of animals: $N_{T1} = 20$, $N_{T2} = 16$, $N_{T3} = 20$.

275 and 2500 Hz, while the corresponding region in turn 2 extends from 2500 to 6000 Hz. The final region, encompassing the highest frequencies, is characterized once again by the equal sensitivity of the SV and ST electrodes. This region begins at 2500 and 6000 Hz in turns 3 and 2, respectively. We have not ascertained the existence or extent of this final region for our usually located (4 mm from the round window) first-turn electrodes.

We conjecture that the reason for the consistent differences in sensitivity between scala tympani and vestibuli electrodes is again the interaction between local and remote potential components. The interactions are facilitated by relatively pronounced cross talk between adjacent cochlear scalae, in other words, by the apparently high conductivity between bordering scalae vestibuli and tympani. Thus, for example, in the second turn at the lowest frequencies the potential conducted from the third turn is greater than that generated in the second-turn. The remote potential is primarily observed in the scala that is closer to its source, which means the scala vestibuli at low frequencies. Thus the SV electrode exhibits an apparently greater sensitivity in each turn over a given low-frequency region. In contrast, above the best frequency for a given electrode location, the activity shifts basally, and as a consequence the electrode closer to the base (ST) picks up an excessive amount of remote CM. Note how clearly this region appears in the second-turn plot (Fig. 5.16), where the best frequency is approximately 1750–2000 Hz. In the third turn the relation is not as clear because there does not appear to be a region of equal sensitivity in the best-frequency band, even though the character of the curves indicates that significant cross talk starts to influence the ST response above 500 Hz and that the region between 275 and 500 Hz is analogous to the equality zone in turn 2. Beyond the frequency band where the remote response has its major effect on the ST electrode, the activity recedes so far toward the base that both electrodes begin to pick up the remote response equally. This final region is the very characteristic segment beyond 2500 Hz in turn 3 and beyond 6000 Hz in turn 2. It is remembered that within this latter segment the differential-electrode recording is most effective in rejecting remote activity and that here the isopotential contour obtained with the differential pair diverges significantly from the single-electrode plots.

Let us now look at the phase transition zones in somewhat more detail. It appears that in the two higher turns, and in turn 3 particularly, the character of phase transition is radically dependent on stimulus strength. To clarify this statement, in Fig. 5.17 the third-turn interscala phase data of one guinea pig are shown in detail at 80, 85, 86, 87, 88, 89, and 90 dB SPL between 1000 and 1500 Hz. Note the orderly transition with increasing intensity. The higher the intensity the steeper the transition, and the 1-dB step from 89 to 90 dB carries the phase from a smooth (albeit rapid) change to an abrupt phase reversal. It is quite illuminating to compare these phase changes with the

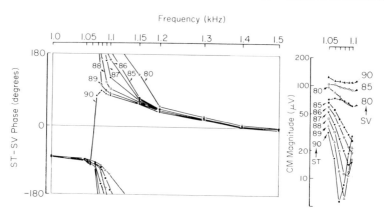

Fig. 5.17. Detailed phase (left) and magnitude (right) CM data from one guinea pig with electrodes in the third cochlear turn. The frequency range is limited between 1000 and 1500 Hz for the ST—SV phase measurements. Very detailed information for both phase and magnitude is given between 1050 and 1100 Hz. The parameters are SPL in decibels. Magnitude data are given for both SV and ST recordings. (From Dallos *et al.*, 1971, p. 1150.)

corresponding magnitude changes in the ST and SV microphonic. In Fig. 5.17 the CM magnitude plots are given over the restricted frequency range of interest of 1050–1100 Hz, with SPL as the parameter over the same range as that in the phase plots. The first obvious observation is that the magnitude of the SV potential is not significantly influenced by stimulus intensity in a frequency-dependent manner. In contrast the ST potential undergoes very rapid and significant magnitude shifts that are radically frequency dependent. Note how a minimum develops at 88 dB and becomes pronounced at 89 and 90 dB. The interpretation of these results must again take the interplay of local and remote responses into account. At 1000 Hz in turn 3 the local response begins to diminish rapidly, whereas it is on the increase in turn 3. Because of the cross talk between the two turns, the scala tympani potential first becomes a mixture of local and remote responses, and then as frequency increases the remote response starts to dominate both scalae. In the frequency range where the rapid phase shift and amplitude minimum develop the exact point of transition from local dominance to remote dominance takes place. A fascinating facet of this phenomenon is the strong influence of intensity. Probably the mechanism whereby intensity influences the pattern of phase transition is tied in with the general basal shift in CM activity that we have already seen to occur with an increase in stimulus strength. Clearly if the relative magnitude of CM potentials between points are influenced by signal intensity then one can fully expect that the interaction between remote and local responses would also be influenced by SPL. This seems to be the case, as the above plots clearly demonstrate.

We noted in Fig. 5.17 the development of an amplitude minimum on the high-frequency side of the third-turn ST plot. In Fig. 5.18 a similar minimum is shown for a second-turn scala tympani recording site. Here the minimum occurs at 4700 Hz; it is very sharp, indicating almost complete cancellation of CM at that frequency. The cancellation again probably takes place between the local and the remote CM component, even though we cannot rule out the possibility that the type of cancellation that Kohllöffel (1971) discussed might be also effective here. It might be worth restating that all the above-discussed evidence indicates that caution must be exercised in the interpreta-

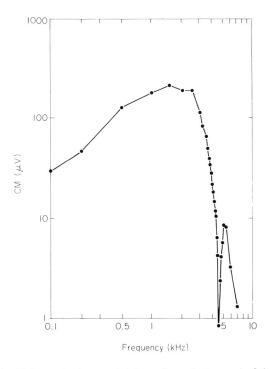

Fig. 5.18. The CM magnitude recorded from the scala tympani of the second turn of one guinea pig as the function of frequency at a constant 70 dB SPL. (From Dallos *et al.*, 1971, p. 1150.)

tion of CM recordings. Due to the fact that the CM is the resultant of the outputs of a multitude of generators, each of which differs in the magnitude and phase of its excitation and consequently in its output, the overall response is a weighted vectorial sum of the outputs of all generators. The weighting function is such that sources in proximity with the electrodes are emphasized but remote sources are not completely eliminated. This weighting function is simply the result of the electrical attenuation of potentials in the cochlea. As we shall discuss in more detail later, this attenuation depends on serial resistance and parallel shunting effects of the electrical pathways in the complex distributed electrical system that the fluid-filled cochlea is. Clearly, if the stimulus conditions are such that the electrodes see activity that is local, thus favorably weighted, and the generators are approximately in phase, then the gross recording reflects the actual outputs of the sources. Conversely, under certain stimulus conditions, in which strongly weighted small and lightly weighted weak (local versus remote) potentials coexist, the recorded CM might not bear any resemblance to either of these components. The almost total null in the CM magnitude in Fig. 5.18 is a good example of this situation. Obviously the generators of the CM did not cease to produce electricity at 4700 Hz in this situation; their outputs simply added up to zero at the electrode location.

It is remembered that when Weiss et al. (1969, 1971) recorded interscala phase in the cat by penetrating a microelectrode through the round window they found highly significant departures from 180° between the CM in scalae vestibuli and tympani. In apparent contrast, our basal-turn recordings in both cat and guinea pig provided nearly perfect phase opposition between SV and ST microphonic over the entire frequency range of interest. In order to seek the cause of the difference in results we performed a variety of additional experiments on both guinea pigs and cats. These experiments involved the recording of phase in cats with micropipettes penetrated through the round window and, in addition, the recording of phase from guniea pigs with micropipettes and with intracochlear electrodes placed in the round-window region. Since in the cat as well as in the guinea pig the phase difference between SV and ST microphonic in the basal turn when recorded with gross electrodes is closely approximated by 180°, it is apparent that the difference between our results and those of Weiss et al. (1969, 1971) cannot be attributed to species differences. There are two remaining possibilities to explain the discrepancies. First, there is a significant difference in location of recording between our placement (4–5 mm from the stapes) and the round-window approach. Second, an unlikely prospect, the methodological difference between gross and microelectrode recordings could be considered.

In order to check these possibilities guinea pigs were prepared with gross electrodes placed across the cochlear partition at the level of the round window. In the same animals the interscala phase was also measured by penetrating the round window with a micropipette. Consequently in these animals the phase was measured at the same location with the two different methods. In Fig. 5.19 the ST − SV phase obtained by both methods is shown for three individual animals. All data were collected at a constant 70 dB SPL. In all three animals normal endocochlear potentials were registered during

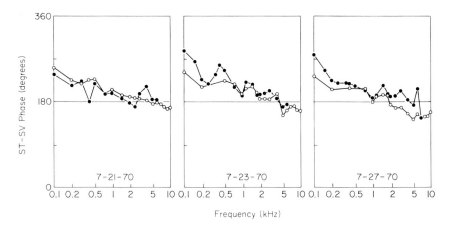

Fig. 5.19. Comparison of ST—SV phase recorded with gross electrodes (open circles) and with micropipettes (filled circles) in three individual guinea pigs. The pipette passed through the round window; phase measurements were made in both ST and SV. The gross electrodes were situated in both ST and SV at the same point along the cochlear partition where the pipette penetrated. Stimulus level: 70 dB SPL. (From Dallos *et al.*, 1971, p. 1151.)

penetration of the scala media. Phase data obtained above 6 kHz with the micropipette are not considered here because of the uncertainty of proper neuralization of the preamplifier at these high frequencies. A number of interesting observations can be made from the plots of Fig. 5.19. It appears that the overall character of the phase response is quite similar from one animal to another, which is in line with our previous observations. In addition, the gross-electrode and microelectrode data are very similar, indicating that the measurement technique does not influence the experimental results. Finally, the response pattern reveals a significantly different configuration than that seen at the 4-mm electrode location (see Fig. 5.3). It is remembered that there the phase response is essentially flat, with a value of 180°. In contrast, the phase pattern at the round-window level shows a definite tilt. At low frequencies the ST—SV phase difference is in excess of 180°, while at high frequencies this phase difference is less than 180°. This configuration is actually quite similar to that seen by Weiss *et al.* (1969) in the cat, even though the departures from 180° are less exaggerated than in their data. Thus it appears that there is a very forceful dependence of interscala phase on the location of the recording electrode. One must conclude that in the "hook" region of the cochlea the interscala phase is systematically different from 180°, in line with the results of Weiss *et al.* This anomalous phase behavior is manifest both in guinea pig and in cat, probably in a somewhat more pronounced manner in the latter species.

It appears to us that the reason for the "improper" electrical properties of the cochlear round-window segment should be sought in the geometrical and electroanatomical properties of this region. As opposed to the elongated, gently curving perilymphatic scalae that characterize the basal turn of the cochlea at the 4- to 7-mm segment (where the phase difference is 180°), the initial portion of the cochlea has a much more complex shape, and here the cochlear partition essentially changes its direction of curvature. While the exact mechanism whereby the geometrical differences exert their influence on the electrical conduction pattern is not at all clear, such a mechanism appears to operate and it renders the round-window regions of cochleae electrically more complex than other portions of the inner ear. It is probably fair to say that this observation adds to the body of information that points toward the inadequacy of round-window CM recording for quantitative purposes.

In continuing the discussion of the relationship between gross CM and the outputs of its generators it is appropriate to quote Whitfield (1967, pp. 43–44), who puts one position on this issue in a very clear light.

> . . . the cochlear microphonic, as normally recorded, is no guide either to the amplitude or waveform of the potentials produced by individual hair-cell generators. The amplitude of potentials produced by the most highly excited hair-cell generators is, in general, much greater than the cochlear microphonic, and may amount to something of the order of 10 mV for intense stimuli. Such potentials will be highly nonsinusoidal.

This position is based on the following theoretical argument. The output of any given hair cell is assumed to be large, certainly much larger than the recorded CM. Furthermore, the waveform of the individual cell potential is probably like a square wave, certainly not sinusoidal. In the interaction between the outputs of a large number of cells a low-pass filtering effect occurs that (a) makes the recorded waveform quite sinusoidal and (b) makes the overall amplitude considerably smaller than the amplitude of the largest individual generator. This low-pass filtering effect operates through the mechanism of cancellation among out-of-phase generators in which it is assumed that the higher the frequency the more rapid the phase change and thus the more severe the cancellation.

Let us examine this posture. First, it is hard to reject the argument that the individual cell output is nonlinear on an a priori basis: We know that nonlinearities abound in the cochlea; effective stimulation is only on every other half-cycle of the stimulus, dc components (SP) are generated from ac stimulus, etc. Thus it is perfectly possible that the cell potential is more a square wave than a sine wave. The question is whether the explanation proposed by Whitfield and Ross is sufficient to explain why strongly nonlinear wave forms are not seen in the gross CM. Our contention is that their explanation is not completely adequate. As we have noted, they assume that phase changes in the spatial dimension are more rapid for harmonics generated in the transducer nonlinearity than they are for the fundamental. While it is true, as we have shown above, that at any given electrode location the phase effect becomes more and more severe as frequency increases it must be emphasized that this is because the phase of the *traveling wave* that corresponds to higher-frequency signals changes more rapidly than the phase of low-frequency traveling waves. As we shall amply demonstrate in Chapter 6, there are no traveling waves associated with frequency components generated in transducer nonlinearities. Consequently, there is no reason to assume that the phase of microphonic potentials that correspond to harmonics generated in a nonlinear transducer (hair cell) would change in space with any more rapidity than does the phase of the fundamental itself. Moreover this argument can be applied to any of the harmonics. We see then that, unless it can be demonstrated that a significant portion of the harmonic components generated in the cochlea are accompanied by traveling waves, the phase cancellation argument does not explain the apparently only mildly distorted waveform of the recorded CM contrasted to the hypothesized nonlinear, harmonic-rich waveform of the hair cell potentials. Evidence is lacking to show that cochlear harmonics at moderate intensity levels are accompanied by traveling waves of their own (Dallos and Sweetman, 1969).

Let us continue the above line of thought a little further. We argued above that, while the Whitfield–Ross model provides very important explanations concerning the relationship between the gross CM fundamental component and the hair cell outputs, it is not as persuasive on the issue of waveform preservation (or lack of it) from hair cell output to gross response. Laszlo (1968) in his significant Ph.D. thesis carried the Whitfield–Ross ideas further. He provided a computer simulation of gross CM production by breaking down a hypothetical guinea pig cochlea into 180 segments, each corresponding to a 100-μ patch of the cochlea. The electrical outputs within any patch were considered to be in phase. He used a mathematical simulation of the middle ear–inner ear transfer function not unlike Flanagan's (1962), and he assumed a markedly nonlinear displacement versus electrical output transfer function for the hair cells. The nonlinear output potentials from all 180 segments were summed after appropriate weighting to account for their distance from the "electrode." Laszlo's scheme is very much like that of Whitfield and Ross (1965) but more formalized. He obtained simulated potential waveforms predicted by the model for a hair cell situated at a particular cochlear site when the stimulus was a 7000-Hz sine wave at various intensities. As the consequence of the assumed transducer nonlinearity the hair cell output is strongly nonsinusoidal at the higher stimulus levels; in fact it is shown to be nearly a square wave at 110 dB. When Laszlo computed the sum of all hair cell outputs, appropriately weighted, for an electrode placed at the same location and for the same stimulus conditions, he obtained a series of waveforms that were significantly more sinusoidal than the outputs of the individual hair cells. As best as I can ascertain, Laszlo's computer technique did not involve a Fourier decomposition of the nonlinear source waveform and the assignment of appropriate spatial magnitude and phase characteristics to each individual harmonic component (in conformity with cochlear dynamics). Consequently the objections that were raised in connection with the heuristic arguments of Whitfield and Ross are apparently not valid here, and we must accept the conclusion that it is *possible* to obtain sinusoidal gross potentials from highly nonlinear source voltages.

Laszlo's results indicate that even more caution is required in the interpretation of gross cochlear microphonic recordings than we have hitherto assumed. It appears that there is a good possibility for the existence of a "spatial filtering" mechanism that, in addition to introducing uncertainties in gross magnitude and phase measurements, creates significant differences between gross potentials and hair cell potentials. We must be cautious of course; the possibility of the existence of such a mechanism does not prove that the process in fact operates. We must look for additional evidence in deciding this issue. It is immediately clear that gross recordings would not provide such evidence, unless we were able to use a preparation in which all hair cells were missing with the exception of a very few concentrated in a narrow strip. Generally the gross recording would be subject to the spatial filtering, if such actually occurs. The answer must lie in obtaining records from individual hair cells.

There are no published reports on recording from mammalian cochlear hair cells, although apparently some investigators may have succeeded in doing so (Peake and Weiss, 1969; Fex, 1970). These investigators did find *sinusoidal* intracellular responses to sinusoidal sound stimulation. In addition they did not find that these intracellular responses were inordinately large; in fact they were in the $100\text{-}\mu V$ range, commensurate with the gross CM. The only relevant published report describes the work of Harris *et al.* (1970). These authors recorded intracellularly from the giant hair cells in the mud puppy lateral line organ. The cupula of a given neuromast was stimulated mechanically by a vibrating pipette. A recording electrode was inserted into a single cell within the neuromast, and another recording electrode monitored neural potentials from the afferent fibers. The first recording electrode was also used to inject dyes into the penetrated cell so that it could be identified in histological sections. Some of the results are shown in Fig. 5.20. Recordings from three cells within the same neuromast are shown. It is known that cells in the lateral line organ are morphologically polarized; that is, they are asymmetrical. About half the cells in a neuromast are polarized so that their kinocilium is toward the caudal end of the animal, while on the other half

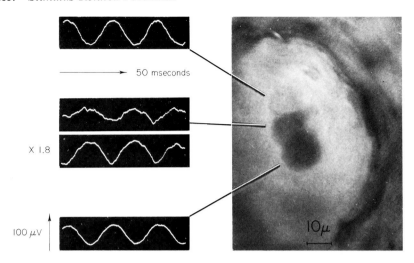

Fig. 5.20. Oppositely phased responses from different hair cells in the same neuromast. Right, stained hair cells in a neuromast. Left, oscilloscope traces of the response from each cell averaged 128 times. The bottom cell and top cell, which hardly stained at all, showed the same phase response. The middle cell showed a response of opposite phase. The trace labeled × 1.8 indicates that the stimulus magnitude was increased by a factor of 1.8. The three penetrated cells were identified *in vivo* as hair cells. The two deeply stained cells retained stain during fixation and were confirmed to be hair cells by histological examination. (From Harris *et al.*, 1970, p. 78.)

of the cells the kinocilium is toward the rostral pole. It is also known that oppositely polarized cells produce microphonics in opposite phase (Flock, 1965). In the figure we see that two of the cells (top and bottom) produce potentials that are in phase, while the middle cell is out of phase. This observation confirms that the recordings do indeed reflect the outputs of single cells. The important result for our purposes is that the outputs are more or less sinusoidal; there is no hint of a potential resembling a square wave. This is in spite of the fact that the stimulus was probably quite intense. The authors note that the ac potentials were invariably small, ranging downward from 800 μV peak-to-peak value. Thus at least the results from the lateral line hair cells are contrary to the notion that microphonics from individual hair cells are highly nonlinear and much larger than the gross CM. Clearly additional results, preferably from mammalian cochlear hair cells, are needed before this important and vexing issue of relationships between hair cell and gross CM can be solved to general satisfaction.

2.   Source of Origin: Theories and Experiments

There are numerous theories designed to explain the mode of generation of the microphonic potentials of the cochlea. Wever (1966) classified the various theories into three groups according to the way in which CM can be generated: (a) by the movements of electric charges, (b) by the movements of ions, and (c) by impedance variations in the path between fixed charges. In the first category is the theory of Gisselson (1960a). In the second category are the theories of Wever (1949), Dohlman (1959, 1960), Christiansen (1963), and Jensen *et al.* (1954). The last three theories are essentially variations on the same theme. In the last category is the theory of Davis (1965). A unique theory was proposed by Naftalin (1965). In a category by itself is the biochemical theory of Vinnikov and Titova (1964), which does not directly address itself to the processes of CM generation and thus will not be treated here.

The various theories might also be categorized on the basis of the magnitude of mechanical motion required to produce adequate stimulation. That displacement magnitude is a critical issue can be demonstrated by some simple considerations. Von Békésy (1948) calculated that the amplitude of vibration of the basilar membrane at 1000 dynes/cm^2 sound pressure is about 10^{-3} cm. Thus at the threshold of hearing the approximate vibratory amplitude of the basilar membrane can be calculated as 10^{-11} cm. The minuteness of this figure can be appreciated if one considers that the thickness of the hair cell membrane is about 10^{-6} cm, the diameter of the hairs is about 10^{-5} cm, and the thickness of the basilar membrane itself is about 10^{-4} cm. Thus, as is emphasized by Lawrence (1965), around threshold the basilar membrane is supposed to vibrate at an amplitude that is 10^7 times less than the thickness of this vibrating membrane. Similarly if one assumes that the vibratory amplitude of the membrane is transferred to the hairs then these hairs are bent with amplitudes of 10^6 times less than their diameter. Considering these inordinate discrepancies one must wonder about the adequacy of the mechanical stimulation provided by the movements of either the basilar membrane or the stereocilia. Three possible considerations can be advanced. First, it might not be legitimate to extrapolate vibratory amplitudes from high-level measures to low-level measures. That is, assuming that von Békésy's figure of 10^{-3} cm at 10^3 dynes/cm^2 pressure is correct it might not be appropriate to assume that 134 dB below this pressure (at threshold) the amplitude is also 134 dB less. If the amplitude versus pressure characteristic of the basilar membrane is highly nonlinear then it is conceivable that a tenfold decrease in pressure produces a much less than tenfold diminution of amplitude. There is some tentative experimental evidence that this might be the case (Rhode, 1971). If the linear extrapolation is inappropriate then of course it is conceivable that structural displacements of various organ of Corti components can occur at threshold which are commensurate with the size of these structures.

If the linear extrapolation is appropriate then in order to rescue the classical theories one must bring in statistical concepts (Davis, 1965) according to which, although the vibratory amplitudes at threshold are subatomic, the concepts of statistical mechanics should nevertheless prevail. While this suggestion is attractive, it should be examined quantitatively to prove or disprove its feasibility. We shall return to this issue in connection with the discussion of the two classical theories, those of Wever and Davis. The third possibility is to abandon the classical theories in which actual mechanical movements of the basilar membrane or the stereocilia are assumed to mediate the electrical response and bring in molecular mechanisms of excitation. Most of the newer theories aim to do just this.

All of the theories to be reviewed below assume that the hair cells are primarily responsible for the production of CM. Some of them consider the hair cell itself more self-sufficient in generating the ac potentials than do others, but all asign a great degree of importance to these structures. Let us consider the evidence indicating that the hair cells are indeed responsible for at least a major share of the CM produced in the cochlea.

Following its discovery the CM was ascribed to just about every structure within the cochlea. Howe and Guild (1933) and Davis *et al.* (1934) first suggested the hair cells as the most likely source. This view eventually became widely accepted, even though it is now clear that practically any vibrating living tissue is capable of producing microphonic-like potentials. Probably the best approach in treating cochlear microphonics is to follow the suggestion of von Békésy (1952) and consider primary and secondary microphonics. The primary potential, which in the living animal largely dominates the response, can be shown to originate in hair cells. This we shall prove below. The secondary microphonic, much smaller than the primary, can be easily discerned only if the dominant primary is artificially reduced. The secondary microphonic could originate at various points within the cochlea.

Von Békésy (1952) sought the origin of the first-order CM by attempting to identify it with either Reissner's membrane or the basilar membrane–organ of Corti complex. He concluded that, while Reissner's membrane is responsible for the production of a small fraction of the total CM, the major potential is generated in the basilar membrane–organ of Corti structure. A further important observation was that upon death of the animal the first-order CM decreased much more rapidly than the second-order CM. As a consequence, some time after death the CM produced in Reissner's membrane became comparable in size with the diminishing first-order microphonic.

Other experiments aimed at determining the site of CM origin were carried out in 1954 by Tasaki *et al.* They utilized microelectrodes in penetrating the various structures within the cochlea and for measuring both dc and ac potential changes. Their now-classic results can be summarized with the aid of Fig. 5.21. In the figure both ac (left side) and dc (right side) potentials

Microphonics   dc Potential
                          0   +50 mV

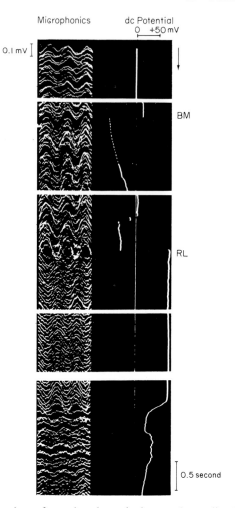

Fig. 5.21. Penetration of a microelectrode into scala media through the basilar membrane. The dc potential and the CM responses to a 500-Hz tone were recorded between the micropipette and a scala vestibuli reference electrode. Penetration sequence is from top to bottom; BM indicates the time at which a large negative potential was first encountered, and RL the moment when the CM phase and the dc polarity simultaneously reversed. In the lowest portion of the picture the withdrawal of the electrode is depicted. (From Tasaki *et al.*, 1954, p. 767.)

are shown in successive time instants as the recording pipette was slowly advanced from scala tympani, through basilar membrane and organ of Corti, and through reticular lamina, scala media, Reissner's membrane, and scala vestibuli. At all boundaries significant changes were noted. First, in ST the dc potential was zero (reference) and the CM relatively small.

As the basilar membrane and the organ of Corti were pierced, irregular negative dc shifts (organ of Corti negativity) were accompanied by an increase in CM. The phase of the CM was the same as in the perilymph. At the instant when the large positive dc potential (EP) appeared the CM reversed its phase. This presumably occurred when the electrode passed through the reticular lamina.* Concomitant with the phase reversal, the CM became much larger and stayed as such as long as the positive EP was encountered. When Reissner's membrane was penetrated the EP disappeared, and the CM was reduced, but its phase remained the same as it was within the scala media. These results strongly suggested to Tasaki *et al.* that the source of the CM is at the hair-bearing ends of the hair cells, i.e., in the region of the reticular lamina.

Let us emphasize again that both Békésy's and Tasaki and colleagues' experiments point to the upper surface of the organ of Corti as the region where the primary CM originates. There is general agreement among present-day students of cochlear physiology that this is indeed the place where CM production is controlled. We are still not quite certain about the site of secondary CM production. Reissner's membrane is certainly involved, but probably not exclusively. The problem of secondary CM, or CM_2, or anaerobic CM, is an interesting one. It can be studied to the best advantage in anoxic or dying animals. It has been known from the earliest days of investigations of CM that upon death the CM first rapidly declines, and then its diminution becomes very gradual so that some response can still be obtained several hours after the animal's death (Davis *et al.*, 1934; Wever *et al.*, 1941). Figure 5.22 shows the time course of the diminution of CM upon the death of the experimental animal. Note that when the heart stops the CM abruptly drops to about 12 dB below its normal value. From this level further decline takes place but at a lesser rate. Several hours after death the CM still persists, but it is only a small fraction of its normal value. Because of the highly dissimilar rates of decline during the first few seconds after death and during later periods, the notion of two different kinds of CM has been accepted (Riesco-MacClure *et al.*, 1949; Davis, 1957). Accordingly, the first, and dominant, type of CM is vitally dependent on adequate oxygen supply. This aerobic microphonic is commonly denoted by CM_1. It would then be CM_1 that declines rapidly upon cessation of heart activity. The second type of CM would not be strongly oxygen dependent, and this anaerobic CM_2 is what one sees persisting after death. In a normal preparation CM_1 and CM_2 presumably coexist and what one records is essentially the resultant of the two potentials. This resultant is hardly distinguishable from CM_1, for

---

* The reader will recall that there is presently some controversy over this matter of whether the critical surface is the reticular lamina or the tectorial membrane. We discussed this issue at some length before.

this potential is of much greater magnitude than CM_2. The "non-oxygen-dependent" CM_2 might arise from completely different source or sources than CM_1. Electrical activity similar to CM can be generated by many biological systems. Thus it is quite possible that CM_1 is the normal primary response of the auditory sense organ, while CM_2 is an incidental response originating in the cochlea in any of a number of ways. It is also possible, however, that CM_1 and CM_2 are generated in the same structure but that, while CM_1 reflects high-level, normal activity, CM_2 is merely a remnant which can be maintained for a long time (Wing as quoted by Davis, 1957). This argument is not at all resolved, although it is more parsimonious not to assume the presence of two different processes in the generation of CM.

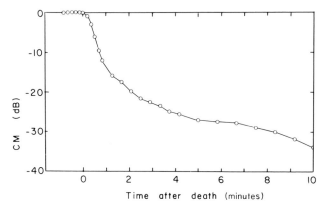

Fig. 5.22. Decrease of CM after death. Zero decibel corresponds to $450\,\mu V$. Recording is with differential electrodes from turn 1 of one guinea pig. The $450\text{-}\mu V$ level corresponds to the maximum of the linear range of the CM in this case.

Let us now return to the primary CM, which is produced in the organ of Corti. There is a great body of literature supporting the notion that the primary CM is intimately tied in with the presence of functioning hair cells within the organ. The early observations were made on animals that are congenitally lacking in hair cells, such as albinotic cats and waltzing guinea pigs (Howe and Guild, 1933; Davis et al., 1934; Lurie et al., 1934). All these observations indicated that, wherever the hair cells were degenerated, no CM could be recorded. Subsequently a voluminous literature was generated on the correlation between the presence of CM and a healthy hair cell population. This literature deals with damage to hair cells due to noise exposure, various surgical traumas, and metabolic and other poisoning agents. We will not even attempt to skim this literature. Suffice it to say that there is a very direct relationship between the integrity of the hair cells and the cochlea's ability to produce CM (Davis, 1957; Wever, 1966). There is one study along these lines, however, that should be specifically mentioned. This is the experiment of Davis *et al.* (1958b) in which they carried out an extensive correlated study of cochlear damage induced by streptomycin poisoning and by venous occlusion, and cochlear potential production. For our present purposes the important observation that grew out of this study was that the primary CM is best correlated with the integrity of the external hair cells. The evaluation of the hair cells was based on light micro-scopy. There were some very clear cases of complete degeneration of the hair cells in the region of the (differential) recording electrodes. In these cases the maximal CM recorded was of the order of 3 μV! In those cases where the inner hair cells were normal but the outer hair cells sustained severe damage the CM was reduced. It can be computed from their data that, in the eight animals where a relatively good inner hair cell population remained while the external hair cells were severely degenerated, the CM sensitivity was reduced on the average by 19.5 dB. In the same animals the maximal CM produced declined on the average from the 800 μV normal value to 136 μV. These results tend to indicate that the outer hair cells are strongly, but probably not exclusively, involved with CM production.

Some of our work (Dallos and Bredberg, 1970) is also pertinent to the discussion concerning the relative roles of outer and inner hair cells in CM production. In guinea pigs exposed to intense, low-frequency sounds for prolonged durations very characteristic and pronounced outer hair cell damage can be produced. A fine example of a cochleogram from this population of animals is shown in the insert of Fig. 5.23. The cochleogram is simply a graphical representation of the integrity of hair cells in the cochlea. The percentage of intact cells is shown as the function of distance along the basilar membrane; the inner hair cells and the three rows of outer hair cells are graphed separately. The hair cell population is determined by examining flat surface preparations of the organ of Corti (Engström *et al.*, 1966) under the phase-contrast microscope and by counting cells. The method is not sensitive to subtle morphological changes within remaining cells; it can merely describe whether a cell is present. Consequently, one must keep in mind that, while a cell might be present, it could have sustained significant structural alterations (Bredberg *et al.*, 1970) and thus it might not function in a normal manner. In the following discussion we shall assume that if a cell is present it is functional, although the reader should keep in mind that this might be an oversimplification.

The pattern of cell damage seen in Fig. 5.23 lends itself to the study of differences between the two major populations. Recordings of CM were made with differential electrodes placed in both first and third turns. The first-turn electrodes produced virtually normal high-frequency CM in all the animals that had the damage pattern illustrated in Fig. 5.23. In some animals with more extensive damage, including inner hair cell loss, and outer hair cell destruction down to the stapes region, high-frequency CM loss was also observed. In the animals that do not fall under this latter category, and that are included in the graph of Fig. 5.23, a clear correlation exists between low-frequency CM loss and the distance between the electrodes and the boundary of the outer hair cell lesion. It appears that, when the lesion invades the basal region as far as the electrodes are, the CM sensitivity shift approaches 35 dB. Note that this decrease in sensitivity occurs when the

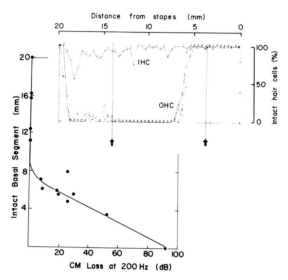

Fig. 5.23. Functional relationship between the shift of the CM pseudothreshold (SPL at 1-μV CM) at 200 Hz for individual animals compared with the median normal value and the extent of intact basal hair cell population. The lesion in the abnormal guinea pigs was created by prolonged exposure to intense low-frequency sound. The cochleogram of an animal that shows a nearly ideal lesion is included. The ordinate in the cochleogram is percent intact hair cells, and the abscissa is distance from the base. Inner hair cells (IHC) are denoted by 0, the three rows of outer hair cells (OHC) by 1, 2, and 3 respectively. The location of the recording electrode pairs is indicated by the arrows. The data shown are obtained from the basal pair. (Cochleogram courtesy of G. Bredberg.)

entire inner hair cell population is apparently normal and when the outer hair cells are likewise normal basal from the electrodes. The normalcy of the high-frequency CM seems to assure that the remaining outer hair cells are functioning in all these cases. Thus there appears to be a strong indication that the CM sensitivity is determined primarily by the outer hair cells and that highly significant losses can be expected without this cell group. The maxima of the input–output functions at the test frequency (200 Hz) were also reduced, but the reduction was slightly but systematically less than that seen for the sensitivity measure. The CM measures from the third-turn electrode location indicate very significant loss of sensitivity. Three animals showed very severe outer hair cell damage in the third turn of the cochlea, coupled with good inner hair cell population and acceptable electrode placement. In these animals the sensitivity of the third-turn differential electrode is reduced by about 50 dB. Thus one can surmise that the change in sensitivity with the virtual absence of outer hair cell population and in the presence of most inner hair cells is of the order of 50 dB.

It is seen on the basis of the above considerations that the production of CM in the cochlea is correlated primarily with the outer hair cells. This contention is of course predicated on the assumption that the inner hair cells that were present in our animals did actually function normally. Only electron microscope examination can suggest that this was indeed the case, and consequently a definitive statement must await such results.*

Now that the hair cells are established as the sources of CM, it is necessary to inquire about the type of stimulation that is appropriate and adequate in exciting these structures to produce the ac potentials. On this issue, as on many others in cochlear processes, we must turn to some of von Békésy's (1951) observations for answers. Von Békésy developed microtechniques for the simultaneous stimulation of and recording from the cochlear partition. He utilized a vibrating electrode that could be used to impart movements on the partition in any direction and simultaneously pick up the electrical response. His first inquiry concerned the problem of whether it is displacement or some time derivative of the displacement of the cochlear partition that is the appropriate stimulus for the production of microphonics. He imparted a trapezoidal time–displacement pattern on his vibrating electrode (Fig. 5.24a) and noted that depending on whether the adequate stimulus is displacement, velocity, or a combination of both one would expect to see very easily discernible response patterns. These patterns are also shown in Fig. 5.24a. When performing the actual experiment, von Békésy noted the waveforms that are given as oscillograms in Fig. 5.24b. It is quite obvious that the response to the trapezoidal displacement pattern of the cochlear partition is a trapezoidal CM potential. Thus the conclusion is inescapable that membrane displacement and not some derivative thereof is the adequate stimulus in CM production. This is a very significant result. Von Békésy then determined which direction of displacement is most advantageous in producing electrical responses. He stimulated displacements in radial, longitudinal, and vertical directions with respect to the basilar membrane

---

* The recent measurements of CM by Wang (1971) from kanamycin-intoxicated cochleae indicate that the sensitivity difference between inner and outer hair cells might not be as pronounced as the discussion above would imply. His data show a sensitivity difference of the order of 35 dB.

to that organ, while the microphonic potentials are not, it is reasonable not to depend on the accessory structures in any theory that purports to explain the CM generation. Instead, as Wever emphasizes, the source of CM should be sought in the hair cell alone.

Wever makes an analogy between hair cells and giant plant cells. The latter are known (Osterhout and Hill, 1931) to produce large electrical responses when mechanically deformed. Normally such cells are negatively polarized in the inside with respect to the surrounding fluid. When a cell is deformed, the apparent positive polarization of the outside of the cell membrane decreases, and large negative-going potentials are observed. In Wever's conception the hair cell of the cochlea is firmly anchored by the cups of Deiters' cells on the bottom and by the reticular membrane at the top. Between these two supports the cell is relatively free. As the basilar membrane moves up and down this motion is transferred to the bottoms of the hair cells by the up and down thrusts of the rigid Deiters' processes. The result is an outward and inward bulging of the cell walls. Note that in this scheme the hairs are assumed to provide anchorage of the upper surface of the cell; that is, when the bottom of the cell is pushed up the rigid hairs hold the top of the cell down and thus the sides of the cell bulge out. It is assumed that the deformation of the wall alters the surface charge. Such alteration is of opposite sign for up and down movement and thus a vibratory motion would generate an alternating change in surface charge concentration. Wever argues against these changes taking place as actual ion movements through the cell membrane. He feels that it would be hard to reconcile the necessarily extremely fast ion movements at high frequencies with the cell's ability to rapidly regenerate its altered ion concentration. Instead he proposes that the ions are bound to the cell membrane, and during membrane deformation only the static field changes.

  b. Davis' (1956, 1958, 1965) *Battery Theory.* We have already alluded to this theory to some extent at various places in this chapter. In this section a brief outline following one of Davis' latest discussions of the subject is given (1965), and then some additional considerations are presented. As early as 1937 Hallpike and Rawdon-Smith and later von Békésy (1952) conjectured that the production of CM in the cochlea could be explained if it could be demonstrated that there is a resting energy pool present that can drive current through some variable resistance. Von Békésy's discovery of the EP provided the required energy pool. Davis formulated the complete theory in what is now known as the "battery theory" or "resistance-modulation hypothesis."

It is assumed that two biological batteries, essentially in a serial arrangement, create a steady current flow across the organ of Corti. These batteries are the endocochlear potential in the stria vascularis and the intracellular polarization of hair cells. The current* driven by these batteries flows through the hair cells. It is assumed that, as sound stimulation sets the basilar membrane in motion, the relative movement of the basilar and tectorial membranes causes the stiff short hairs to bend. The hairs act as microlevers; they probably do not really bend but instead exert lateral pressure on the top of the hair cells (Hawkins, 1965). The region of the top of the hair cell which might be the likely site of ion transfer (i.e., current flow) between endolymph and the interior of the hair cell is the small area of plasma membrane surrounding the basal body (Hawkins, 1965) or that which is substituted in place of the basal body in those species in which the latter disappears during development (Spoendlin, 1966). The basal body (Flock *et al.*, 1962; Engström *et al.*, 1962) fits into a round opening of $1.5\text{-}\mu$ diameter in the cuticular plate. It is then assumed that the graded lateral deformation of the top of the hair cell, brought about by the force exerted by the hairs, changes the electric resistance of the region of the basal body. Since the hair cells are in the path of current flow, a change in resistance is coupled with an inherent change in total current. In this scheme current flow is the critical variable. Microphonic potentials are merely a manifestation of this changing current flow; voltage drops due to this current on a given resistance. Because of the asymmetry of the arrangement of hairs on the upper surface of the hair cells, it is natural to assume that deformation of that surface by the hairs in opposite directions would cause opposite changes in resistance, i.e., increase or decrease about a resting value. Clearly then to and fro bending of the hairs can give rise to resistance changes around a normal (no stimulus) value, and the consequence is the production of a modulation of the resting current, which modulation is of course reflected in the measured CM. The scheme can naturally provide for the generation of SP also; the only requirement is a one-way bending component of the hairs.

The extremely small size of movements that ought to provide adequate mechanical deformation in the vicinity of threshold is somewhat troublesome. The amplitude of vibration of the basilar membrane appears to be around 10^{-11} cm at threshold (if linear extrapolation of von Békésy's high-intensity measurements is utilized), while the thickness of the hairs that are supposed to work as levers at that amplitude is 10^{-5} cm. As we have seen the opening in the cuticular plate is about 1.5×10^{-4} cm, and even the diameter of a membrane pore is of the order of 3×10^{-8} cm. Opponents of the classical theories are fond of emphasizing these enormous discrepancies, and admittedly it is hard to visualize how a hair can be moved or bent with an amplitude that is a million times less than its diameter when such movements are clearly on a subatomic scale. Davis invokes statistical concepts, namely, that while the motion of any hair is indeed subatomic there are many hairs stimulated,

* The current is likely to be a K^+ current, flowing from endolymph into the hair cells.

and thus some average effect might occur. He quotes a study by Miller *et al.* (1964) in which the electrical output of a condenser microphone was detected at pressure levels corresponding to the human hearing threshold. The analogy is provocative, for the diaphragm of the microphone at that pressure does move with amplitudes that are subatomic and clearly much smaller than the thickness of the microphone diaphragm. We do not have a generally accepted, clear-cut theoretical structure that reconciles the difficulties of extremely small movements with effective stimulation. Nevertheless we must keep in mind that the proposed scheme can operate in a number of modes, such as (a) linear hair cell transducer coupled with nonlinear basilar membrane mechanics, (b) linear basilar membrane mechanics coupled with nonlinear transducer, (c) linear operation enhanced by statistical effects, and (d) nonlinear operation enhanced by statistical effects. Actually any of these schemes could reconcile the difficulties. It is worthwhile to examine the scheme of resistance modulation in detail with the aid of simplified circuit analysis and to present some experimental data directly relevant to this scheme.

In Fig. 5.25 a schematic cross section of a cochlear scala is shown overlaid with its electrical equivalent circuit. The three points M, V, and T signify electrode locations in scalae media, vestibuli, and tympani where potential

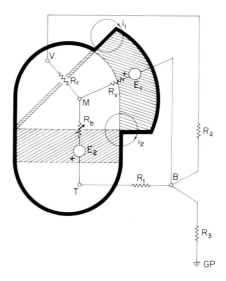

Fig. 5.25. Schematic of the cochlear circuit. Points V, T, and M indicate the recording locations in the three scalae, B is the node corresponding to the blood vessels, and GP denotes the animal ground. The symbols E_1 and E_2 represent dc potential sources corresponding to the stria vascularis source and the intracellular negative polarization respectively. The organ of Corti resistance R_b, is assumed to be the only variable quantity. Kirchoff's equations are set up in terms of the circulating currents i_1 and i_2.

measurements can be made. The two voltage sources correspond to the endocochlear potential originating in the stria vascularis (E_1) and the intracellular hair cell negativity (E_2). The resistors R_r, R_v, and R_b denote the membrane resistances associated with Reissner's membrane, the wall of the stria, and the basilar membrane. Actually, the latter, R_b, is the effective resistance of the cuticular plate of the hair cells, and it is assumed to be a variable. The resistances R_1 and R_2 signify connecting resistances to the blood supply, and finally R_3 is the resistance from the latter to an area in the animal's body where any reference electrode would be located during electrical measurements. This scheme corresponds to that treated quantitatively by Johnstone *et al.* (1966). We shall use their numerical values wherever appropriate and shall also discuss their considerations of this circuit in Section IV. This circuit should be construed as the *overall* electrical representation of the cochlea as seen by measuring electrodes introduced into the scalae at points *M*, *V*, and *T*. In other words, this is not an incremental circuit for one hair cell or for one narrow segment of the cochlea. Such incremental circuits could be constructed with topological features similar to those of the one shown, but interconnections would need to be supplied to adjacent and far circuit elements also. In addition the values for the circuit elements would be different in an incremental circuit.

Our immediate interest is to compute the potential variation at points *V*, *M*, and *T* when R_b changes. Specifically let us assume that $R_b = R_0 + R \cos \omega t$, where R_0 is the resting value of the basilar membrane resistance and R is the magnitude of the resistance change, which is of course dependent on the displacement magnitude of the membrane and thus on stimulus strength. Note that we are dealing with a purely resistive circuit. This is clearly an oversimplification, for significant capacitive effects due to the various membranes might be expected to influence the behavior of the circuit, especially at higher frequencies. For the time being, however, our only interest is to demonstrate the relationship between potentials in the various scalae and resistance variation; consequently it is unnecessary to complicate the derivation with reactive components.

One can write two Kirchoff equations for this simple circuit in terms of circulating currents i_1 and i_2:

$$i_1(R_r + R_v + R_2) - i_2 R_v = -E_1$$
$$-i_1 R_v + i_2(R_b + R_v + R_1) = E_1 + E_2 \tag{5.2}$$

The system determinant D and the determinants for i_1 and i_2 can be written as

$$D = (R_r + R_v + R_2)(R_0 + R_v + R_1) - R_v{}^2 + (R_r + R_v + R_2)R \cos \omega t$$
$$D_{i_1} = -E_1(R_0 + R_v + R_1) + (E_1 + E_2)R_v - E_1 R \cos \omega t$$
$$D_{i_2} = (R_r + R_v + R_2)(E_1 + E_2) - E_1 R_v \tag{5.3}$$

The circulating currents then can be written as $i_1 = D_{i_1}/D$ and $i_2 = D_{i_2}/D$. Furthermore, the voltages at points V, M, and T can be expressed with the aid of i_1 and i_2 as follows:

$$E_V = -i_1 R_2 \qquad E_M = -i_1(R_r + R_2) \qquad E_T = -i_2 R_1 \qquad (5.4)$$

After substitution and some simplification we obtain

$$E_V = \frac{E_1(R_0 + R_1) - E_2 R_v + E_1 R \cos \omega t}{(R_r + R_v + R_2)(R_0 + R_v + R_1) - R_v^2 + (R_r + R_v + R_2)R \cos \omega t} R_2$$

$$E_M = \frac{E_1(R_0 + R_1) - E_2 R_v + E_1 R \cos \omega t}{(R_r + R_v + R_2)(R_0 + R_v + R_1) - R_v^2 + (R_r + R_v + R_2)R \cos \omega t} (R_r + R_2)$$

$$E_T = \frac{E_1(R_r + R_2) + E_2(R_r + R_v + R_2)}{(R_r + R_v + R_2)(R_0 + R_v + R_1) - R_v^2 + (R_r + R_v + R_2)R \cos \omega t} R_1 \qquad (5.5)$$

Probably the most advantageous method of proceeding is to substitute some numerical values that are reasonable approximations for the actual overall resistances in the cochlea. We can borrow such values from the work of Johnstone et al. (1966), who obtained them by actual measurement. Accordingly, $R_r = 46$ kΩ, $R_0 = 24$ kΩ, $R_v = 13$ kΩ, $R_1 = 1.8$ kΩ, $R_2 = 2.4$ kΩ, and $R_3 = 4.7$ kΩ. These values are rounded. For the voltage source E_2 that represents the common intracellular polarization, a value of 70 mV is assumed. We know that the EP is usually measured as 70 mV; this value should be equivalent to E_M with $R = 0$. If one substitutes all numerical values into the expression for E_M then the magnitude of the second voltage source E_1 can be readily computed. The result of such computation yields $E_1 = 160$ mV. Thus the stria vascularis voltage source, which is commonly said to have a value of approximately $+70$ mV, is seen to be more properly considered as a source with a voltage of $+160$ mV. The $+70$ mV is that which is measured in the scala media as the result of voltage drops in the cochlear circuit; this voltage drop is what was designated as endocochlear potential, or EP. We have values now for all circuit elements and after substitution the following three expressions can be obtained for the three voltages, E_V, E_M, and E_T.

$$E_V = \frac{7.723 + 0.384R \cos \omega t}{2213.3 + 61.4R \cos \omega t}$$

$$E_M = \frac{155.232 + 7.718R \cos \omega t}{2213.3 + 61.4R \cos \omega t}$$

$$E_T = \frac{21.6756}{2213.3 + 61.4R \cos \omega t} \qquad (5.6)$$

These expressions provide the three resting voltage values, with the $R = 0$ substitution, of $E_V = +3.49$ mV, $E_T = +9.8$ mV, and of course $E_M = +70$ mV.

Let us compute the values of E_V, E_M, and E_T as the functions of $R \cos \omega t$; in other words, let us inquire how the voltages in the three scalae change with the variation of the basilar membrane resistance. The computations are carried out in the range $-10 < R \cos \omega t > +10$. Johnstone *et al.* (1966) found that the change in R_b was approximately 2.2kΩ in respect to a 5000-Hz tone pip at 95 dB SPL. Consequently a $\pm$ 10-kΩ change provides a reasonable range for computation. The computations are tedious but straightforward. The results are shown in Fig. 5.26, where the *change* in the three potentials is plotted as the function of the change in resistance (i.e., $R \cos \omega t$). The

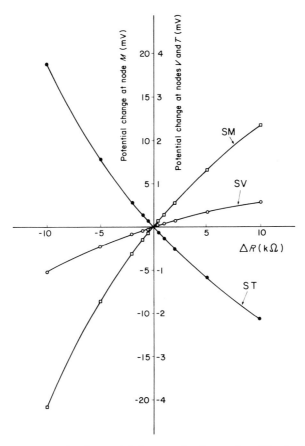

Fig. 5.26. Magnitude of potential change at the three nodes of the circuit of Figure 5.25 as a function of the change in the resistance R_b.

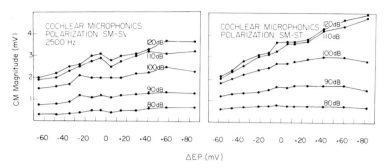

Fig. 5.28. Graphic representation of the cochlear microphonics produced by a 2500-Hz stimulus at different SPL's and at different levels of polarization. The current was passed between scala media and scala vestibuli (left), or scala media and scala tympani (right). The abscissa indicates the change in EP and the ordinate the magnitude of the CM. (From Honrubia and Ward, 1969b, p. 390.)

to zero) they would have needed such high polarizing currents that it would have destroyed the normal functioning of the cochlea due to electrolysis. Consequently Honrubia and Ward employed a clever trick. It is known (von Békésy, 1952; Konishi *et al.*, 1961) that during asphyxia the EP naturally reverses polarity. It achieves a value of approximately − 20 mV about 5 minutes after the commencement of oxygen deprivation. It is also known that, while the negative organ of Corti potential is concurrently reduced during asphyxia, its reduction is at a much slower rate (Butler, 1965). As a result of these changes the dc potential difference across the reticular lamina is significantly reduced during asphyxia. This reduction is great enough that if assisted by moderate polarization the gradient can be reversed. This is exactly what Honrubia and Ward did. Their pertinent results are shown in Fig. 5.29. Here polarization began 45 minutes after asphyxia when the EP was − 17 mV; this is the first point on the graph. Further changes in EP, due to polarizing currents, are shown on the abscissa, while the ordinate shows the CM magnitude. The inserts are the actual CM waveforms. The crucial finding is that when the EP was changed to − 53 mV the CM disappeared. In addition, as the EP was made more negative, the CM started to increase again but it *reversed its phase*. These findings strongly support the hypothesis that CM is generated by the modulation of resting current through the organ of Corti.*

c. Dohlman's (1960) *Molecular Theory.* This theory is based partially on the observations of Vilstrup and Jensen (1961) that endolymph contains

---

* It is of course well to remember that these experiments were actually done on the anaerobic CM, or CM_2. While they are indicative of the mechanism of CM_1 production as well, they do not constitute a complete proof that this normally dominant component is also generated by the resistance-modulation process.

been the
many pr
concerns
tion. The
did exte
SP, over
Ward, 1
culmina

App;
nonuniti
is proba
logical s
two cor
summat
Davis *e*
electric;
ted acti
They n
or-none
It was r
in the o
In 1952
of thre
They s
resistar
the twc
either
generat
but un
It is al
with va
versus
and in
contai
tions c
matior
the SF

In
of wh
merely

    * T

scala t

pas
(su
Bé
for
du
rel
to
ne
his
the
ac
cu
dis
to
an
tia
ex
vc

th
ac
at
in
m
lil
is
p
ga
w
fr
b
e
tl
p
r

a
a
c
c
t

hyaluronic acid, and on those of Jensen *et al.* (1954) that upon displacement
of a fluid containing hyaluranate solutions electric potentials can be produced.
Hyaluronic acid is a mucopolysaccharide, a long negatively charged molecule
which, as demonstrated by Dohlman, is present in the endolymph around
and in the cupular structures. Dohlman assumes that the cupula of the
semicircular canals as well as the tectorial membrane of the cochlea are
highly similar structures. Moreover, he asserts that all such cupular structures
make intimate contact with the top plate of the ciliated epithelium and that
the cilia are essentially embedded in fine canals in the cupular substance.
He considers the apparent separation of cupula and tectorial membrane
from the underlying structures as fixation artifacts. Thus the hairs are
presumed to lie in canals of the superstructure, and it is further assumed that
mucopolysaccharide molecules adhere to the walls of the canals and also to
the surface of the hairs. Relative movement of these long charged molecules
originating either in fluid displacement or in the relative displacement of the
cupular structure and the hairs would create relative movement of the negatively charged molecular chains and the positive potassium ions of the endolymph. Such movement results in "displacement potentials," as was shown
by Jensen *et al.* (1954). The polarity of this potential depends on the direction

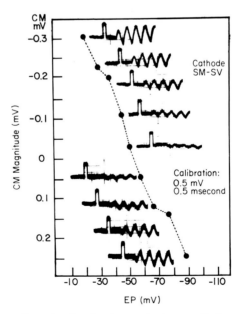

Fig. 5.29. Recordings showing the changes in the magnitude and polarity of CM produced by cathodal polarization of the scala media of an anoxic guinea pig. (From Honrubia
and Ward, 1969b, p. 391.)

292

pic
ric
ga
sei
thi
to
"t
cr'
tec
Su
co
de
in
th;
to
pr'
Cl
m'

m'
by
ap
tia
m'
pr'
m'
as
po
th'
be
th'
sm
sta
po

B.

1.

de
Dι

the fundamental CM component, and even more so compared to higher harmonic components in CM, made the acceptance of the straightforward distortion hypothesis tenuous. In order to deal with this difficulty these authors postulated their mechanism of phase cancellation, which we have already discussed in detail. In this scheme, it is remembered, since the CM voltages sum vectorially at the electrode location, high-frequency responses suffer an apparent diminution due to cancellations among out-of-phase generators. Such cancellation of course does not affect the SP. Thus it is conceivable that the apparent size of the distortion component (SP) might be observed as being bigger than the distorted signal (CM) from which the former is derived in the process of nonlinear distortion. This ingenious argument certainly makes it possible to accept the distortion hypothesis for the genesis of SP.

The distortion hypothesis was further espoused by Johnstone and Johnstone (1966) and by Engebretson and Eldredge (1968). The former authors derived a mathematical model for the generation of the SP. They showed that sinusoidal motion of the basilar membrane would always yield asymmetrical displacement of the cilia and thus the means of producing SP. Another contribution was made by the latter authors, who studied simple electrical models and demonstrated that a number of nonlinear electrical phenomena that are known to exist in the cochlea (SP, combination tone production, and the interference effect) can be accounted for by the same nonlinearity. Engebretson and Eldredge also emphasize, which we believe is a key point, that several nonlinear processes probably coexist in the cochlea, and these processes can account for the various (hard to reconcile with a single source hypothesis) properties of the SP. Kupperman (1966, 1970) further elaborated on the nonunitary nature of SP. He recorded from the scala tympani of all four turns of the guinea pig cochlea and focused his attention on the interaction between, and the nature of, the positive and negative SP. He demonstrated that the positive SP recorded from scala tympani shows strong localization to the site of maximum excitation. This potential is regarded by Kupperman as a manifestation of current flow between scalae media and tympani in the region of maximum stimulation. He regards the negative SP in the scala tympani as a sign of summated asynchronous neural potentials.

Davis, the discoverer of SP, now regards it ". . . as an incidental byproduct arising from asymmetry in the mechanism that produces cochlear microphonic rather than as a major physiological mechanism" (Davis, 1968, p. 652). Others are not so pessimistic about the possible function and significance of the SP. Honrubia and Ward (1969a) have completed a significant parametric study of the SP, and they surmise that the negative SP is likely to act as a stimulus to the 8th nerve while the positive SP is probably inhibitory. These authors recorded SP with fine pipettes from the scala media in all four turns of the guinea pig cochlea. They varied signal intensity, frequency, and duration. It was found that SP magnitude increased linearly with log duration. The authors provided a number of plots giving the longitudinal distribution of SP as the function of stimulus duration and intensity. The familiar relationship again emerged that in the region of maximum stimulation the SP is negative. It was noted that the maximum SP⁻ remained at the same point at all intensities, in contrast with the usually observed basal shift of CM maxima. In all turns the SP was elicited by tones whose frequency was considerably below that favorable to the electrode location, the SP started out positive, went through a maximum with increased sound intensity, decreased toward zero, and finally turned negative at very high intensities. Frequencies that were favorable to the electrode location elicited negative SP's, even at relatively low intensities. One of the major limitations of this study is that for technical reasons no data were obtained at low sound intensities.

b. The Dependence of SP on Stimulus Parameters.* With the previous review in mind we can now proceed to a more complete description of the properties of the summating potential. It should be kept in mind that the SP is extremely sensitive to the parameters of the eliciting stimulus and to the recording site, and, with relatively minor alterations in these, its characteristics can change rather drastically. First we shall explore the spatial distribution patterns of the SP in the two perilymphatic scalae and then these will be contrasted with that in the scala media.

The characteristics of the SP when recorded from scala vestibuli (SV) and scala tympani (ST) can be expressed four ways. One can simply record the potentials from SV and ST with an indifferent electrode as the reference and talk about the distribution pattern of SP as obtained from such recordings. The other two possibilities arise when the ST and SV potentials are combined to yield $DIF = SV - ST$ or $AVE = (SV + ST)/2$. We became acquainted with the meaning of these combinations in Chapter 2. We also saw the limitations inherent in utilizing such techniques, including the possibility of obtaining false registrations if either local or remote potential components overdominate the response and if the recording conditions are not highly symmetrical. We also noted, however, that such recording techniques can be highly informative if appropriately handled, and they do provide more information than recordings with a single electrode. It is remembered that the combining of the ST and SV responses comprises the classical differential-electrode recording method (Tasaki *et al.*, 1952) that was invented to minimize either CM (AVE) or AP (DIF).

For our purposes the potentials DIF and AVE are construed as follows.

* Based on Dallos *et al.* (1972).

The DIF potential is proportional to the potential difference across the cochlear partition, and to a good approximation this quantity describes the *locally generated voltage*, that is, one whose source is located between the electrode tips. The AVE response is proportional to the *common potential* of the two scalae. Ordinarily this response is associated with remote activity but, aside from this, we tend to look at this potential as either being proportional to a voltage drop created by longitudinal current flow, which is in the same direction in both scalae vestibuli and tympani, or one that reflects the asymmetry of cochlear electroanatomy, or both. Both operations, $DIF = SV - ST$ and $AVE = (SV + ST)/2$, can be and have been performed either electronically during experiment or graphically or arithmetically from the SV and ST data. Either method yields essentially the same result. We shall present data on the pages to follow in both forms: SV and ST or DIF and AVE. When either form is given the other can be obtained by simple computation.

The relative independence of the DIF and AVE components was considered in detail in Chapter 2. It was emphasized that it is difficult to reliably record one of these components if it is small, provided that the other component is very large. We shall see for example that the DIF component recorded from the higher cochlear turns at high frequencies is quite small and does not seem to show a clear pattern of change with signal parameters. At the same time the AVE component is rather large. In this situation the DIF component that one records is probably nothing more than an artifact resulting from imperfect electrode balance. The greater the disparity is between DIF and AVE in a given recording situation, the more reliable the recording is for the larger and the less reliable it is for the smaller component.

Unless otherwise indicated in the discussions that follow the plots depicting SP magnitude as the function of various parameters are median plots. Data points are obtained as the median value of individual data that are available for a given experimental condition. The number of experimental animals that contribute to a given median datum is not the same; fewer points are available at the extremes of the intensity range, for example, and fewer points from the third cochlear turn than from the first. The range of the number of animals whose responses were used for obtaining a given point was between 3 and 19, the majority being between 5 and 7.

Let us first consider the response patterns in the form of input–output functions, that is, SP magnitude versus sound intensity at any given frequency and electrode location. In Fig. 5.30 a set of such functions is shown for basal-turn electrodes; both SV and ST responses are included. The eight pairs of plots depict the variation of SP as the frequency changes from 200 to 10,000 Hz and as the signal intensity changes between 40 and 100 dB sound pressure level. Note that these are log–log plots. The ordinate gives the SP magnitude in microvolts over a ± 80-dB range, while the abscissa is expressed in decibels re 0.0002 dyne/cm^2. At 200 Hz, below 70 dB SPL, *both* SV and ST electrodes register negative potentials. Moreover, below 60 dB they see approximately the same potential magnitude. Above 70 dB the SV potential turns positive, while the ST potential remains negative. Above approximately 80 dB the absolute value of the SV potential exceeds that of the ST potential. If the sound intensity is further increased beyond 100 dB SPL, another polarity reversal can be seen: At approximately 110 dB the ST

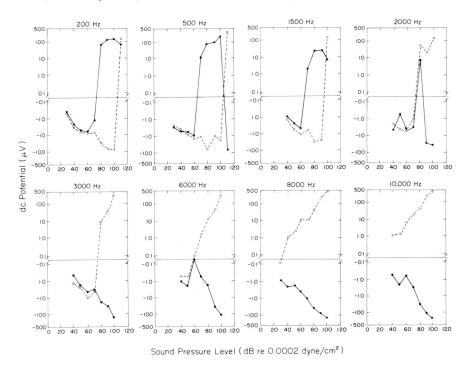

Sound Pressure Level (dB re 0.0002 dyne/cm²)

Fig. 5.30. Median SP input–output functions at various frequencies from scala vestibuli (●) and scala tympani (○) of the first cochlear turn. (From Dallos *et al.*, 1972, p. 15.)

potential goes positive and at even higher SPL's the SV potential would go negative. The picture then would be similar to that seen for 500 Hz. At this frequency the character of the response is quite like that at 200 Hz; at very low SPL's both electrodes see about equal negativity. Around 70 dB the SV electrode becomes positive, but here a second reversal occurs within the depicted range. At approximately 105 dB both scalae reverse their polarity. As stimulus frequency further increases, the pattern seen for 500 Hz undergoes a gradual change into the pattern shown for the 3000-Hz condition.

This change involves the disappearance of the positive hump for the SV electrode, which is now negative at *all* SPL's, and the gradual lowering of the crossover point of the ST potential. Note that here as well as in the following plot (for 6000 Hz) we still see *both* scalae at the approximately identical negative potential level at the lowest intensities. Attention is called to the very consistent slight inflection or reversal in the SV potential plot at approximately 60 dB, which is of course the level at which this scala turned positive at lesser frequencies. The overall pattern seen at 3000 Hz continues at 6000 Hz, the only difference being that the ST crossover occurs at a lower intensity. This process continues as frequency is raised until, as shown in the 8000-Hz plot, the SV is negative while the ST is positive at all intensity levels. The 10,000-Hz plot is almost identical—at least it appears so. Actually there are important albeit subtle differences between them, as will be seen in the DIF and AVE plots of these same data.

The plots of Fig. 5.30 reveal a very consistent and systematic shift in the SP pattern from low to high frequencies and from low to high intensities. The following salient features are worth mentioning. At very high intensities, irrespective of frequency, the basal SV potential is negative, and the basal ST potential is positive. This observation is in harmony with descriptions of the SP in the literature. In fact it is this potential, positive in ST and negative in SV, that is traditionally regarded as the SP^-. It is often said that the SP is positive (i.e., SV is positive re ST) at low intensities. Our plots show that this is correct but not universally. We see the SV-positive–ST-negative combination at the midintensities and only at low frequencies. We further see that, except at the highest frequencies, both scalae of the basal turn are negative at the lowest intensities. This observation is significant on two counts; first, it is a new observation not hitherto noted and, second, it is contrary to the very common assumption in the literature that the polarities of the two scalae are always opposite.

Let us now recast these data into the $DIF = SV - ST$ and the $AVE = (SV + ST)/2$ components. These plots are shown in Fig. 5.31. It is remembered that we identify the DIF component as the local response and the AVE as the common potential of the two scalae. Note first that the AVE pattern is somewhat similar at the lower frequencies. At very high intensities the AVE potential is positive in the base at all frequencies, but at lesser SPL's it turns negative and stays negative. The exceptional frequency is 10,000 Hz, where the average potential of the two scalae is positive at *all* intensities. The DIF plots depict a complete and orderly transition from low to high frequencies. At 200 Hz the local response is positive at all SPL's, while it is negative at all SPL's at the highest frequency tested. In between, a transition takes place in that at high intensities the DIF potential turns negative. This occurs at lower intensities as the frequency increases. It should be noted that even

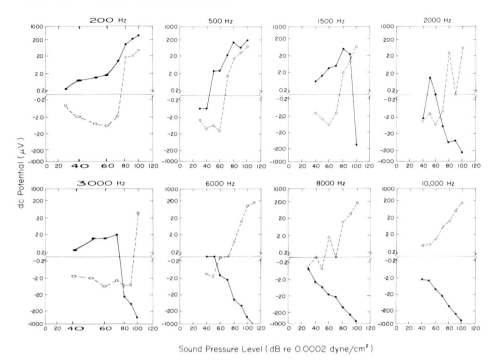

Sound Pressure Level (dB re 0.0002 dyne/cm²)

Fig. 5-31. Median SP input–output functions at various frequencies from the first cochlear turn. Plots are given for the DIF (●) and AVE (○) components. (From Dallos *et al.*, 1972, p. 16.)

at 200 Hz if we had shown the situation at much higher SPL's the DIF response would have been negative. This transition at 200 Hz would have occurred at approximately 110 dB (at higher intensities for lower frequencies). One can summarize by saying that the local potential (DIF response) is negative at *all* frequencies if the intensity is high enough. This negativity is seen at lesser and lesser intensities with the increase in frequency. The local response stays negative at all intensities at high frequencies, but it turns positive at lower frequencies and at lower intensities. This low-level positivity and high-level negativity corresponds to the traditionally expressed SP⁺ and SP⁻. Some important new observations arise from the data shown in Fig. 5.31. These observations involve primarily the AVE potential that has not been paid any attention in the literature. This potential, as we now see, is always negative at low intensities, except (as we shall see in more detail) in a narrow frequency range near the "best" frequency of a given electrode location, where it is positive at all SPL's. It is also seen that at high intensities the AVE potential is always positive.

Let us now turn our attention to SP data recorded from the higher turns

sources and mechanisms of generation. Experiments specifically designed to selectively influence some of the suspected sources are required to ascertain the true composition of the response.

It is the contention of Davis (1960) and Davis *et al.* (1958a) that SP^+ and SP^- do not originate within the same structures; in fact they identify the external hair cells as the source of SP^+ and the internal hair cells as the source of SP^-. Assuming that as direct consequence of the geometry of the cochlear partition the external hair cells are more sensitive, then the shape of the SP input–output function in turn 1 for a moderate-frequency stimulus is easily explained. At low sound levels only the external hair cells would be stimulated effectively; thus the SP^+ produced by them would predominate. With increasing stimulus strength the internal hair cells would also become active and would produce increasing amounts of SP^-. First, the presence of SP^- would merely slow the growth of SP^+ (the recording electrode simply picks up the algebraic sum of the potentials present), but then the presumably faster growing SP^- would completely counteract the SP^+, producing zero SP at a given intensity level. Beyond that the SP^- would dominate. This argument of course is based on the assumption that SP^+ and SP^- do not originate from the same source. One problem with this interpretation which is clearly apparent from our extensive data is that at the best frequency for a given recording location there is no positive local SP component at any intensity: the steady-state DIF SP is all negative.

An interesting series of experiments by Davis *et al.* (1958b) is the basis for the contention that the generators of SP^+ and SP^- are distinct. Davis and his colleagues injected streptomycin into the bullae of guinea pigs and examined the electrical responses from the cochlea from 4 to 7 days after the injection. All tests were followed by histological workup, which suggested that streptomycin affected primarily the external hair cells. The internal hair cells, the supporting cells, and the stria vascularis were not so strongly involved. The most serious destruction occurred near the round window, through which the drug presumably entered the cochlea. Another procedure used by Davis and co-workers was the surgical obstruction of the cochlear vein. From 5 to 8 days postoperative, the animals were tested for their cochlear response and then histological tests on the inner ear were performed. The primary effect of venous obstruction was the degeneration of the stria vascularis in the vicinity of the round window. Secondary effects were observed on the external hair cells and the supporting structures of the organ of Corti.

This series of experiments resulted in many important conclusions regarding EP, CM, and SP. The conclusions regarding EP and CM are quite clear-cut and reliable. Unfortunately, the implications of the experiment regarding the SP, while very suggestive, are not completely unequivocal. Summating potential was absent in *all* cases (eight animals) where the inner hair cells of turn 1 were destroyed (in all eight of these animals the outer hair cells were also missing). With the exception of two animals, some SP^- was present (in 20 animals) whenever the inner hair cells were not severely damaged. In all 20 of these animals the outer hair cell population was *not* completely absent in either turn 1 or 2. If it were not for the exceptions, for the relatively gross histological methods employed (i.e., only light microscopy, no hair cell counts), and for the relatively strong correlation between inner and outer hair cell damage, a very strong case could be made for the internal hair cells being the generators of the SP^-. As it is, an interpretation of the data could be that the internal hair cells might be the source of this dc potential, but the case is not at all tight. Nonetheless, Davis *et al.* feel that the exceptions are only that, and that they can be explained by other mechanisms. In passing Davis *et al.* also state that the SP^+ most likely originates in the external hair cells, for the potential and the cells alike display high vulnerability to injury.

An important counterargument against associating SP^- with the internal hair cells and SP^+ with the outer hair cells comes from the work of Stopp and Whitfield (1964), who found summating potentials not unlike those recorded from mammalian cochleae in the inner ears of pigeons. Since in avian cochleae there are no different inner and outer hair cells, it is unlikely that the two different polarity SP components would be produced by different hair cell groups.

An interesting contrast with Davis' association of the internal hair cells with the production of SP^- and the external hair cells with that of SP^+ is the theory of Johnstone and Johnstone (1966). These authors derived a geometrical model of hair displacement and concluded that the basilar membrane displacement to hair displacement transfer function is nonlinear and that as a result a dc distortion component (SP) can be produced. Their theory assigns SP^+ to the internal and SP^- to the external hair cells. A more complete exposition and criticism of this scheme is given in Chapter 6.

Some information on the sources of the various SP components was obtained in the study by Dallos and Bredberg (1970) that we have already mentioned. The SP data generated in this study are considered preliminary and thus they are discussed quite briefly. Since the various SP components do not have such easily characterized input–output functions as the CM responses, it is difficult to utilize some quantitative description (sensitivity shift or reduction in maximum) for the assessment of the effect of hair cell loss on this potential. Accordingly we adopted a rating scale so that correlations between SP and hair cell population could be made. It was found that all correlations, both for DIF^- and DIF^+, are very strong with outer hair cell damage but very weak with the state of the inner hair cells. While both hair cell groups might produce these SP components,* in a normal ear the observed response appears to be determined to a very large degree by the outer hair cells alone. Since this finding is contrary to the now-classic experiments of Davis *et al.* (1958b) more work on this subject is required before final statements can be made. The positive AVE SP was evaluated on the basis of responses to the 8000-Hz tone bursts from the basal turn. The input–output function of Fig. 5.31 clearly shows that in the normal case the 8000-Hz signal frequency is just below that which would produce the most clear-cut positive AVE response. The fluctuations in the low-level median response indicate that in some animals the response starts negative at low SPL and then it turns positive at higher levels, while in other animals the response is positive at all levels. Thus 8000 Hz is not an ideal frequency from the standpoint of homogeneity. Because of the variability of the low-level normal response, evaluation of the abnormal SP was made on the basis of the high-level segment alone and consequently a less detailed three-point rating scale was indicated. On the basis of this less precise rating we noted a rudimentary correlation between outer hair cell damage and SP response.

One can make the preliminary statement that the AVE^+ response is apparently much less fragile than either of the DIF components. From the animals in the study that showed the most severe damage one can glean the information that the inner hair cells might produce a negative AVE component, while the outer hair cells generate the positive response. In the normal animal the positive component is strongly dominant. These observations should be considered as very tentative; they must await further confirmation. Our results indicate that the AVE^- response is not strongly determined by the condition of the hair cells in the immediate vicinity of the recording electrodes, but in remote regions of the cochlea. Thus for example, the AVE^- component recorded from the third turn seems to be related to the degree of normalcy of the first-turn outer hair cell population and not the degree of damage in the third turn. This component can be quite normal when the local hair cell population is very severely depleted. The converse is also true; the low-frequency, low-intensity negative AVE response in the first turn is missing in almost all cases in spite of the excellent local hair cell population.

2. General Considerations†

At this stage of our understanding of the properties of the SP it is difficult to draw a comprehensive picture of the phenomenon. A great deal of new information is being produced that restricts the utility of the available

* Recent observations on kanamycin-intoxicated cochleae suggest that inner hair cells do not produce significant DIF^+.

† Based on Dallos *et al.* (1972).

data and adds considerable complexity to the description of the phenomenon. We can merely attempt to make a few, very tentative suggestions about the origin and interrelations of the various SP components.

In considering the origin of the various constituents of the SP, the first important problem concerns the independence of the AVE and DIF components. Let us, for example, consider the relatively pure DIF and AVE responses that are seen from the basal turn at high frequencies. Here we can deal with phenomena that are related to a hydromechanical disturbance that is confined to the vicinity of the electrodes. Thus it is unlikely that the electrical responses would be confounded by remotely located active sources. The question to be answered is, are the AVE and DIF components the result of the operation of two independent mechanisms, or are they the manifestations of the same process? In the latter case one would have to assume that the potential gradient would be the primary response; it would originate in the organ of Corti in some asymmetrical distortion process. The common potential would have to be construed as a resultant of the first potential; it would be produced by a simple electrical asymmetry between the scala tympani and scala vestibuli. Such asymmetry is actually suggested by the circuit model proposed by Johnstone *et al.* (1966); we have shown in Section III, A, 2, *b* that linear resistance change in the element stimulating the organ of Corti resistance in that model does yield an asymmetrical potential change at the two nodes simulating the scala vestibuli and tympani. The result of this is a possibility for a common-mode potential to appear in the two scalae.

We have seen (Chapter 2, Section II,A,1,*c*) that as the result of cochlear asymmetries in the electrical network one can obtain significant DIF and AVE components from both intra- (E_D) and extrapartition sources (E_A). Let us concern ourselves with estimating the expected AVE component when the only source is E_D, the generator within the organ of Corti. The equivalent electrical circuit of the cochlear cross section, as shown in Fig. 5.25 with resistive values obtained by Johnstone *et al.* (1966), can serve as the basis of the computations. The values used are $R_r = 46$, $R_b = 24$, $R_v = 13$, $R_1 = 1.8$, and $R_2 = 2.4 \, k\Omega$. The solution of this simple circuit problem yields the following relations: $E_V = 0.014E_D$; $E_T = -0.05E_D$; DIF $= 0.064E_D$; and AVE $= -0.018E_D$. Clearly the circuit analysis predicts that the scala tympani voltage (E_T) is considerably in excess of the scala vestibuli potential, and as a consequence of this asymmetry there is a sizable AVE component. The computations moreover predict that the polarity of the AVE component is opposite to that of the DIF component. The ratio of the magnitudes of the predicted DIF and AVE components is 3.56. These computations indicate that there is a very real possibility that the AVE component that we measure in the stimulus-related response is a simple manifestation of the organ of Corti source, produced by the asymmetry of the cochlear network.

A good analog of the above computation is the situation in which recording is made from the basal turn with high-frequency stimulation. In this case all hydrodynamic activity is confined to the basal region of the cochlea, and thus we do not have to contend with remote potential sources. We remember that in this situation there is a sizable AVE SP component of positive polarity that coexists with the negative DIF component. The magnitude ratio between these two potentials is of the order of 3–5, the DIF component being larger. These numbers are probably not significantly different from the predicted ratio. It is instructive to consider at this point the behavior of CM. In the situation of interest, namely, when recording is in the basal turn and the stimulus is of high frequency, all evidence at hand indicates that the CM has virtually identical magnitude and opposite phase in ST and SV (Dallos *et al.*, 1971). We have obtained a considerable amount of data to compare the relative magnitudes of CM and SP, DIF and AVE components. One can simply state that in situations when the AVE CM component is 40–60 dB below the DIF CM component, the AVE and DIF SP components can be of the same order of magnitude. In other words, the recordings indicate that virtually complete ac symmetry can go hand in hand with very significant dc asymmetry. The former is manifested by the fact that the common-mode CM potential is only a hundredth or a thousandth of the CM gradient. The latter is of course indicated by the fact that the AVE and DIF SP components are commensurable.

There are two possible explanations for the difference between symmetry properties in the cochlea for ac and dc signals. The first, and more obvious, explanation is that there are significant capacitive effects operating that would provide ac pathways between ST and SV and the potential source and also to ground, and they would thus equalize the ac potentials without affecting dc imbalances. The other explanation is that the circuit asymmetries are not significant and that one must seek the source of generation of the AVE component in other cochlear processes. There is no conclusive experimental evidence either for or against the presence of strong capacitive effects operating in the outer scalae of the cochlea. Some considerations, however, might militate against assigning a significant role to capacitive reactances. Consider that if it is indeed capacitive equalization of the CM that yields virtually identical ST and SV potentials at high frequencies in turn 1, then one should be able to discern a gradual increase in CM disparity between these scalae as frequency is lowered, and at very low frequencies the ST/SV microphonic ratio should approach that for SP. The latter is of the order of 1.5–5; that is, the ST potential is larger by that factor. Even cursory study of CM versus frequency plots obtained from ST and SV reveals that there is a disparity between the potentials in the two scalae at low frequencies. The invariable result is, however, that the CM is *larger* in SV than in ST below approximately 2000 Hz (see, for example, Fig. 5.16a). The disparity is of the order of 1.6 : 1. We have stated previously (Dallos *et al.*, 1971) that such differences (which are even more pronounced in the higher turns) are most likely the result of cross talk between turns. It is thus possible that the circuit asymmetries are overshadowed by the opposite asymmetry provided by cross conduction between turns. This would, however, require a very sizable amount of cross conduction to completely reverse the effect. The resolution of this problem must await accurate reactance measurements in the cochlea. Lacking these, one cannot rule out the possibility that the AVE SP component is a manifestation of electroanatomical asymmetries of the inner ear. One must keep in mind, however, that our data on correlation between SP and hair cell damage (Dallos and Bredberg, 1970) indicate that there might be some independence between the DIF and AVE components. Thus, in sound-damaged ears a considerably larger intact cochlear segment is necessary for the production of normal DIF responses than for normal AVE responses.

Aside from the hypothesis that the AVE component is a result of the electrical network asymmetries of the cochlea, one must consider another quite feasible mechanism for the generation of this component. A major portion of the AVE potentials could reflect voltage drops that result from longitudinal current flow between strongly and weakly excited cochlear regions. In this scheme the AVE^+ potential would reflect the source region, which would correspond to strong excitation, while the AVE^- would be associated with the sink of the longitudinal current flow, that is, with areas of weak or nonexisting excitation. It should be realized that if two regions in the cochlea demonstrate different potential levels with respect to indifferent tissue, as segments corresponding to strongly and weakly excited regions clearly do, then current flow between these regions is inherently present. Thus our measurements do indicate the presence of longitudinal currents in the cochlea, and the only question is whether it is the current or the voltage differences that constitute the primary factor. In the former case one can assume resistance changes to exist in the strongly excited zone, with the consequence of the development of a current source (or sink) there. The current is supplied by neighboring segments where resistance changes do not occur. As a consequence of the current flow voltage differences develop and these are measured as the AVE components, both positive and negative, the two being complementary. In the second case, the voltage differences develop due to the previously discussed electrical asymmetries, and the current patterns are set up as the consequence of these potential drops. Clearly the two cases depict different phenomena, but at this juncture we do not possess enough information to firmly decide which possibility is more likely.

All SP components, being dc responses to an ac stimulus, are the products of nonlinear distortion. One of the central problems in dealing with the SP is the determination of the nature and site of the involved nonlinear processes. A fair number of mechanisms have been suggested by various investigators. These have been confined to the explanation of what we now recognize as the DIF component and, more particularly, the negative DIF potential. Some of these proposed mechanisms are treated in Section II, E of Chapter 6.

A few properties of the negative AVE response need to be considered next. Cursory examination of the AVE$^-$ component might suggest that this potential is merely a remote response in analogy with the similarly recorded AP. Indeed, this potential can be recorded in all regions of the cochlea that are distant from the maximum of the traveling wave envelope for a given stimulus; the response is strikingly present even far apically from the region of strongest excitation, i.e., in a segment where there is no excitation at all. This potential thus could be the reflection of distant activity—a passively conducted response. Some observations must be explained, however, before this view of the negative AVE component can be safely adopted. First, we noted that the slope of the AVE$^-$ input–output function is one-half, as opposed to the unity slope of the functions of those potentials whose remote reflection this AVE$^-$ is supposed to be. Second, the relationship between the magnitudes of the AVE$^-$ and the DIF$^-$ components is such that the concept of assigning a mere remote response character to the AVE$^-$ is not completely straightforward.

To explore these ideas, simultaneously recorded first-turn DIF and third-turn AVE responses were collected at various intensity levels for four high frequencies, 6, 8, 10, and 12 kHz. Even the lowest of these frequencies generate a traveling wave that is completely extinguished far basally from the third-turn electrode location. The four input–output functions for the AVE components can virtually superimpose. In other words, over this 6-kHz frequency range, the third-turn AVE response does not materially change with frequency. Highly significant changes do occur in the magnitude of the DIF components, however. As frequency increases this response becomes larger in the first turn. The relative magnitudes of the two components at various frequencies are very revealing. At 12 kHz the DIF component is larger, except at the lowest intensity, while in contrast at 6 kHz the AVE component is larger, except at the highest intensity. If the AVE component were a mere remote reflection of the DIF component, it is unlikely that its magnitude would stay constant as the region of DIF activity were constricted to ever-diminishing segments in the basal portion of the cochlea. It would also be unlikely that its magnitude would be bigger than that of the DIF$^-$ response that arises much closer to the point of maximum excitation, such as in the 6-kHz case. If we assume, however, that the AVE$^-$ component is not simply a conducted remote response, but the actual counterpart of the AVE$^+$ component, these difficulties are somewhat alleviated.

The one remaining problem that we have no immediate explanation for is the peculiar slope of the AVE^- input–output function, namely one-half. In the narrow region where the AVE^+ component is positive at all intensities (in other words, in the region where this component is maximum) its input–output function possesses unity slope. The question of why the potential drop in the source and sink regions (that is, the AVE^+ and AVE^- components) would grow at different rates can probably be explained by the nonlinear spread of the region of excitation with increasing intensity and thus by a nonlinear growth of current density. The hypothesized longitudinal current would be controlled by an active region in the vicinity of maximum excitation and it would flow into all inactive regions. This way the AVE^+ would reflect the active region, while AVE^- would prevail in all inactive regions. Our study on cochlear damage (Dallos and Bredberg, 1970) indicated that there was excellent correlation between the integrity of the AVE^+-producing active region and the normalcy of distant AVE^- potentials. For example, in cases where there was almost complete damage of the third-turn hair cell population and still a good first-turn population existed, the AVE^- potential recorded from the third turn in response to high-frequency signals was virtually normal. Conversely, in this situation the low-frequency, low-intensity negative segment of the first-turn input–output function of the AVE potential was almost invariably missing.

One additional possibility that is worth mentioning is that some portion of the negative AVE response might reflect cochlear generator potentials. In the original report on the SP phenomenon Davis and colleagues (1950) did assume that they were recording the postsynaptic potential arising in the dendritic region of the auditory nerve. A generator potential is certainly present in the auditory sense organ (Davis, 1961a), but it has not been experimentally identified as yet. It is possible that we do record this generator potential in those cases where at low signal intensity the AVE component is much greater than the DIF component, such as when recordings are made from the first at relatively low frequencies. We have some preliminary evidence indicating that these negative AVE potentials are indeed the manifestations of generator potentials. Thus, for example, these potentials disappear immediately after death, while other SP components persist; they can also be masked.

As we have noted there is a general similarity between SP patterns reflected by the DIF and SM components. Apparently both are dependent primarily on the potential gradient across the organ of Corti and are the manifestations of the same nonlinear processes. The differences between the DIF and SM patterns are probably attributable to the differing electrical circuit elements that are involved in the registration of these potentials at their respective recording sites. One difference involves the wider spread of the

SM component around its maximum. This is probably related to the fact that the insulating properties of the cochlear duct are better than those of the perilymphatic channels. The scala media is essentially a core conductor and potentials are expected to spread farther in it than in the more lossy scala vestibuli–scala tympani complex. Another, related difference is the appearance of negative SP in the scala media at low intensities and at all frequencies. Apparently, remote negative activity is conducted in the scala media with such small losses that it can overcome a generally small, positive local response. Finally, the waveforms of the SP in the scala media are radically different from those in the perilymph. From the presence of both slow and fast response components one can surmise that the electrode "sees" the scala media SP through a circuit involving both resistive and capacitive elements. Apparently, such capacitance is not involved to any significant measure in the registration of SP from the two outer scalae.

Our final consideraiton is directed toward establishing some relationships between CM, SP, and the traveling wave pattern. To facilitate the discussion in Fig. 5.36 a composite graph based on data from one animal is presented. Included in the graph are CM and SP recordings from the third turn of the cochlea. The CM magnitude (obtained with differential-electrode recording) at constant 50 dB SPL, the DIF and AVE SP components at constant 50 dB SPL, all as functions of stimulus frequency, are compared with the schematic tuning curve of basilar membrane displacement for the cochlear location where the electrodes are situated (approximately 14.5 mm from the stapes). From von Békésy's (1944) frequency map one obtains a best frequency of 400 Hz, and the tuning curve is constructed by assuming its basal slope to be 6 dB/octave and its apical slope to be −100 dB/octave (Johnstone et al., 1970). We first note the good agreement between the frequency of the maximum CM and the maximum mechanical displacement. In this case the maximum of the DIF^+ response almost coincides with the maximum of the CM response; its frequency is about 300 Hz. It is striking that the DIF^- component peaks at a considerably higher frequency than the CM-traveling wave maximum. The difference is approximately 1 octave. This is a highly consistent finding. The AVE^+ peak is more variable. In some animals it occurs at the same frequency as the DIF^- maximum, and in others it is at a lower frequency. The fact that the DIF^- component peaks at higher frequencies than the CM at a given location indicates that this potential has its maximum on the apical slope of, and beyond, the traveling wave envelope. We have shown that intermodulation components in the CM are similarly located with respect to the displacement pattern of the cochlear partition (Worthington and Dallos, 1971). These observations suggest that the nonlinearities that produce microphonic distortion at moderate sound levels and those responsible for the production of the DIF SP are related. It also appears that the positive DIF SP is best correlated with the point of maximum and the proximal slope of the traveling wave envelope, at least at low sound levels. As intensity increases, the DIF⁻ and AVE⁺ components expand much further basally and become the dominant responses over the entire spatial extent of the traveling wave.

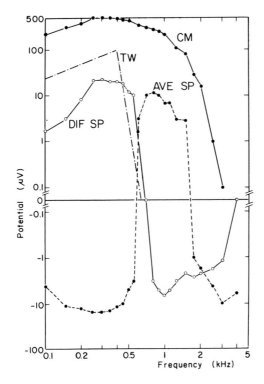

Fig. 5.36. Various recordings obtained from third-turn electrodes in one guinea pig. All these data were collected at a constant 50 dB SPL. The CM potential magnitude as recorded with differential electrodes is given in the top graph; the DIF and AVE SP components are also shown. The mechanical tuning curve (TW) for the cochlear location (14.5 mm) is schematized for comparison with the potential functions. The peak of the mechanical tuning curve is placed at 400 Hz in accordance with von Békésy's cochlear map (1960, p. 504). The low-frequency slope is drawn as 6 dB/octave and the high-frequency slope as −100 dB/octave. (From Dallos *et al.*, 1972, p. 70.)

IV. Electroanatomy of the Cochlea

We have already examined several facets of the line of investigation that was termed electroanatomy of the cochlea by von Békésy (1951). The electroanatomy of an organ describes the distribution and spread of electrical potentials within that structure as well as the distribution of other electrical parameters (resistance, capacitance) upon which the former depends. Specific issues that received attention in earlier discussions were the relative magnitudes of various potentials from scala to scala, distribution patterns of the different potentials, the measurement of these potentials, and factors that affect the measurements. In this section our primary concern is to bring together evidence concerning the pattern of electrical resistance in the cochlea and thus determine the expected rate of attenuation of potentials from their source to their site of recording. Few investigators have direct studies of the potential spread in the cochlea. Their results as a rule are not directly comparable because of the difference in experimental technique and orientation. There are two essentially contrary views. According to one, potentials spread widely in the cochlea, with relatively moderate attenuation (Wever and Lawrence, 1954). According to the opposite opinion (Tasaki, 1957; Davis, 1957) the attentuation of potentials along the length of the cochlea is very rapid, and thus there is no appreciable spread of potentials. As we shall see below these divergent viewpoints based on different experimental results are the direct consequence of dissimilar experimental techniques. In order to evaluate the available experimental data, we must decide first what sort of potential distribution is of essential interest to us. Since the generators of stimulus-related potentials are presumed to be the hair cells, and since these electrical sources create a potential difference across the organ of Corti (perpendicular to the basilar membrane) which is communicated to the endolymph of the scala media on the one hand and the perilymph of the scala tympani on the other, it stands to reason that the spread of potentials should also be measured across the organ of Corti, that is, between scalae media and tympani.

The first systematic measurements of the electrical conductivity of the cochlea were made by von Békésy in 1951. These measurements are also the most extensive and probably the most sophisticated. Von Békésy's first concern was to determine the total of the effective resistances across which a voltage, introduced between scalae vestibuli and tympani near the window region, develops. Figure 5.37 shows schematically that such a potential is developed across a resistance r, corresponding to the total series resistance of the cochlear partition, and that the potential is influenced by the resistances between "ground" (i.e., the indifferent tissues of the animal) and the vestibular (R_1) and tympanic (R_2) measuring points. Von Békésy measured three ratios from which these lumped equivalent resistance values could be computed directly. His values are $r = 2250 \, \Omega$, $R_1 = 3700 \, \Omega$, and $R_2 = 8500 \, \Omega$. These values are the means obtained from 12 guinea pig ears. He noted that, at least at 1000 Hz, there was no reactive impedance component, and thus the voltages developed across essentially pure resistances. The primary grounding

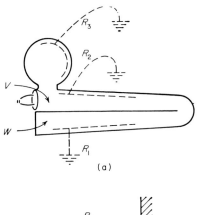

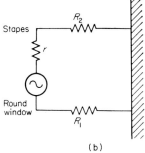

Fig. 5.37. Schematic drawing of the inner ear, showing the resistances between it and the body of the animal. Resistance *r* is that between points *V* and *W*. (From von Békésy, 1960, p. 658.)

path was shown to be formed by the endolymphatic space through the cells of the organ of Corti through the nerve fibers in the modiolus to the brain. The bony shell of the cochlea proved to be a good insulator when compared to the grounding path through the auditory nerve.

Von Békésy's next concern was to determine whether the cochlear partition possesses appreciable insulating properties or if it is electrically transparent. The two extreme situations are depicted in Fig. 5.38, where two fluid-filled tubes are shown, one without and the other with a perfectly insulating partition, which divides the latter into two channels. Assuming that electrical potentials are transduced into the fluid in either case with a dipole source, the dependence of the potential on the source–electrode distance is shown in the accompanying plots. If the potential is measured in a homogeneous medium then it decreases in inverse proportion with distance. As a consequence the decrease between two points near the source is much greater than between two other, equidistant points far from the source. This can be seen by comparing the change of potential between points *A'* and *A''* with that between *B'* and *B''* shown in plot (a) of Fig. 5.38. In contrast, if an insulating

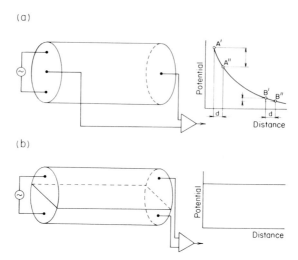

Fig. 5.38. Change of potential with distance in a volume conductor. (a) Homogeneous medium; (b) the medium is divided by an insulating partition.

partition is interposed between the two poles of both the source and the measuring electrodes, then there is no potential drop with increasing distance, as is indicated in plot (b) of Fig. 5.38. Von Békésy considered that these theoretical arguments could be tested in a physiological preparation, and thus one could decide whether the insulating properties of the cochlear partition are of any significance. He drilled a series of equidistant holes through the cochlear bone of guinea pigs into the scala tympani and also holes placed symmetrically into the scala vestibuli. The hole pairs were numbered 1, 2, ..., 6 from the round window. Potential difference was measured from the number one hole pair (E_1) and also from the number two hole pair (E_2). It was observed that the ratio E_1/E_2 was invariant with the site of the electrical source. In other words, E_1/E_2 did not change from the condition in which the stimulus was delivered between the number three holes to that in which voltage was applied between the number six holes. This finding indicated that the cochlear partition does possess appreciable resistance and that the electrical behavior of the cochlea is better described as a transmission line than as a homogeneous conductor.

The same method was used by von Békésy to measure the actual attenuation of an electrical signal applied between scala tympani and scala vestibuli along the length of the cochlea. Let us emphasize again, the measurement is as follows. Holes are placed symmetrically around the cochlear partition in the guinea pig cochlea. These holes form a series from base to apex. Stimulation is introduced between one hole in the scala tympani and the corresponding hole in scala vestibuli. These holes are either the first or the last of the series. Potentials are measured between corresponding holes at various distances from the location of the stimulating electrodes. The resultant attenuation versus distance plot (Fig. 5.39) is reported to be independent from the site of the stimulation. Stated differently, the electrical transmission in the cochlea appears to be symmetrical. From Fig. 5.39 one can see that the average attenuation along the length of the cochlea is approximately 6.7 dB/mm. Thus a potential generated in a given spot decreases to about half of its value 1 mm away, to one-fourth of its value 2 mm away, and so forth. These results clearly indicate that, while the cochlea cannot be considered as a homogeneous conductor (in which case the attenuation would be considerably greater), it is also improper to assume that the cochlear partition provides infinite insulation. In reality the resistance pattern of the cochlea is highly complex and can best be visualized as a distributed system, or transmission line.

Von Békésy's method provides a clear-cut figure for attenuation of potentials which develop across the cochlear partition and which are measured across the cochlear partition. The figure of about 6–7 dB/mm indicates rapid attenuation and thus a rather confined electrical activity. It is imperative to consider, however, how realistic this figure of attenuation is from the physio-

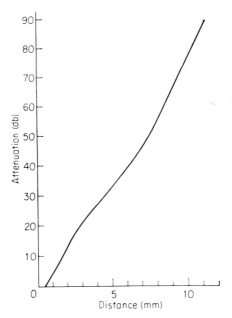

Fig. 5.39. Attenuation of a voltage across the cochlear partition as a function of distance along the cochlea, measured from a point 0.5 mm from the basal end of the basilar membrane. (From von Békésy, 1960, p. 666.)

logical viewpoint. Clearly our best method of measuring cochlear potentials is the differential-electrode technique in which electrodes are placed symmetrically in scalae tympani and vestibuli. This measuring condition is actually duplicated in the von Békésy experiments, and thus his method provides an excellent basis for comparison with a large and informative segment of pertinent literature. Consider, however, that during actual measurements of cochlear potentials the source is not neatly placed across the cochlear partition but is inside that partition, whereas during measurements with differential electrodes these are across the partition. The two situations would be analogous only if Reissner's membrane were electrically transparent, a condition that is disproved by von Békésy's own experiments (1952). In these experiments he measured ac potentials during the penetration of the cochlear partition with a microelectrode. He observed that the potential changed very little while the electrode traversed either the perilymphatic or endolymphatic space, but large potential changes were seen when the electrode penetrated through either the organ of Corti or Reissner's membrane. These potential jumps were of equal magnitude, indicating that the insulation of the perilymph from the endolymph is the same on both sides of the scala media, i.e., that the insulation provided by Reissner's membrane is about the same as that offered by the basilar membrane–organ of Corti complex.

In addition to the essential nonequivalence of the site of the source in the previously discussed experiments and in the actual differential-electrode recording situation, another important consideration should also be mentioned here. As Tasaki (1957) and Misrahy et al. (1958) point out, the two perilymphatic scalae are connected by the low electrical resistance of the spiral ligament. Thus there is an effective shunt for all potentials measured between these scalae. We now know that the potential difference between scala media and scala tympani is always considerably greater than the potential difference between scala vestibuli and scala tympani. Consequently electrical potentials are expected to spread farther within the scala media than within the perilymphatic channels. If this argument is correct then the 6.7 dB/mm attenuation factor derived by von Békésy is too high in describing the physiologically significant situation, i.e., when the source is within the cochlear partition. It is interesting to note that the quantitative information provided on attenuation rate by Misrahy et al. (1958) indicates a tenfold potential drop between second and third turns, with an approximately 5-mm interelectrode distance. This of course provides an attenuation of 4.0 dB/mm, lower than von Békésy's figure. It should be noted that Misrahy et al. placed both the stimulating and recording electrode pairs between scala media and scala tympani, and thus theoretically their attenuation factor should be lower.

Tasaki (1957) briefly mentions that he obtained attenuation rates of 4–6 dB/mm with sinusoidal voltages applied between scala media and scala tympani. Unfortunately it is not stated between which scalae the measurements were taken. It is, however, likely that Tasaki's usual differential-electrode technique was used; i.e., the measuring electrodes were in scala vestibuli and scala tympani. If this is the case then Tasaki's experiments most closely approximate the usual physiological situation, namely source between scalae media and tympani while measurement is between scalae vestibuli and tympani. It appears then that, if one considers all the above evidence, the attenuation factor of 4–6 dB/mm is probably a good approximation for the usual intracochlear measuring situation. It is of great importance to emphasize that this high attenuation is strongly dependent on the method of measurement. Such rates are obtained if the differential-electrode technique is used. Clearly much lower attenuation rate is to be expected if single intra- or extracochlear electrodes, referred to an indifferent ground electrode, are used for measurement. My own experience with differential recording of CM is also closely in line with the above observations. The distance between our routinely placed first- and third-turn electrode pairs (guinea pig cochlea) is approximately 10 mm. It will be recalled that the sensitivity difference at 10 kHz (which is close to the best frequency for our first-turn electrode location) is about 40–60 dB between the two electrode pairs. We have shown (Dallos, 1969a) that the small response at high frequencies which is recordable from the third turn is actually not a local response but a propagated remote CM. This implies that the basal-turn CM is attenuated by at least 40–60 dB when measured in the third turn. As a consequence the rate of attenuation is of the order of 4–6 dB/mm, in complete agreement with Tasaki's suggestion.

All previous discussions pertained to experimental situations in which the stimulus was delivered between two points within the cochlea and propagated potentials were measured between two points, again both of which were within the cochlea. Such measurements yield relatively high attenuation figures. Wever and Lawrence (1954) used a somewhat different experimental technique for the measurement of cochlear attenuation, and not surprisingly their results are not like those discussed above. Wever and Lawrence introduced their stimuli between electrodes placed on the round-window membrane and on the stapes footplate. This stimulus placement is similar to that of von Békésy in that potentials are introduced between the two perilymphatic scalae. The voltages were measured with a needle electrode placed on the cochlear bone either near the round window or at the apex. The reference electrode was placed into the masseter muscle. It was found that the voltage difference between the near (round window) and far (apex) electrodes was a relatively constant 19 dB for stimulus frequencies between 100 and 15,000 Hz. This attenuation figure is equivalent to a rate of potential decline of about 1 dB/mm. It is important to keep in mind that this technique measures the potential difference between a single point on the cochlear bone and the animal's body, which is presumably at some average potential. Consequently this method does not reveal local potential differences to the same extent as does the differential-electrode technique. Again our own experience corroborates the results of Wever and Lawrence. If one compares the isopotential curves obtained with single intracochlear electrodes (Figs. 2.9 and 2.10) for first and third turns, then a sensitivity difference of 20 dB at 10 kHz is evident. Ten kilohertz is a frequency component that is generated primarily in the vicinity of the basal electrode. The response picked up by the third-turn electrode at that frequency is primarily a remote response. Since the two electrodes are approximately 10 mm apart, the attentuation is of the order of 2 dB/mm. This figure is higher than the Wever and Lawrence data indicate, the reason for which must undoubtedly lie in the fact that their pickup electrode was on the outside of the cochlear bone, while ours was intracochlear. It is to be expected that the mucous lining of the cochlea would have high conductivity, and thus electrical activity could propagate in it with relatively low attentuation.

An extensive investigation of the resistance patterns in the basal turn of the guinea pig was completed by Johnstone et al. (1966). These investigators noted that the pattern of current flow between two electrodes within the cochlea is complex, involving several parallel current paths. In order to estimate the electrical resistance of various membranes and paths one must first devise an electrical model of the cochlea and based on that one must perform an appropriate series of resistance measurements. The model Johnstone et al. chose is shown in Fig. 5.25. The letters M, V, and T have their customary meaning; they correspond to nodes in the equivalent circuit; B, another node, signifies the vascular plexus within the cochlea and GP corresponds to indifferent tissue of the animal. The various resistances between the nodes denote the various membrane and path resistances. There are six resistances in the equivalent circuit. In order to determine them six independent measurements must be made. There are a very large number of possible combinations of measurements, and Johnstone et al. took particular pains to choose a set that they considered optimal. Measurements of dc resistance were performed, square current pulses were injected, and the ensuing voltage drops were measured. In table 5.1 the results of a representative set of experiments are shown. The first column indicates the two points between which the current was injected, and the second column indicates the two points between which the resulting voltage was measured. The ratios of voltage and current provide resistance values, and from the set of six such values the resistance parameters shown in Fig. 5.25 can be computed. The authors' best estimate of parameters (which, the reader will recall, we have used in our computations of circuit properties before) are $R_b = 24.2$, $R_r = 46.1$, $R_v = 12.6$, $R_1 = 0.62$, $R_2 = 0.81$, and $R_3 = 1.58$ kΩ. Johnstone *et al.* assumed that the first three values represent the effective resistance of a segment of the basal turn that is equal in length to approximately one length constant, which they found to be about 2 mm. On the other hand, they assume that the latter three values represent the entire first turn, that is, about three length constants in parallel.

TABLE 5.1

REPRESENTATIVE RESISTANCE VALUES OBTAINED BY MEASURING VOLTAGE DROPS BETWEEN THE INDICATED NODES IN RESPONSE TO CURRENT DELIVERED BETWEEN TWO OTHER NODES [a]

Current between[b]	Voltage between[b]	Typical results (kΩ)
V–G	*T–G*	1.6
T–M	*T–G*	0.25
V–M	*V–G*	0.5
V–M	*T–G*	−0.1
V–M	*M–G*	−5.0
T–V	*M–G*	0.0

[a] From Johnstone *et al.* (1966, p. 1401).
[b] The nodes are *T*, scala tympani; *V*, scala vestibuli; *M*, scala media; *G*, ground.

The central problem of how resistances in the cochlea change when sound stimuli are presented has received only cursory attention so far. Johnstone *et al.* made some measurements; they estimated that R_b decreased by about 10% when a 5000-Hz tone was present at 95 dB SPL. Kurokawa (1965, in Japanese) also measured resistance changes in the presence of sound. He found an approximately 13% drop in the effective resistance of the organ of Corti when a 4000-Hz tone was present at 95 dB sound level. Similar qualitative observations were made by Misrahy *et al.* (1958). Since the resistance-modulation hypothesis is enjoying wide acceptance, the time is certainly ripe for a thorough examination of the problem of resistance changes in the cochlea due to sound stimulation. On the basis of the few observations cataloged above, it is clear that resistance change does accompany acoustic stimulation. It is also clear from our computations in Section III, A,2,*b* that these resistance changes are probably sufficient to explain CM and partly SP generation. This is underscored by some observations by Misrahy *et al.* (1958) and Kurokawa (1965) indicating that the time course of resistance change is very closely matched by the time course of diminution in EP, which is a component of the SP. The entire problem of resistance change versus stimulation needs to be examined in a systematic fashion, with particular attention to the linearity of the change and to the effect of frequency of stimulation. Another very important problem that has not received any systematic scrutiny is the reactance pattern of the cochlea. There are indications that significant reactive components accompany the resistive elements

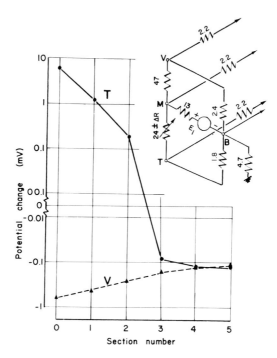

Fig. 5.40. Measurements on a three-dimensional model of cochlear electroanatomy. The magnitude of the voltage change at nodes *ST* and *SV* are plotted as measured at the various circuit sections. The stimulus is a 4-kΩ change of the "organ of Corti resistance" in section 0. The insert shows the configuration of the first section and the coupling paths leading to the second section.

in the cochlear circuit (Johnstone *et al.*, 1966; Weiss *et al.*, 1969). Our observations concerning high-frequency ac symmetry contrasted with a dc asymmetry (manifested by the presence of an AVE SP component in response to a high-frequency stimulus when recorded from the basal turn where the resulting CM is the same in both SV and ST) also point to the possibility of the existence of very significant reactive components in the cochlear electroanatomy.

It is appropriate to close this section by describing the results of some of our experiments on a three-dimensional network model of the cochlear electroanatomy. The lumped-parameter model was built on the basis of Johnstone and Johnstone's (1966) resistance measurements. It consists of a set of five resistance networks serially interconnected with coupling resistances. The individual networks are in the configuration shown in Fig. 5.25, with the exception that for simplicity only E_1, the stria vascularis dc source is included. The configuration of the first network (section 0) is shown in the insert of Fig. 5.40. In this network segment the controlling organ of Corti resistance was so fabricated that a set amount (ΔR) could be added to or subtracted from the resting value of 24 kΩ. In all other segments only the 24-kΩ constant resistance value was incorporated. Voltage changes as a result of the resistance change were measured at all three nodes (SV, ST, and SM) of all sections. These measurements on the first section were in complete accord with our computations, which have been presented before. With an increase of the controlling resistance the voltage levels of SV and SM increased, while that of ST decreased. The voltage change in SV and ST was highly asymmetrical. However, as the data points for section 0 in Fig. 5.40 show, the ST voltage change is about ten time as great as the SV change. This tends to indicate that some of the prototype resistance values (Johnstone and Johnstone, 1966) are inaccurate. The important result, the reason for presenting these data, is the change of voltage at various nodes distant from the segment in which the resistance change takes place. In both ST and SV nodes with increasing section number the potential change due to resistance change in section 0 decreases. The striking observation is that this decrease is much more rapid for the ST nodes. In fact at a certain distance away the polarity of the ST voltage change reverses and beyond this the two nodes (ST and SV) are at approximately the same potential level. This behavior is a clear-cut correlate of some observations on "remote" CM and SP in physiological preparations. It is remembered that in situations where the recording electrodes and the active cochlear regions are distant (for example, in a case of high-frequency stimulation and recording from the apical region of the cochlea) both scala tympani and vestibuli electrodes record about the same amount and same polarity (or phase) summating potential or microphonic. Thus, for example, as Figs. 5.16 and 5.3 demonstrate, at high frequencies in the third turn the CM magnitude in scalae vestibuli and tympani is the same and the CM phase between the two scalae is zero. Similarly, the fact that the high-frequency SP response in the higher turns is the same negative voltage in both scalae (for example, the 10,000-Hz panel in Fig. 5.32) seems to correlate well with the measurements on the model.

V. Whole-Nerve Action Potential

When Wever and Bray (1930) first recorded electrical potentials from the cat auditory nerve, they noted that the gross activity followed the sound pattern up to relatively high audio frequencies, approximately to 3000 Hz. The activity was first thought to represent purely neural responses, but it soon became clear that this "Wever–Bray effect" constituted a mixture of whole-nerve action potentials and what became known as cochlear microphonics. The whole-nerve, or compound, action potential itself can be recorded with various techniques so that it is relatively free from an overlay of CM. In this section we shall examine the nature and properties of the compound auditory action potential.

A gross electrode on the auditory nerve, or in the vicinity of the cochlea, is capable of recording a series of negative potential changes that are linked with discrete auditory events. These negative voltages reflect summated activity in the auditory nerve. The acoustic conditions that are favorable for their elicitation are usually associated with rapid temporal changes in stimulus pattern, such as the onset of noise or tone bursts, clicks, and individual cycles of low-frequency tones. Common among such stimuli is the presence of sharply defined events in time, which are apparently the most important prerequisites for the simultaneous firing of a large number of auditory neurons. Such synchronized discharge of an entire neuronal population is manifested by the compound action potential.

In Chapter 2 we discussed at considerable length the differential-electrode technique, which can be used to good advantage in separating AP from CM. We noted that for the intracochlear electrodes the AP appears as a "remote" potential. It is in phase at the location of both ST and SV electrodes, and thus when the outputs of these are added the AP is emphasized, while the CM (being in phase opposition) is rejected. While the AP is clearly the response of the auditory nerve trunk, a legitimate question, which has been raised often, concerns the exact point in space at which the AP originates. At one time it was thought that this potential is most intimately associated with the cell bodies of the spiral ganglion (Davis et al., 1950). It is now more apparent that the axons contribute to this response, while the cell body performs primarily metabolic functions. Several investigators ventured opinions on the exact site of origin of the AP (Davis et al., 1952; Tasaki, 1954; Pestalozza and Davis, 1956; Teas et al., 1962). The early investigators suggested that the whole-nerve AP is registered as the activity passes through the internal auditory meatus. Teas et al. (1962) refined this assertion and pointed to the emergence of the activity from the internal meatus as the event that is signified by the AP. This latter suggestion appears to be most valid to us, and it is developed in a semiquantitative manner below.

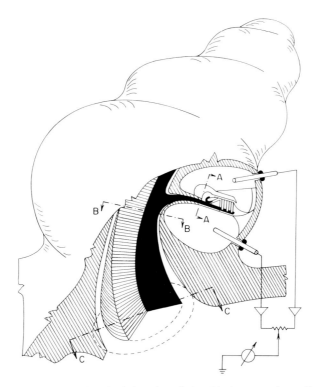

Fig. 5.41. Schematic drawing depicting the relationship between the auditory nerve, the cochlear bone, and the recording electrodes. The three surfaces, marked by *A–A*, *B–B*, and *C–C*, are the potentially important spatial regions in the genesis of the whole-nerve action potential.

Fig. 5.41 a schematic representation of the guinea pig cochlea is shown. The drawing indicates the course of the auditory nerve from habenula perforata (*A–A*) to the medulla. The bony cochlea is shown split up so that the cross section of a single turn as well as the outline of the internal auditory meatus can be discerned. The cochlear bone is shaded to emphasize how it envelops the nerve between the habenula and the central entrance to the internal meatus. Two recording electrodes, one in scala tympani and the other in scala vestibuli, are also shown. As is customary for AP recording, the electrode outputs are added, and the combined signal is registered in reference to an indifferent electrode. Three cross sections of the nerve that are important in our succeeding discussions are indicated by the lines *AA*, *BB*, and *CC*. It is notable that between *AA* and *BB* the bone separating the nerve trunk from the scala tympani is extremely thin (of the order of microns). The question arises as to whether such a thin bony layer can act as an effective insulator. If even this thin bony divider behaves as a good electrical insulator, the entire peripheral segment of the nerve between AA and CC is effectively shielded from the cochlear electrodes. If, however, the insulation is poor the propagated neural activity does not disappear from the electrodes' "sight" until it reaches BB. As we shall see below, there is a significant difference between the two cases, as would be manifested in the waveform of the AP recorded by the intracochlear electrodes. In order to consider recorded waveforms of neural activity, we must digress briefly and give a relatively cursory treatment of electrical potentials in a volume conductor. Our discussion is based on the treatment of this subject by Woodbury (1960).

An axon is generally surrounded by other axons and interstitial fluid. Since both the intercellular fluid and inactive neurons are good conductors, it can be said that an active nerve fiber is surrounded by a medium of high electrical conductance. This medium is normally equipotential; this is altered only when there is current flow in the medium. The source for such current flow must be sought in the activity of the nerve fiber, specifically in the potential difference between adjacent active and inactive segments of the axon. In regions where an axon is inactive its membrane is polarized so that the inside is negative with respect to the outside. Wherever a nerve spike occurs this polarization is momentarily reversed, and thus in the active region the outside is negative and the inside of the fiber is positive. The current flow between active and inactive regions depolarizes the inactive region immediately adjacent to an active one. When depolarization reaches a critical magnitude a full-blown action potential spike develops and the previously inactive region becomes active, while the previously active region slowly repolarizes. This of course is the well-known sequence of spike propagation in nerve fibers. For our purpose it is important to remember merely the charge separation across the fiber membrane and the changes in charge separation concomitant with the presence of a spike.

Electrically, this situation of charge separation across a thin insulating membrane is analogous to a so-called electric dipole layer. A dipole layer consists of opposite electrical charges separated by a very small distance. The charge on the surface of the membrane is proportional to the potential difference across the membrane, since the latter acts as a capacitor. As a consequence the dipole moment per unit area is proportional to the trans-membrane potential. It is a relatively straightforward matter to derive a formula for the potential at a point P in the medium due to the presence of an electrical double layer. Here we simply present the simplified final results, according to which the potential at point P is proportional to the product of the membrane potential that sets up the double layer and the *solid angle* that is subtended by the surface at point P. The solid angle expresses how

large an object appears to be when viewed from a certain point. Thus this
measure depends on both the actual size of the object and its distance from
the viewer. The closer a given object is to the point from which it is viewed,
the larger it appears to be. To compute the solid angle subtended by an object
at point P, one projects the object on the surface of a sphere of radius r,
drawn around P. If the surface area of the projection of the object on the
sphere is denoted by A, then the solid angle (Ω) is equal to A/r^2.

Let us now consider the potential at a given point that is generated by
an inactive nerve cell. To compute the potential at a given point P, one can
subdivide the cell into two segments along the perimeter of sight. The near
segment produces a positive potential at P in the amount of $+E_m K\Omega$,
since from the point in question the outside positive charges are "seen".
The far segment produces the same amount of voltage at point P as the near
segment since the spatial angle is the same, and so is the membrane potential
E_m. The only difference is that the polarity is now negative since the negative
charges are closer to the point P. Clearly the total potential generated by the
cell in its quiescent state is zero.

Let us now consider an extension of this example. If a nerve fiber is not
quiescent but a segment of it is active, then in a given instant it can be depicted
as shown in Fig. 5.42, where the cross section of the fiber is shown with an

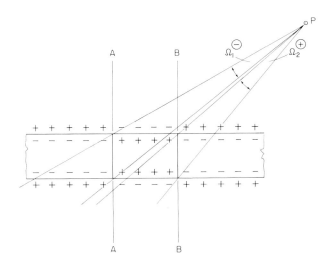

Fig. 5.42. Schematic of an active nerve fiber at a given instant. The active region is
contained between A–A and B–B. From point P the negative contribution of the active
region is seen through spatial angle Ω_1, while the positive contribution is seen through Ω_2.
Since in this instance $\Omega_1 > \Omega_2$, the resulting potential at P is negative. The portions of the
cell that are outside A–A and B–B are assumed to extend far in both directions. These
portions are quiescent and thus do not contribute a potential at point P.

active region between lines AA and BB and inactive regions extending on both sides of the active segment. The two inactive segments behave as independent, quiescent cells in that their near and far membranes contribute charges of equal magnitude but opposite polarity, with the result that the net potential at point P is zero. The active region, however, is different. Consider the contributions of the two portions of the cell that are delineated by solid angles Ω_1 and Ω_2. In the first case point P sees negative charges on the proximal sides of both the near and far membranes, and thus the potential due to them is negative at P. In the second case the charges seen are positive, and thus this segment produces a positive potential at P. Since $\Omega_1 > \Omega_2$ we can assume that the overall potential at P is negative. In the case of a propagated discharge (spike), we can construct a simplified picture of the potential variation at point P by simply repeating the type of reasoning that was employed above as the active region moves along the fiber. Consider first that the active region is far away. Then the nearer demarcation between active and inactive zones subtends a greater solid angle than the farther one, and consequently the net potential is positive. As the active region approaches the electrode the two solid angles become more similar and at a particular point the angle corresponding to the distal boundary becomes greater. At this point the potential reverses and becomes negative. As the active region passes under the electrode the potential remains negative, but when it moves to a sufficiently far distance so that the solid angle of the now-proximal boundary becomes greater the potential reverses again. Thus a $+ - +$ potential sequence is expected as a spike passes an electrode. This so-called triphasic potential is indeed the typical event that can be recorded with an extracellular electrode from a propagating spike.

Let us now consider the situation, depicted in Fig. 5.43, in which the fiber is immersed in two media, one conductive and the other insulating. Let us also place the electrode (point of measurement) at the boundary between the two media. Assume that a local depolarization travels from left to right toward the electrode. The time course of the recorded potential can be deduced from our previous arguments. It will first be positive as the spike approaches the electrode, and then it becomes negative as it arrives in the close proximity of the recording point. The difference is, however, that the negative phase is not followed by a third, positive phase. This is simply due to the fact that as the first front disappears into the nonconducting medium it ceases to produce a potential at the electrode location. Thus, as the second front approaches the boundary, the negativity decreases toward zero potential, and as it disappears beyond the dividing line the potential becomes zero, for the rest of the electrically visible cell is inactive and thus externally neutral. Note then that in the situation in which the activity propagates from a conducting into a nonconductive medium, a positive–negative $(+ -)$

sequence is expected. The converse is also true. When the spike propagates in the opposite direction, i.e., when the propagation is from insulating to conducting medium, the first potential seen by the electrode is negative, and this is followed by positive polarity. Thus in this case we have a − + potential sequence.

Let us now utilize these arguments in deducing the wave shape of the compound action potential seen by intracochlear electrodes. Figure 5.41 is a useful reminder of the geometry of the situation. If we first assume that the entire bony envelope between *AA* and *CC* is good insulator, and if we further make the entirely reasonable assumption that the initial segment of the auditory nerve fibers (location of spike initiation) is at or more central from the habenula perforata, then it is clear that the only possibility for the electrodes to register an AP is to record the activity as it leaves the bony cavity at the internal meatus. Thus this situation corresponds to the case

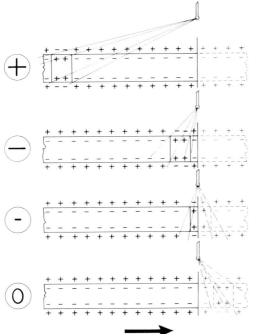

Fig. 5.43. Sequence of potential changes seen by an electrode when the nerve fiber passes from one medium into another. To the left of the electrode the fiber is surrounded by a conductive medium, while to the right it enters an insulating medium. When the activity is far away, the electrode sees a positive potential. As the activity approaches the electrode the potential turns negative. As the active segment passes into the nonconducting medium the negativity decreases and it completely disappears as the active region propagates beyond the boundary. The + − potential sequence is not followed by a final + potential since the active region within the insulating medium is not "seen" by the electrode.

in which activity travels from nonconducting to conducting medium and consequently a minus–plus potential sequence is expected. The second possibility corresponds to the situation in which the initial bony divider, between *AA* and *BB*, is not a good insulator. Under these conditions the insulating tube would correspond to the *BB* to *CC* segment. Here we would expect to see first a positive–negative potential change corresponding to the propagation of spike activity from *AA* to *BB* and to its disappearance from "sight" at *BB*. In addition we would expect to see, after some time delay corresponding to propagation time between *BB* and *CC*, the emergence of the activity from the insulating tube at *CC*; i.e., the first $+ -$ sequence would be followed by a second $- +$ sequence. The diameter of the myelinated nerve fibers in the internal meatus is approximately 2 μ, and the spike propagation velocity for fibers of this diameter is approximately 10 m/second. The length of the *BB–CC* canal is about 2 mm, and consequently the propagation time in this segment is of the order of 0.2 msecond. This is probably too short a time for two distinct negative potentials to be discerned; thus it is likely that in this situation one would see a positive–negative–positive sequence describing the compound AP. These are the two possibilities, and it is relatively easy to choose between them. Careful study of action potentials reveals that they are clearly biphasic and consist of a negative–positive sequence (Teas *et al.*, 1962). In Fig. 2.4 we demonstrate such an AP, and if the second negative peak, designated as N_2 (about which more will be said below), is ignored then it is clear that the potential is first negative and then becomes positive. There is no sign of an initial positivity. It is then reasonable to accept the hypothesis that the AP as recorded in the vicinity of the cochlea reflects neural activity emerging from the internal auditory meatus.

We have already intimated that the compound action potential is a manifestation of the *synchronous* firing of a large number of nerve fibers in the 8th nerve trunk. It was also mentioned that, in order to elicit such synchronous firing, relatively sharply defined temporal stimulus characteristics are required. It is appropriate to enlarge upon these concepts here and to refer to some considerations and studies by Goldstein and Kiang (1958). These authors pointed out that the firing of any given neuron is a probabilistic event. That is, at any given instant and under any given stimulus condition whether a neuron fires cannot be stated deterministically; instead, one can deduce a probability that a response would occur under the given condition. The actual probability depends on the past history of the neuron. Some heuristically derived probability density functions for different stimulus conditions are shown in Fig. 5.44. In section (a) the probability of firing as the function of time, $P(t)$, is shown following an impulselike stimulus. After a given latency there is a very high probability of response, manifested by the sharp peak in $P(t)$. After this peak there is a reduced probability of firing due to refractoriness of units that responded during the initial activity. After the refractory period the probability assumes a steady value, the same as it was before the stimulation. This value corresponds to the probability of spontaneous responses and is generally greater than zero. In panel (b) of the figure the probability of response to an abruptly turned on tone or noise burst is shown. Here the initial onset constitutes an event not unlike the click itself in that this sharp stimulus event is capable of synchronously exciting many neurons. As a consequence there is an initial sharp rise in the

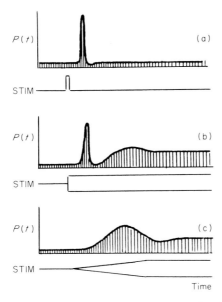

Fig. 5.44. The probability of firing, $P(t)$, for three stimulus time patterns. The upper function in each case is $P(t)$, and below this function, on the same time scale, there is a schematic representation of the stimulus. The time patterns are (a) click, (b) bursts of noise with fast onset, and (c) bursts of noise with slow onset. (Adapted from Goldstein and Kiang, 1958, p. 112.)

probability of response, again followed by a dip due to refractoriness. Here, however, the probability of firing does not return to the resting level but is maintained at a higher value as long as the stimulus is on, since the presence of the acoustic excitation does raise the probability of firing above the spontaneous level. In panel (c) of Fig. 5.44 the probability function associated with a gradually rising tone or noise burst is presented. Here the initial sharp stimulus event is missing, and consequently there is no abrupt rise in the probability of response at the onset. Instead there is a gradual increase in the probability of the firing as the acoustic conditions change from no stimulus to full stimulus strength.

If the waveform of the unit response (i.e., the potential change picked up by the recording electrode from a single active nerve fiber) is denoted by $U(t)$, and we make the assumptions that there are N units that contribute with equal weight at the electrode site, then the compound response can be computed with the aid of the convolution integral.

$$A(t) = N \int_{-\infty}^{t} P(\tau)U(t-\tau)d\tau \qquad (5.7)$$

The integration is performed over time and τ is a dummy variable. Teas et al. (1962), using an argument similar to the one just presented, have shown theoretical AP responses to clicks and to tone bursts. They assumed that the unit response $U(t)$ is biphasic and that the area under the negative phase is the same as that under the positive phase. With this assumption they deduced that AP activity should be observed in response to bursts of tones only at the onset and at the cessation of the stimuli. The potential should return to the base line during the presence of the stimulus. Had they assumed a monophasic unit response, they would have had to predict sustained AP activity during the duration of the stimulus in addition to the on and off transients. They actually demonstrated that no sustained activity could be found and considered this to be proof of the biphasic nature of the unit response. Actually Teas and colleagues used ac-coupled amplifiers with 0.01-second time constants, and it is rather questionable whether such a system could actually demonstrate sustained dc responses. As a matter of fact, dc level shifts can be clearly demonstrated with dc-coupled systems when the intracochlear electrode outputs are added to provide the average response (CM-canceling, AP-enhancing mode of recording) during tone bursts. It is highly unlikely, however, that what one sees under these conditions is AP. We have discussed this response in the previous section. It is the now-familiar AVE SP component that is positive in the highly excited region of the cochlea in opposition to the normal negative polarity of the AP.

Goldstein and Kiang (1958) provided experimental verification of their contention that sharply structured events in time are required to elicit significant AP. In Fig. 5.45 some of their results are shown. Here AP responses at the onset of tone bursts are presented for various rise times of the burst. Rise times ranged from 10 μseconds to 5 mseconds. One can very clearly see from the response traces that the AP magnitude decreases as the rise time increases. In fact when the rise time exceeds 5 mseconds there is no discernible onset AP. We know from single-unit studies (Kiang, 1965) that there is a great deal of spike activity during the presentation of a tone burst. Thus the ingredients of an AP are present in all stimulus conditions of Fig. 5.45, but these ingredients do not add up to a composite for the case with the long rise time because there is no synchronization of the unit activities in the many fibers of the nerve trunk.

We have mentioned that the AP is considered to be the summated activity of hundreds of nerve fibers firing essentially in synchrony. It is evident that from a circuit theory viewpoint the individual sources are connected in parallel. On that basis one would assume that the magnitude of response obtained from the entire parallel population would be equal to or somewhat less than the voltage output of a single generator. Since the outputs of all generators are essentially identical (the neural spike) one would expect to have on this basis a compound potential whose magnitude is largely inde-pendent of the number of contributing sources and hence independent of stimulus intensity. In reality the AP magnitude is finely graded and is a very direct function of stimulus strength. Davis (Stevens and Davis, 1938) addressed himself to this apparent contradiction and gave a most cogent explanation, which is presented here.

Davis pointed out that the fiber diameter in the auditory nerve is quite

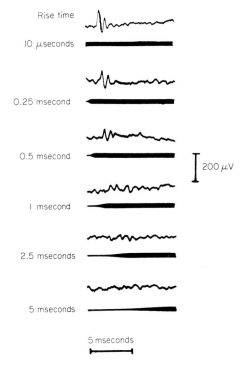

Fig. 5.45. Peripheral responses as a function of rise time of tone bursts. The intensity of the 8000-Hz tone bursts was 25 dB above visual detection level of the response. (From Goldstein and Kiang, 1958, p. 110.)

uniform, leading to uniform propagation velocity. As a consequence spikes traveling in all active fibers reach the point where AP is registered from at about the same instant. If the contributions of the individual fibers do summate, the magnitude of the AP is proportional to the number of active fibers. How do the responses summate? Davis cites two mechanisms. First, an active fiber travels in a bundle of other fibers. When these neighboring fibers are passive, their resistances are low and consequently they effectively shunt the electrical output of the active source. As more and more surrounding fibers become active they cease to act as passive shunting resistances and consequently the effective output of any one of the active fibers is increased. A more significant effect is due to the fact that in a volume conductor potential drops are observed and are directly proportional to current flowing in the conducting medium. The AP registered by the electrodes is a voltage drop across some effective cochlear resistance, and it is a consequence of current driven through that resistance by the source of the AP: discharges in the auditory nerve. The effective cochlear resistance is relatively low, certainly much lower than the source resistance of an elementary generator of AP, that is, of a nerve fiber. When more and more fibers are active the actual source resistance is reduced, with the consequence that the combined source is capable of delivering increased current to the external load. In fact, the ability to produce current is proportional to the number of active parallel sources, and thus the voltage drop across the effective resistance is also proportional to the number of parallel sources.

To put this argument on a somewhat more quantitative basis, in Fig. 5.46 a schema of parallel generators is shown. The internal resistance of any generator is r and the load resistance on the parallel combination is R. If the source voltage is e, then it is a relatively straightforward job to show that the voltage drop across R, which is denoted by E, can be expressed as

$$E = e \frac{n}{(r/R + n)} \tag{5.8}$$

where n is the number of parallel sections. Let us take the following not unreasonable values as an example: $r = 10^7 \Omega$, $R = 10^3 \Omega$, $n = 10^4$ V, $e = 10^{-3}$ V. These values correspond to a full-blown AP generated by the simultaneous firing of a very large fraction of the auditory nerve when the output of an individual fiber (extracellular potential) is taken as 1 mV. Substitution yields $E = 500 \mu$V, which is, as we shall see, of the appropriate magnitude. In Fig. 5.46 the magnitude of E is also plotted as the function of n, with the same arbitrary parameters as in the above example. It is notable that the registered compound voltage E is proportional to the number of active sources up to the highest numbers, where it asymptotically approaches the individual source voltage. We can apparently accept the general contention that the compound action potential magnitude is an excellent measure of the number of simultaneously active nerve fibers.

We have now seen some semiquantitative relationships between the magnitudes of single-unit discharges and the compound AP. Let us now inquire into timing relations between these two classes of potential. It is very widely assumed that the AP reflects the simultaneous firing of nerve fibers that innervate the basalmost portion of the cochlea. The reasoning behind this assumption is relatively simple. In order to build up a sizable AP, time synchrony among the individual sources is required. It is the basalmost portion of the basilar membrane that tends to vibrate in phase

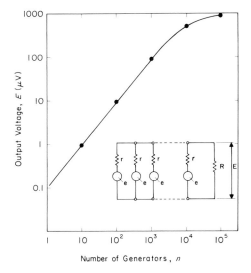

Fig. 5.46. Schema of parallel voltage sources feeding a common load resistance (*R*). Each source is assumed to have the same internal resistance, *r*, and the same nominal output, *e*. If the values $e = 10^{-3}$ V, $r = 10^7 \Omega$, and $R = 10^3 \Omega$ are assumed then the voltage across the load resistance as the function of the number of generators is shown in the graph.

for most effective stimuli, and consequently it is the nerve fibers originating in that region that tend to get stimulated in synchrony. Fibers originating from more apical regions are activated only after an appropriate traveling wave delay, which, as we have seen in Chapter 4, can be quite sizable, up to about 5 mseconds. This of course is considerably longer than the entire duration of the AP. On this basis it is reasonable to compare the firing patterns of fibers originating from the basal turn with the time course of the AP. The earliest such comparison was provided by Tasaki and Davis (1955). They noted clear correlation between N_1 and N_2 and unit responses. In a similar vein, but with more advanced recording and data processing techniques, Kiang (1965) has shown that it is the discharge of single fibers having high characteristic frequency (i.e., originating in the basal turn) that occur together with N_1. In Fig. 5.47 a series of poststimulus time histograms (number of spikes at any instant after the delivery of a stimulus) are compared with AP recordings obtained from the round window. For fibers having low characteristic frequency (originating far from the stapes) the unit discharges occur much later than the AP. The time delay is clearly associated with travel time on the cochlear partition. As the fiber's characteristic frequency is increased, there is closer and closer correspondence between the peak in the

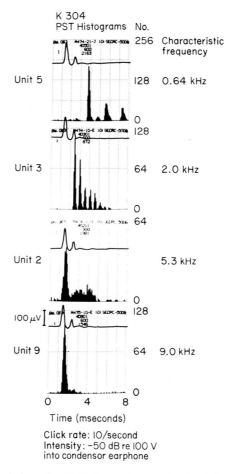

Fig. 5.47. The relation of unit discharges to neural potentials recorded at the round window for four units of differing characteristic frequencies. (From Kiang, 1965, p. 31.)

histogram and N_1. It is notable, however, that even the discharges of a fiber whose best frequency is 9000 Hz occur somewhat later than the peak of N_1. Kiang provides other examples as well. For example, in a fiber whose best frequency is 15 kHz, outstanding correspondence between the timing of the N_1 and the first peak in the histograms is seen for a wide variety of stimulus conditions. These examples strongly indicate that it is the initialmost segment of the cochlea whose response is primarily reflected in the N_1 component of the compound AP.

While the above-cited evidence indicates that it is probably a relatively narrow cochlear segment that is the primary contributor to the AP, there is evidence that more than the initial few millimeters of the cochlea are required for normal AP to develop. Davis (1961b) estimated that about half of the cochlea could be excited synchronously and thus might contribute to the AP. This would mean that approximately 10,000 fibers deriving from the initial 10 mm of the cochlea might fire more or less in unison in response to a very strong stimulus of appropriate frequency spectrum. Some interesting correlations between hair cell population and AP response can be gleaned from studies on sound-damaged guinea pig ears (Dallos and Bredberg, 1970). When guinea pigs are subjected to prolonged exposure to low-frequency tones of very high intensity then significant outer hair cell damage ensues with very little deterioration in the inner hair cell population. Hair cell counts obtained from surface preparations reveal damage configurations exemplified by Fig. 5.23. Note that in this cochlea the inner cells are almost 100% intact, while the outer hair cells are almost 100% missing between 6.0 and 18.4 mm. The sharpness of transition between intact and missing outer hair cell populations is particularly striking. Compound AP data in response to 8000-Hz tone pips were obtained from 15 animals with various degrees of hair cell loss. When compared to sensitivity norms (SPL at 10-μV AP magnitude) established on normal animals, excellent correlation between sensitivity shift and hair cell loss was found. In Fig. 5.48 the relationship is graphed. On the ordinate the length of the intact basal segment of outer hair cells is given, while on the abscissa the SPL required to elicit 10-μV AP is shown. We note that with the exception of one animal all data points scatter around a straight line. The median normal SPL required to reach the criterion AP magnitude is indicated by the dashed vertical line.

The important conclusion that one can draw from these data is that it requires an intact basal outer hair cell segment of 15 mm to achieve normal AP sensitivity. It should be emphasized that 15 mm is approximately three-fourths of the total length of the guinea pig cochlea. It would thus seem that a remarkably large segment of the cochlea must be intact if normal AP sensitivity is to be assured. Because of the previously discussed timing considerations, it is highly unlikely that all fibers originating from the first

15 mm do actually contribute to the AP response. It seems necessary, however, that all hair cells in these initial 15 mm that are innervated by the fibers be present. One is tempted to speculate that in order for the fibers from the first few millimeters, which probably do provide the actual voltage that is signified by the compound AP, to function normally, this segment must somehow be facilitated by the rest of the operating hair cells. In other words, the results indicate that there is a strong possibility that longitudinal interaction among hair cells or dendritic zones is in existence over wide cochlear regions.

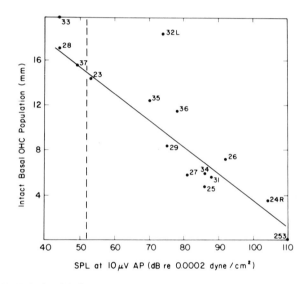

Fig. 5.48. Relationship between the SPL required to generate a 10-μV AP at the onset of 8000-Hz tone bursts and the extent of intact basal outer hair cell population. Outer hair cells were destroyed by prolonged exposure to a loud low-frequency tone. The type of damage that occurs is demonstrated in the cochleogram of Fig. 5.23. The animal whose cochleogram is shown in Fig. 5.23 is identified in this figure as no. 27. The vertical dashed line is the median SPL at 10-μV AP for a group of normal guinea pigs. (From Dallos and Bredberg, 1970.)

We have established the identity and likely source of the N_1 component of the compound AP, and it is appropriate now to consider the later components, N_2 and N_3. In response to clicks and at the onset of tone or noise bursts, after the characteristic N_1 response, additional negative potentials can often be seen. These negative deflections have essentially the same waveform as N_1 but they are smaller in magnitude. Between N_1 and the second negative potential N_2, there is a time delay of approximately 1 msecond, and if a third deflection follows, designated as N_3, it is separated from N_2 by an additional 1 msecond. The magnitude of N_3 is invariably smaller than that of N_2, and this third component is quite often absent from the response. There has been a great deal of speculation concerning the source of origin of N_2 and N_3; these have been considered to be either the compound responses from the cochlear nucleus or the results of multiple firing of the primary neurons. The second explanation appears to be more realistic. Tasaki (1954) presented some correlations between single-unit discharges and AP. He noted a parallelism between the size of N_2 and the probability of obtaining double discharges from single primary neurons. When the stimulus condition was such that more than one spike was frequently elicited from the nerve fibers, the size of N_2 was considerable. Conversely, when most responses from the single fiber consisted of one spike per stimulus presentation then the N_2 was small. It is noteworthy that the time delay between N_1 and N_2 (approximately 1 msecond) corresponds well with the refractory period of neural units.

In the following pages the dependence of the AP on stimulus characteristics is discussed. First, the magnitude and latency of the N_1 component as the function of signal intensity is examined, and then the AP magnitude is considered as a function of stimulus repetition rate. The waveform of the N_1–N_2 complex is quite similar when the eliciting stimulus is a discrete click, or the onset of noise or tone bursts. The following discussion of AP input–output functions thus could be based on any of these stimuli. It is important to note, as we shall demonstrate in detail later, that when the stimuli cannot be considered discrete, that is, when they are repeated with relatively small interstimulus interval, then both waveform and magnitude changes are seen in the AP. Consequently the discussion assumes discrete stimulation.

In Fig. 5.49 a typical input–output function for N_1 is given together with the interquartile ranges obtained from 18 normal animals. These data represent responses obtained from guinea pig basal-turn recordings (AVE mode, i.e., CM-canceling arrangement) with 8000-Hz tone bursts as the stimuli. The abscissa is stimulus sound pressure level, while the ordinate is N_1 magnitude. The first observation is that there is a very real threshold for the AP below which no response is detectable. For our representative animal this threshold occurs at 33 dB SPL. Above threshold the response rises quite rapidly but decelerates and reaches a plateau approximately 50 dB above threshold. Beyond the plateau there is an actual dip in the magnitude for many animals. The response, however, recovers and a secondary rise is then seen.

The shape of the input–output function strongly suggests that two independent processes might contribute to the response. To demonstrate this possibility, Davis (1961b) replotted one of his AP input–output functions in

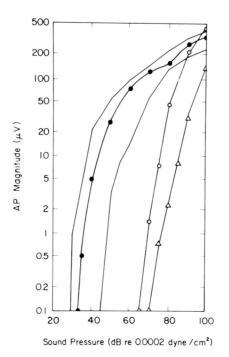

Fig. 5.49. Whole-nerve action potential magnitude as the function of stimulus level. Interquartile range and the response of one representative animal (●) are shown. The stimulus is a tone burst of 8000 Hz and rapid rise time. Recording is from a pair of electrodes; AVE = (SV + ST)/2 is given from the basal turn of guinea pig cochleas; $N = 18$. Also included are two "recruiting" AP input–output functions. One pathological animal (sound-damaged ear, ○) has a cochleogram very similar to the one shown in Fig. 5.23; it is designated as no. 29 in Fig. 5.48 (from Dallos and Bredberg, 1970). The second animal (kanamycin intoxication, △) has no outer hair cells over the basal 10 mm of the cochlea; its inner hair cells are virtually normal.

a semilogarithmic coordinate system. His plot is reproduced in Fig. 5.50. In the top segment of the figure the voltage increments obtained over successive 5-dB steps in the stimulus are also plotted, and this graph clearly reveals that the total response is made up as the sum of three component populations (remember that AP magnitude is proportional to the number of active units). The first population represents a group of sensitive neurons that respond at low intensities and thus determine the AP threshold. This group saturates and ceases to provide any incremental contribution by 75–80 dB SPL. At that level, however, a second less sensitive group begins to contribute substantially to the total response. This less sensitive group is apparently composed of a larger number of fibers than the first group, for it is seen to provide the large voltage magnitudes that characterize the high-intensity response. There is apparently even a third group of neurons that becomes active at extremely high levels, above 100 dB SPL. Davis assumes that these neurons are representative of fibers not originating in the basal half of the cochlea and thus normally are of no significance in the AP response. In Fig. 5.49 this third response region is not evident since we did not show responses above 100 dB SPL.

The two neural populations, showing low and high thresholds, respectively, have been identified both with outer versus inner hair cells and with row 1

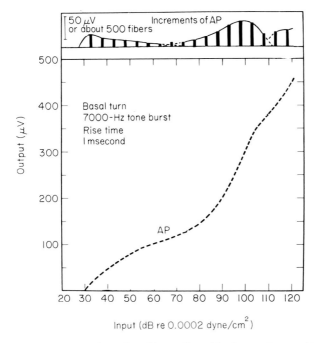

Fig. 5.50. Input–output data plotted in semilogarithmic coordinates. Above are shown the increments of AP voltage for successive 5-dB increases in SPL. Three populations of neurons seem to be present. The population with very high thresholds (above 110 dB SPL) undoubtedly contains many neurons that do not arise in the basal turn. The calibration bar for voltage (50 μV) is estimated to correspond to about 500 nerve fibers. (From Davis, 1961b, p. 134.)

versus rows 2 and 3 of the outer hair cells (Davis, 1961b). Some of our data on sound-damaged guinea pigs support the differentiation according to outer and inner hair cells (Dallos, and Bredberg, 1970). We have noted that concomitant with the deterioration of the basal outer hair cell population the AP threshold shifts toward higher and higher intensities. This is demonstrated in Fig. 5.48. At the same time the maximal AP magnitude is not significantly affected. In Fig. 5.49 a demonstration of this phenomenon is given by comparing the AP magnitude function obtained from a damaged ear (virtually normal inner hair cells, severe outer hair cell loss beyond the first 7 mm of the cochlea) with a characteristic normal curve and normal interquartile range.

We can observe that considerable threshold shift occurred in this animal, but once threshold is reached the AP magnitude undergoes an accelerated growth and it reaches normal size around 90 dB SPL. In this preparation all three outer hair cell rows suffered essentially identical damage, while the inner hair cells were in excellent condition (as determined by light microscopy). Thus it is logical to assign the low-threshold population (more or less missing in this example) to fibers that are innervating the outer hair cells, and the high-threshold population to those connected to inner hair cells. The threshold difference between the two populations appears to be of the order of 40–50 dB. The maximal voltages provided by the two populations are approximately in a ratio of $1:5–1:6$. This might be taken as a crude estimate of the ratio of the number of fibers that innervate outer and inner hair cells. This ratio points in the direction of some findings of Spoendlin (1966), who estimated that in the cat about 90 % of the fibers innervate inner hair cells and only 10 % innervate outer hair cells. This ratio is most likely to be smaller in guinea pigs. Thus the electrophysiological measure seems to support the unexpected result that the majority of fibers that compose the 8th nerve do innervate the inner hair cells.

In addition to the AP input–output function obtained from a sound-damaged ear, in Fig. 5.49 another abnormal function from a kanamycin-intoxicated ear is included. The histological workup on this ear revealed that the inner hair cells were all virtually normal but that the outer hair cells were completely missing in the basal 10 mm of the cochlea. The AP input–output function shows a threshold shift similar to that from the sound-damaged ear and it grows at a similar accelerated rate. The major difference between the two types of pathological functions is that in the kanamycin-damaged ear the AP magnitude does not achieve normal values at the highest intensities, while in the sound-damaged ear it does. Apparently threshold changes of the AP are very well correlated with basal outer hair cell population. Moreover, it seems that if some outer hair cells do remain intact and the inner hair cell population is in good condition, then complete "recruitment" of the AP function can be achieved, while only partial "recruitment" is possible if no outer hair cells remain in the basal segment of the cochlea.

To complete the discussion on the dependence of N_1 on stimulus intensity we shall now examine the effect of stimulus strength on response latency. Figure 5.51 shows a combined input–output and latency function taken from the work of Kiang *et al.* (1962). The magnitude function shows the familiar two segments, and interestingly so does the latency function. In general as stimulus intensity is increased the time lag between N_1 and the onset of the sound decreases. The decreasing function clearly possesses two ranges, which meet where the high-threshold process begins to dominate the response.

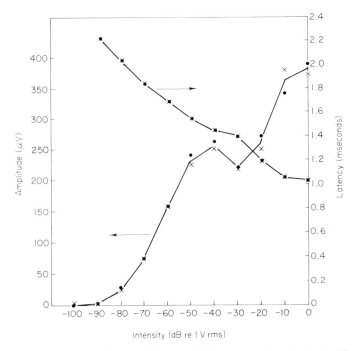

Fig. 5.51. Amplitude and latency of averaged N_1 responses to noise bursts. Magnitude is measured between first negative and first positive peaks, and latency is measured from stimulus onset to the peak of N_1. Measurement taken as intensity increased, ● ; decreased, X. (From Kiang *et al.*, 1962, p. 119.)

Thus far we have been considering the properties of AP in response to discrete stimuli, that is, in a situation where the presentation of stimuli is so arranged in time that there is no interaction between the responses to adjacent input signals. A very legitimate and important question concerns the case in which stimuli are presented in such proximity that their responses interact. How do the waveform and magnitude of the compound AP change with stimulus repetition rate? In Fig. 5.52 averaged AP responses to 0.1-msecond noise bursts at various repetition rates are presented. The top trace, obtained with one burst per second, can be considered as the baseline to which other responses are to be compared. With this low repetition rate the individual stimuli can be considered as truly discrete. The response shows the now-familiar N_1 peak followed by a positive peak (P_1) and by N_2. The latter in this case is composed of two subpeaks, a situation often seen. The waveform and magnitude of the response at a repetition rate of 10/second are in no way different from the 1/second AP. At 100/second, however, the response magnitude is diminished, even though the waveform is virtually unchanged. As one further increases the repetition rate, profound changes in both waveform and magnitude occur. The response at 1000/second clearly illustrates the point: The magnitude is down (note the increased number of samples) and the interaction between adjacent response complexes renders

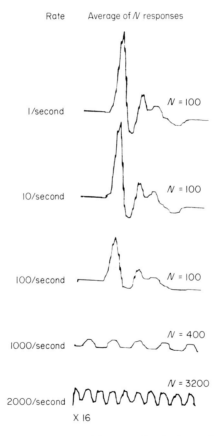

Fig. 5.52. Averaged responses to 0.1-msecond noise bursts for several repetition rates. Number of responses averaged, N; sweep duration, 5 mseconds; peak-to-peak amplitude of the 1/second response, approximately 100 μV; stimulus intensity, 35 dB re visual detection. Note that the gain is increased by 16 in the bottom trace. (From Peake *et al.*, 1962, p. 566.)

the waveform almost sinusoidal. At even higher repetition rates the waveform does not alter substantially, but the magnitude rapidly diminishes. For the trace shown at 2000/second both the number of samples and the system gain had to be increased as indicated to make the trace presentable. In general the upper limit of resolvable AP response is under 3000 repetitions per second, but occasionally responses are as high as 5000/second.

The study of the functional relationship between AP magnitude and stimulus repetition rate provides more than just theoretical interest. One must realize that one of the most important "repetitive" signals is comprised of pure tones, and the AP response to these can be inferred from the previously discussed data. The individual cycles of a sinusoidal stimulus do act as discrete stimuli if the frequency is low enough, and compound action potentials that appear in response to every cycle of the stimulus have been identified as long as the AP itself has. We gave some examples of such stimulus-locked AP in Chapter 2 (Fig. 2.6). The AP can normally be recorded together with CM in response to pure tones. It can clearly be recognized at very low frequencies, but between approximately 700 and 1500 Hz the AP and CM waveforms are quite similar and purely visual separation of the two is tenuous. In this frequency region the AP can considerably influence both magnitude and phase of the composite potential that is recorded from the round window or from intracochlear electrodes. It is very important that this fact be realized by experimenters who wish to study either CM or AP but not the indiscriminate mixture of the two.

The fact that neural responses can be observed up to 3000–4000 Hz gave rise to voluminous speculations on both the mechanism of this high-rate neural potential and its significance in auditory theory. The mechanism was subject to speculation, for it was well known that single auditory nerve fibers cannot sustain discharge rates in excess of approximately 200/second. The question thus arose as to how a nerve trunk can perform a feat that none of its constituent fibers can, that is, how it can respond repetitively at rates in excess of a few hundred cycles per second. A widely accepted explanation was provided by Wever (1949) in his famous "Volley" theory. Single auditory neurons that are responding to low-frequency sinusoidal stimulation tend to discharge on a particular phase of the cycle. This phenomenon is examined in more detail below; here only the simple fact is of importance. The phase locking of any given fiber to the stimulus insures that even if the fiber does not respond on every single cycle, when it does respond, the interspike interval is always an integral multiple of the signal period. Assuming that a large number of fibers are responsive to a particular sinusoidal signal, one can immediately see that there are always some fibers that respond on any one particular cycle. To explain, any given fiber might respond only to every fifth or tenth cycle of the stimulus, but there are always a sufficient number of fibers that respond in a given instant. In fact there is some reason to assume on a statistical basis that the population of responding fibers group fairly evenly and that in any given cycle the number of active fibers is about the same as that in any other cycle. The response is thus contributed by an "alternation" (Pumphrey and Rawdon-Smith, 1936) of active fibers.

Clearly, as the frequency of the stimulus is increased, the total population must be divided into more and more subgroups of periodically discharging fibers. The result of this is the reduction in the magnitude of the compound action potential, which as we have already seen is simply proportional to the number of simultaneously active neurons. At higher frequencies not only the magnitude of the AP decreases, thus contributing to the disappearance of the response, but in addition the synchrony between single-unit responses and stimulus also deteriorates. This phenomenon is not unexpected since the single neural spike is not a mathematical impulse in appearance but possesses a finite width. Clearly when this width becomes commensurate with the signal period, precise synchronization between the two might be difficult. Even more important is the fact that neural discharges do not constitute a deterministic mechanism; instead, a neuron fires with a certain probability for a given stimulus. There is in consequence some jitter in the timing of the spikes in relation to the point in time on the stimulus when firing is expected. Such indeterminacy in time is not very significant when the range of jitter is small compared to the stimulus period. When the two are comparable, however, it is not possible to maintain synchronism.

These considerations indicate that volleying in the auditory nerve should cease at a certain frequency; the experimental evidence places the frequency limit between 4000 and 5000 Hz. The fact that groups of nerve fibers are capable of providing phase-locked discharges at low audio frequencies provides the basis of the frequency theory (Wever, 1949), or of the duplex theory (Licklider, 1951), of hearing. According to these, at least at the lower portion of the audio range frequency information is conveyed to the higher auditory centers by the 8th nerve in the *timing* of neural volleys.

Not only is it possible to show that AP responses are time locked to the cycle of low-frequency sinusoidal stimuli, but it has been determined that excitation of AP occurs when the CM generated by the stimulus goes negative in the scala vestibuli (Rosenblith and Rosenzweig, 1952; Tasaki, 1954) or, the equivalent, when the acoustic wave at the eardrum is in its rarefaction phase (Davis *et al.*, 1950). Peake and Kiang (1962) verified these findings by comparing responses to condensation and rarefaction clicks. They noted that the latency of N_1 was shorter for rarefaction clicks, at least at high stimulus levels.

Rarefaction at the drum and negative CM in scala vestibuli can be thus considered the excitatory phase of the stimulus. Under these excitatory conditions the current through the organ of Corti that generates the CM flows from scala media to scala tympani. Tasaki and Fernández (1952) showed that when the quiescent current flow is enhanced by electrical polarization of the cochlear partition (i.e., by making scala vestibuli positive with respect to scala tympani) then both CM and AP are enhanced. If motion of the basilar membrane that corresponds to rarefaction at the drum leads to excitation of auditory nerve fibers, it is likely that motion in the opposite direction would yield a reduction in neural activity. Kiang (1965) actually demonstrated this by studying the changes in single-unit responses with rarefaction and condensation clicks. It could be shown that the condensation phase actually inhibits spontaneous neural activity in primary fibers.

The last topic to be discussed in this section pertains to the influence on the AP, elicited by a given acoustic stimulus, of the presence of another, so-called masking stimulus. Actually, this inquiry is very important since pure tones or clicks are rather abstract auditory signals. In nature input signals are always present as mixtures of a variety of components, and thus it is rather important to know how our responses to the usual standard stimuli are influenced by the presence of other input signals. It was noted very early in the study of auditory neural responses (Derbyshire and Davis, 1935) that the presence of a tone or a hiss can very effectively reduce the magnitude of click-evoked action potentials. Since the relative frequency compositions and intensities of the masked and masking signals profoundly affect the degree of masking, it is not very productive to review in detail the many experimental findings in this area. Teas *et al.* (1962) and Teas and Henry (1969) did extensive parametric studies on selective masking procedures using narrow bands of noise as the masker and brief transients as the maskee. The results indicate that the AP, or segments of it, can be reduced or completely eliminated by masking noise.

To explain the physiological substrate of masking, the early experimenters assumed that a "line busy" effect was operating. This was meant to describe a phenomenon whereby responses to the masking noise would preempt the available fibers, which consequently could no longer respond to the primary stimulus. In other words, it was assumed that the general activity in the nerve was raised by the noise and that this activity overshadowed that due to the signal. Experiments on single-unit responses conclusively disproved this contention (Kiang, 1965; Hind *et al.*, 1967; Brugge *et al.*, 1969). It was found that activity due to the masker does not increase to overshadow the response to the signal; instead the latter response decreases with increasing of the masker intensity. The effect is very similar to one that would be caused by a simple reduction in the stimulus strength. For example, in Fig. 5.53 PST histograms are shown in response to tone bursts at various background noise levels. Note that as the masker intensity is increased the activity corresponding to the tone burst is gradually diminished. This change takes place without an increase in spike rate in the fiber and without an overall increase in the total number of spikes. The line busy effect thus cannot operate. Apparently masking is brought about, not by a saturation of the nerve fiber by responses to the masker, but by the fiber assuming a response

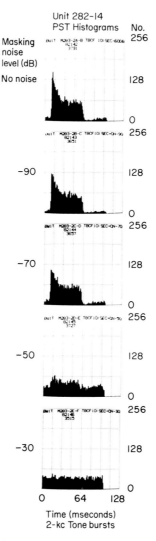

Fig. 5.53. Masking of single-unit responses to tone bursts by broad-band noise. Each histogram represents 1 minute of data. (From Kiang, 1965, p. 109.)

pattern that is characteristic of the masker as opposed to the maskee. That this is the case can be seen with great clarity in cases of two-tone interaction (Hind *et al.*, 1967). When a low-frequency tone is presented, an auditory nerve fiber responds periodically, in a phase-locked fashion with the stimulating tone. The response of this fiber to another low-frequency tone is similar, and the average periodicity now corresponds to this second tone. When both tones are present together the response simply reflects the algebraic summation of the two component tones. If one is considerably bigger, the neural periodicities correspond to it alone. Here then masking is produced by the masker preventing the fiber from producing its time-locked response to the maskee.

VI. Experimental Manipulation of Cochlear Potentials

The number of reported studies on various alterations of the responses of the inner ear by means of experimental modifications of cochlear function is truly astounding. In this section, only a minute, and probably quite capriciously selective, portion of this literature is reviewed. Topics of interest are the effects of anoxia, pressure and changes in cochlear temperature and in ionic concentration of the cochlear fluids.

A. ANOXIA

Oxygen deprivation radically affects all cochlear potentials Anoxic conditions can be created a variety of ways such as clamping the trachea, having the animal rebreathe the expired air, respiration with air having reduced oxygen concentration or with pure nitrogen. All these methods create an oxygen deficiency and affect cochlear potentials. Probably the best method of inducing anoxia in the cochlea allows the maintenance of the general physiological state of the animal undisturbed. Clearly the above techniques do not conform to this requirement. Anoxic conditions can be produced locally by occluding the anterior inferior cerebellar artery and thus interrupting the cochlear blood flow (Perlman *et al.*, 1951). Such a technique was used by Konishi *et al.* (1961) in their study of cochlear anoxia. The effect on the various potentials of inhibiting the blood flow is quite rapid and dramatic. On the average it takes 36 seconds for the EP to drop from its high positive value to zero. Upon reaching zero the EP does not stay at this level but reverses polarity and becomes increasingly negative. This negativity reaches its maximum value about 5 minutes after the onset of arterial occlusion; this value can be as great as -70 mV, but the median negative maximum is -47.5 mV. After the potential reaches a negative maximum it slowly returns to zero.

After the oxygen supply is reestablished the EP completely recovers.

Such complete recovery was seen by Konishi *et al.* (1961) even after arterial occlusion lasting 50 minutes. The recovery curve is quite interesting. As Fig. 5.54 shows, the initial recovery is rapid and is accompanied by a period of supernormality. The occurrence of supernormality seems to correlate well with the duration of occlusion; that is, after the return of oxygen it takes longer to reach supernormal EP if the occlusion was of longer duration. However, the magnitude of supernormality apparently does not correlate well with the duration of oxygen deprivation. It is interesting that supernormality can follow even 50 minutes of arterial occlusion.

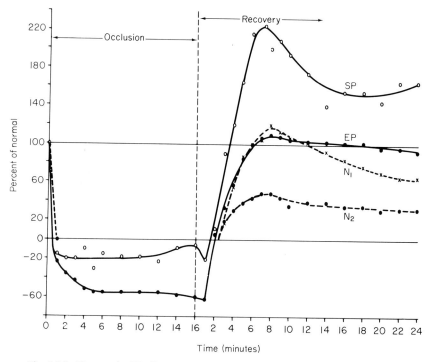

Fig. 5.54. Changes in EP, SP, N_1, and N_2 that occurred during and after a 16-minute anoxic interval. (From Konishi *et al.*, 1961, p. 354.)

Changes in the measured EP can occur through either of two mechanisms. First, the alteration of cochlear function can directly affect the source of the EP, the stria vascularis, and, second, the alteration can modify the load resistance on the source and thus change the measured voltage. It appears that anoxia influences both the source and the load. The radical changes in both magnitude and polarity of the EP under anoxic conditions are difficult to explain with simple resistance changes alone. It is most likely that in interfering with the metabolic functioning of the stria the anoxia radically influences the source. On the other hand, we know (Johnstone *et al.*, 1966) that the effective load resistance as measured in the scala media does change during anoxia. Interestingly, this resistance first decreases, then as EP turns negative it begins to increase again, and in fact it becomes supernormal. The overall change in EP under these conditions is likely to manifest the simultaneous alteration in both source output and load resistance. It is quite possible that the apparent supernormality of EP after anoxia is correlated with increased load resistance and smaller load current.

We have already acquainted ourselves with the course of CM after death. The most conspicuous feature of the change in CM is an initial precipitous drop followed by a very slow decrease in the residual CM. The component that decreases immediately upon the expiration of the animal is thought to be of different origin (CM_1) than the component that lingers on (CM_2). The two components are often designated as aerobic and anaerobic. The study of Konishi *et al.* (1961) on local cochlear anoxia also provided interesting information on the behavior of CM and SP under such conditions. They studied the CM magnitude in response to an approximately 90-dB-SPL 9400-Hz tone pip, recorded from the first turn of a guinea pig cochlea with differential electrodes as the function of time of anoxia and time of recovery. It was observed that the CM plateaus at about 10% of its normal value within 2 minutes after the initiation of occlusion. When the blood flow is reinstated the CM returns close to its normal value but does not always reach it. This observation is significant, because *all* other potentials, EP, SP, and AP, show varying periods of supernormality after the return of normal oxygen supply. The CM recovery apparently depends on the duration of occlusion; the shorter it is the better the possibility of a full CM restoration.

The experiments of Konishi *et al.* (1961) investigated the effect of anoxia on the negative SP. It is important to keep in mind here, and in the discussions on experimental modifications of the SP, that in virtually all reported experiments the stimulus parameters were such that only one aspect of the complex SP phenomenon was investigated. In general, high-intensity, "standard" stimuli produce a negative potential drop across the cochlear partition, and this SP^- has been the subject of most investigations. In the results of Konishi *et al.* (1961) the behavior of the SP^- during anoxia proved to be somewhat erratic and less uniform than that of the other potentials. Upon occlusion of the blood flow the SP immediately declined and in most instances its polarity changed from negative to positive in about 40–60 seconds. During long-term anoxia, the SP, unlike EP and CM, did not reach an asymptotic value; instead it fluctuated around the zero point in a seemingly random manner. As Fig. 5.54 demonstrates, the rapid recovery of SP during the first few seconds after the restoration of oxygen availability parallels that of the other potentials. In contrast with EP and CM the SP shows large but variable supernormality. The magnitude of the SP reaches 6–10 times its normal value on occasion. The most interesting observation on the effect of anoxia, first noted by Goldstein (1954), is undoubtedly the polarity reversal during the early state of anoxia. While such polarity shift was also seen for EP, the time courses for the two potentials are poorly correlated. It is important to remember that these findings apply to the SP produced in the basal turn by the standard 9400-Hz, approximately 90-dB-SPL tone pip. There is apparently no information available on whether the SP^- polarity reversal during anoxia is accompanied by an SP^+ polarity change. There is of course no information as yet on the behavior of the AVE SP component under such experimental conditions.

Among the many experimental modifications of inner ear function that influence the AP, cochlear anoxia (in extreme form, death) has the most profound effect. Within seconds after the onset of the anoxic period the compound AP disappears completely. This is in contrast with the behavior of various cochlear potentials, all of which are changed by oxygen deprivation but not with such abruptness. All other potentials, CM, SP, and EP, undergo gradual changes and alterations during anoxia; these are systematic varia-tions, lasting many minutes. When oxygen supply is restored to the cochlea, the AP, along with other cochlear potentials, returns to near normal value. In Fig. 5.54 the time course of the change of N_1 and N_2 is also included. The N_1 component, after a brief supernormality, stabilizes at about 60% of its preocclusion value, while N_2 is apparently more fragile, its final value being approximately 30%. Apparently some recovery of N_1 can be seen even after long periods of oxygen deprivation, lasting up to 40 minutes (Konishi et al., 1961). The profound influence of oxygen availability on AP is most likely a manifestation of the sensitivity of the spike initiation process to oxygen lack, as opposed to that of the ability of fibers to maintain propagated discharges.

B. INTRACOCHLEAR PRESSURE

Small pressures (10 cm H_2O), whether static or dynamic, cause very little change in the CM. According to Butler and Honrubia (1963) such changes amount to reductions of less than 20%. Allen et al. (1971) studied both short- and long-term effects of static pressure changes at higher levels upon the CM. They increased pressure by forcing saline into the perilym-phatic space without providing an outflow hole in the cochlea. When pressure is repeatedly applied and removed, significant magnitude changes in the CM occur but these decrements are completely reversible. The pressure effects are frequency dependent. As Fig. 5.55 shows, low frequencies are more influenced than the higher frequencies. In fact the results appear to be dichotomized in that the three lower test frequencies show a level shift with pressure change of approximately 2.4 dB/cm Hg, while the three higher frequencies shift only 1.2 dB/cm Hg. When increased perilymphatic pressure is maintained for significant time duration, CM sensitivity gradually diminishes and this process becomes irreversible. In Fig. 5.56 results are shown for one cat during and after prolonged application of 10 cm Hg pressure. The major loss occurs immediately after pressure application, and

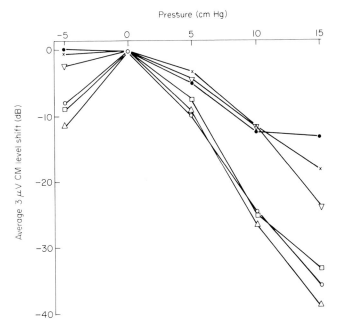

Fig. 5.55. Average shift in the SPL that is required to elicit 3-μV CM in the cat at different frequencies as a function of intracochlear pressure. Frequency (hertz): ◯, 250; △, 500; ▢, 1000; ▼, 2000; X, 4000; ●, 8000. (From Allen *et al.*, 1971, p. 390.)

this loss has the previously discussed property of being more marked at the low frequencies. During the maintenance of pressure the loss curves parallel one another at all frequencies. After 60 minutes the losses vary from 60 dB at low frequencies to 30 dB at high frequencies. When pressure is removed, some recovery is usually seen at all frequencies but it is always more pronounced at the low frequencies. It appears that the prolonged pressure application results in a frequency-independent loss of about 30 dB in this case.

It is likely that the short-term effects that are frequency dependent and that do recover completely are the consequences of simple mechanical modification of the cochlear hydrodynamics. The pressure probably results in an overall increase in stiffness, particularly in the window region. The long-term effects do not seem to be frequency dependent. They are probably correlated with hair cell damage, conceivably due to anoxia resulting from blood vessel collapse. It is certain from histological findings that prolonged pressure application does not cause any dramatic changes, such as membrane ruptures, and that the causes of the losses are more subtle.

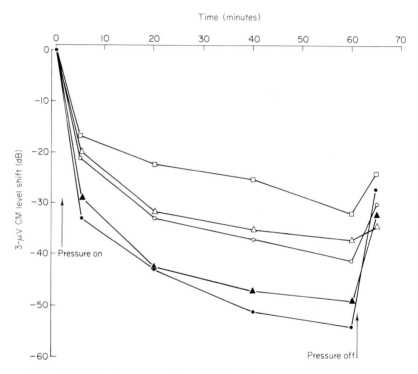

Fig. 5.56. Shift in the SPL that is required to elicit 3-μV CM in one cat at different frequencies as a function of time during the sustained application of 10 cm Hg intracochlear pressure. Frequency (hertz): ●, 500; ▲, 1000; △, 2000; ○, 4000; □, 8000. (From Allen *et al.*, 1971, p. 394.)

Tasaki *et al.* (1954) investigated the effect of increased perilymphatic pressure on the dc resting potential by pushing Ringer's solution into either scala tympani or scala vestibuli through a hole in the cochlear wall and letting the fluid escape through another hole in the contrary scala. Thus they produced dynamic pressure in the perilymph. Such momentary pressure increase in either scala has the effect of displacing the entire cochlear partition toward the other scala. Tasaki *et al.* noted that when fluid was injected into scala vestibuli the endocochlear potential increased (became more positive), but upon injection into scala tympani the EP was reduced. When isotonic KCl solution was forced into the scala media through a micropipette, an increase in EP was noted. These experiments indicated that the magnitude of the EP was clearly correlated with the displacement of the cochlear partition; that is, movement toward the scala tympani increased EP, while movement toward scala vestibuli decreased it. From this evidence Tasaki *et al.* concluded that the EP must originate in a structure that moves with the basilar membrane. They specifically ruled out the vascular stria since it is not displaced by pressure application. We now know that these conclusions are not correct, but the findings of course still stand.

The simplest explanation, which has been suggested as a possible mechanism in SP and CM generation also, appears to be as follows. The stria vascularis is the source of the EP. This biological battery sets up an electrical current flow pattern through the scala media, organ of Corti, basilar membrane, and scala tympani, with the blood stream as the return circuit. As Hallpike and Rawdon-Smith (1937) and von Békésy (1952) suggested, if a biological battery is available and a membrane can be found which changes its resistance upon mechanical stimulation, then the production of stimulus-related potentials in the cochlea can be explained. Davis perfected this resistance modulation scheme (1965); he assumed that the EP is the battery and that the variable resistance elements are the hair cells. We can consider the stria vascularis as a voltage source of finite internal resistance that provides a potential difference across an external load resistance. This load is of course the combined resistance of the entire organ of Corti, basilar membrane, scala tympani, etc., connecting path and also includes many shunting resistances. We measure the EP in the scala media, which is the junction point (point M in Fig. 5.57) between the internal source resistance and the load resistance. Now consider the potential at this point M when the load resistance R_L changes. From Ohm's law we can easily compute that

$$E_M = E_S \frac{R_L}{R_L + R_S} = E_S \frac{1}{1 + R_S/R_L} \tag{5.9}$$

In Fig. 5.57 the value of E_M/E_S is also plotted as the function of R_S/R_L. It is very clear that the measured voltage can be grossly influenced by the load on the source. We do not a priori know the value of either E_S^* (remember that the approximately $+70$- to $+100$-mV EP is denoted by E_M) or R_S, but most likely in the quiescent state the system is at a point on the steep initial section of the curve; assume that this is point Q. Then if R_L varies

---

* See, however, Section III,A,2,*b* for more information.

about its resting value, E_M will change with it. The variation in both is relatively small, probably only a few percent, as indicated by the ranges drawn in the figure. The important idea is that, if *anywhere* within the cochlea there is a structure or membrane that is in the current path and whose resistance changes with sound stimulation or with artificial deformation of the basilar membrane, then the measured EP will change due to the load change on the stria vascularis source. This simple scheme shows that it is perfectly acceptable to have the potential source in the stria in spite of the experimental evidence of Tasaki *et al.* The critical issue is that the apparent potential measured in the scala media changes, depending on the loading effect of the cochlear resistance.

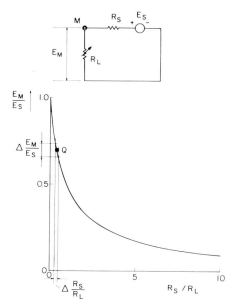

Fig. 5.57. Top: A simple network model depicting the relationship between a voltage source and the measured voltage across the load resistance. Bottom: Plot of the ratio of load voltage and source voltage (E_M/E_S) as a function of the ratio of the source resistance and load resistance (R_S/R_L). It is assumed that the system is operating around the quiescent point Q.

If pressure is applied to the cochlear fluids then significant changes in SP can be noted. Davis and colleagues (1958a) summarized experimental findings obtained when pressure changes were effected by intraaural muscle contraction, increased air pressure in the ear canal, or fluid injection into a cochlear scala, by stating that increased pressure in scala vestibuli causes an increase in the positivity of the scala media, while increased pressure in scala tympani reduces the positivity of the scala media. Butler and Honrubia (1963) corroborated these findings. These authors created a hydrodynamic pressure increase in the cochlea by forcing fluid into one scala and letting it escape through a small hole drilled into the other scala. The flow of fluid displaced the cochlear partition in a direction that depended on the inflow and outflow positions. When measured in scala media the SP increased up to 10 cm H_2O pressure in scala vestibuli and decreased for higher pressures. With the pressure applied to the scala tympani the SP decreased with increasing pressure and reversed its sign at about 10 cm H_2O. Changes in SP magnitude with pressure are quite similar to changes in EP. Misrahy *et al.* (1957) made several observations on factors that affect the SP. They concluded that the major influence on the summating potential is distortion within the cochlea. They noted than any alteration in the cochlear fluid dynamics created changes in either the magnitude or sign of the SP or in both. One interesting observation of Misrahy *et al.* was that when small holes were drilled in the cochlea of the guinea pig the SP^- was effectively sensitized. Allen and Habibi (1962) noted reversal of SP polarity in cats under conditions of pure intracochlear pressure increase (increased cerebrospinal fluid pressure) without concomitant displacement of the cochlear partition.

C. TEMPERATURE

Butler *et al.* (1960) studied the effect of temperature changes on various cochlear potentials. They found that in response to brief tone bursts (approximately 80 dB SPL, at 8000 Hz) the CM magnitude decreased in an orderly fashion as cochlear temperature was lowered. When plotted against log temperature, the CM change gave a straight-line plot. Over a 10°C range the drop in CM amounted to some 6 dB. The shape of the CM input–output functions was not changed by hypothermia; all values merely shifted down by approximately the same amount. One important consideration is that temperature changes were obtained by reducing the entire body temperature with an ice pack. Coats (1965) carried out a similar experiment, but he maintained constant body temperature and reduced only the cochlear temperature with the aid of a small cold probe. He found very minimal changes in CM over a wide (50°C) temperature range. He recorded from the round window of cats and his stimuli were clicks. Since the click intensity used was apparently relatively low and produced a small CM to begin with, it is difficult to tell how easily changes in the CM could have been detected. At any rate, the Coats study shows very minute effects of temperature on CM; the Butler *et al.* study does show more systematic, but still small, effects. Significantly, both studies show greater effects on AP, and Butler *et al.* also indicate qualitatively different effects on SP.

Apparently hypothermia changes the AP in a relatively complex manner In Fig. 5.58 data from Butler *et al.* (1960) are shown. The AP (N_1) input–output functions are given for three cochlear temperatures, normal, 5°, and 10°C below normal. The normal function is in the now-familiar two-segment configuration indicating the interaction of two processes. When the temperature is lowered 5°C, the low-level segment of the function remains virtually unchanged, while a portion of the high-level response shows supernormality. An additional 5°C reduction in temperature leaves the high-level pattern unchanged, but it virtually eliminates the low-level response.

The mechanism of the differential effect on the low-level (associated with outer hair cell response) and high-level responses (associated with inner hair cell response) is not at all clear, but the phenomenon is mentioned since it

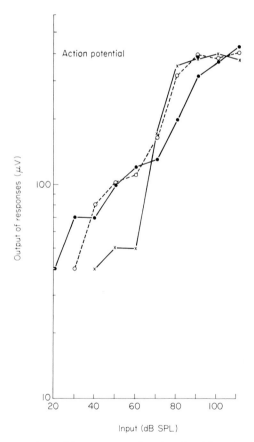

Fig. 5.58. Comparison of input–output function for AP at 35.8°C (●), 30.8°C (○), 25.8°C (X). Data shown for one animal. (Adapted from Butler *et al.*, 1960, p. 690.)

supports the hypothesis that there are indeed two different regions of response as manifested by N_1 at low and high intensities. Apparently AP amplitude is a linear function of temperature, at least within 0° and 45°C (Coats, 1965). The slope of the function is about 3.5 $\mu V/°C$. The AP latency was also measured and it too is dependent on temperature, and a linear function is again adequate to describe the relationship. The latency decreases with increasing temperature at a rate of 0.06 msecond/°C. It is unfortunate that we do not know the SPL at which the measurements were taken, but it is a safe guess that it was relatively high. It was emphasized by the author that changes in AP and in CM are very different when cochlear temperature is altered. It would be interesting to examine this correspondence at low levels, where both AP and CM are at least indirectly mediated by the same hair cell group, the outer hair cells.

D. CHEMICAL ENVIRONMENT

Tasaki *et al.* (1954) demonstrated that the introduction of isotonic KCl solution into the scala tympani of guinea pigs did not affect the EP, while it largely abolished the CM. In an experiment that is essentially the counterpart of the Tasaki *et al.* (1954) study, Konishi *et al.* (1966) replaced the endolymph with a variety of perfusates. They used isotonic KCl, perilymph, and Ringer's solution (low K, high Na concentration) to replace the endolymph in the guinea pig cochlear duct while monitoring cochlear potentials including EP. They noted a clear-cut difference in the results of perfusion between the potassium-poor perfusates (Ringer or perilymph) and the KCl solution. The EP was much more severely reduced in the former cases than in the latter, although in neither case was there an abrupt diminution in EP magnitude. The fact that the EP is more severely affected by the perfusion with potassium-poor solutions was interpreted by Konishi *et al.* to mean that, while the stria vascularis produces EP, high potassium content in the scala media is necessary for its proper functioning and thus for the maintenance of normal EP.

Konishi and colleagues in later experiments investigated the effect of other chemical manipulations on the EP. They found (Konishi and Kelsey, 1968b) that the introduction of tetrodotoxin into either scala tympani or media did not affect the EP, and neither did sodium deficiency of the perilymph (Konishi and Kelsey, 1968a). These findings indicate that the above changes did not affect either the oxidative metabolism of the stria vascularis or the resistance of the membranes that line the scala media, for if either of these had been altered a concomitant change in EP would have been expected. Konishi and Kelsey (1968b) noted, however, that the perfusion of the scala tympani or media with 0.1 % procaine solution resulted in a slight increase in the EP. This fact is probably tied in with an increase in membrane resistance due to reduced potassium permeability caused by the procaine. The same authors (1968a) also noted that when the K^+ concentration of the perilymph was increased a temporary increase in the EP also occurred. This phenomenon is most likely the result of the decrease in the potassium diffusion potential across the membranes that line the scala media. The decrease is simply a consequence of the reduction in the K^+ gradient.

Konishi and colleagues (1966) also studied the influence of endolymphatic K^+ concentration on the CM. They perfused the scala media of guinea pig cochleae with potassium-poor perfusates while recording cochlear potentials with differential electrodes from the basal turn. Control experiments, during which the perfusion was made with isotonic KCl solution, showed some reduction in potentials, but the effects were mild, particularly during the initial time segment of the perfusion process. In marked contrast, when the perfusate was either perilymph or Ringer's solution (both are of high Na^+ and low K^+ content) the effect on CM was pronounced. Within approximately 12 minutes from the start of the replacement of the endolymph, the CM was reduced to its usual postmortem value, that is, CM_1 had disappeared. The low-level residual CM was maintained at a fairly steady level during the prolonged perfusion. It appears from these results that high potassium concentration in the scala media is essential for the maintenance of cochlear function as manifested by CM production. It is of additional significance that the reduction in CM is irreversible. A companion experiment was performed by Konishi and Kelsey (1968a). In this study, instead of altering the chemical composition of endolymph they modified that of the perilymph. When the scala tympani was perfused with sodium-free solutions (choline chloride or sucrose) the CM was virtually unaffected.

Tasaki and Fernández (1952) demonstrated that CM can be promptly depressed if the scala tympani is perfused with fluid containing high levels of potassium. Thus we can summarize by noting that CM is strongly dependent on the high K^+ content of the endolymph, but it is insensitive to the removal of Na^+ ions from the perilymph. On the other hand, the CM cannot be maintained if the ionic content of the perilymph is so altered that K^+ ions are dominant.

Of the many chemical modifications of the functioning of the peripheral auditory system that can have an effect on the AP, only a few are mentioned here, and even these are treated very briefly. It is well known (Loewenstein *et al.*, 1963) that tetrodotoxin effectively eliminates propagated spike activity in nerve fibers without an influence on the generator potential. Similarly, it was shown (Katz, 1950) that procaine blocks propagated potentials but does not significantly affect the receptor potentials. Katsuki *et al.* (1966) and Konishi and Kelsey (1968b) found that tetrodotoxin indeed depresses auditory AP, and apparently if properly low concentrations are used the CM is not affected. The latter authors also noted that procaine has the expected effect of greatly reducing AP while the CM is only moderately affected. Konishi and Kelsey (1968a) also observed that when scala tympani was perfused with sodium-free solutions the AP was significantly reduced without any effect on CM or EP. This effect on AP is not surprising since apparently the Na^+-free solution diffuses into the intercellular spaces of the organ of Corti and thereby causes a deficiency of vital Na^+ ions around the nonmyelinated segment of the auditory nerve fibers.

Just as we have called attention to the differential effect of temperature on low- and high-intensity segments of the AP input–output functions, we must emphasize similar observations for drug-produced AP reduction. With tetrodotoxin and procaine intoxication, and especially when the scala tympani Na^+ concentration is reduced, the low-level response is more severely affected than the high-intensity N_1. In Fig. 5.59 an example of normal AP input–output function is compared to that obtained when sodium ions were removed from the perilymph. Note that the high-level response is barely affected while the low-level response segment is effectively eliminated.

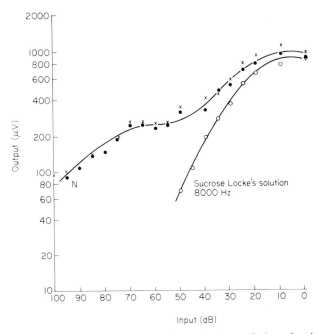

Fig. 5.59. Input–output curve of N_1 before and after perfusion of scala tympani with sucrose Locke's solution. Control ● ; immediately after perfusion ○; and 31 minutes after end of perfusion X. (From Konishi and Kelsey, 1968a, p. 466.)

This picture is strikingly similar to the one that we presented (Fig. 5.49) for animals whose outer hair cells were damaged. It is also somewhat similar to functions seen when the cochlea is cooled. All these conditions reveal that the high-level response, presumably mediated by fibers that innervate inner hair cells, is a very robust one. This response is surprisingly resistant to manipulations of the cochlear environment, suggesting that its initiation might depend on a somewhat different mechanism than that of the sensitive low-level response.

VII. Transducer Processes

A. The General Transducer Scheme: Sensory Receptors

A sensory receptor organ is formed by a conglomeration of sensory receptor cells and an accessory structure. The former are specialized neurons that are capable of interacting with the environment and that are particularly responsive to specific factors in the environment, such as particular forms of energy. The accessory structure is a framework for the sensory cells; it has multiple functions. In general the accessory structure strongly influences the operation of the sense organ by performing distribution and preanalysis of the stimulus. More specifically, these structures can direct and funnel the stimulus to the receptor cells; they can perform filtering of the environmental stimulus; and in most cases they contribute to the dynamic response of the receptor mechanism. Accessory structures can be defined broadly or narrowly to include all or only certain portions of the structures that intervene between the sensory cell and the environment. For example, a broad definition would include the pupil mechanism of the eye or the middle ear muscles of the ear. A narrow definition would exclude the more peripheral portions of the sense organ and would admit only the actual supporting matrix of the sensory cells, for example the retina or the organ of Corti. The broad definition is probably preferable. Chapter 4 was devoted entirely to the description of the most elaborate accessory structure developed in nature, the cochlear partition. It is quite clear that the functional properties of the basilar membrane–organ of Corti system do determine to a great extent the sensitivity, the dynamic range, and the frequency range over which a particular auditory organ can function. It is also clear that via the traveling wave mechanism the accessory structure (the basilar membrane) performs a high-level distributive and filtering function in determining which groups of sensory cells receive excitation under any stimulus condition. Clearly then a good understanding has now been developed of the nature, purpose, and operation of the auditory accessory structure. Our task now is to examine the other major component of the sense organ, the sensory receptor cell.

All receptor cells are considered to be specialized neurons and thus they fit schemes that were developed to describe and classify the general functioning of neurons (Bodian, 1962). The general scheme defines portions of a neuron according to function rather than morphology. The typical neuron can be described as having three main functional parts. These are the receptive pole or dendritic zone, the transmission apparatus or axon, and the distribution apparatus or presynaptic zone. In this scheme the location of the cell body (perikaryon) is incidental, since this structure is considered to be the center of protein synthesis and as such its function is to maintain the metabolic integrity of the neuron and not necessarily to participate in signal transmission. The receptive pole and the presynaptic region are defined functionally as the input and output regions of the neuron. These two regions are at opposite ends of the neuronal structure, and thus both a functional and structural polarization of the neuron, both sensory and nonsensory, exists. This functional polarization is the crucial common factor in all neurons. The actual organization, spatial arrangement, and even the absence or presence of particular portions of the usual neuronal elements are of little consequence. Examples are shown in Fig. 5.60, as sketched after Thurm (1969).

In the figure the relative spatial arrangement is shown between the two important poles of the sensory neuron: the receptive region and the pre-

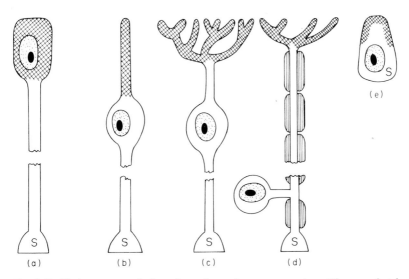

Fig. 5.60. Various geometrical configurations of sensory receptors. The cross-hatched segment corresponds to the receptive region, while S indicates the presynaptic region. (a)–(d) Primary sensory neurons; (e) sensory receptor cell of a secondary sensory receptor system. (Adapted from Thurm, 1969, p. 46.)

synaptic region. In all five examples the former region is indicated by cross-hatching, while the latter is denoted by the letter S. In example (a) the receptive region and the cell body are united, an organization seen in certain invertebrate photoreceptors. Example (b) shows the receptor region developed as a single distal process of a bipolar neuron, which is analogous to a dendrite. This arrangement is exemplified by the vertebrate chemoreceptor. In example (c) the situation is similar but the arborization of the receptor region is similar to the most common appearance of dendrites. Example (d) is similar in organization but here the axonal segment is myelinated and the cell body forms a side branch. This organization is most common for vertebrate receptors in the skin. Finally, in example (e) we see the ultimate specialization of the receptor neuron. Here the perikaryon, the receptor region, and the presynaptic region all form a tightly organized package from which the axonal part is most conspicuously absent. This latter type is most important for our purposes, for the auditory receptors are of this variety. One can develop a general classification of the sensory cells on the basis of their morphology. According to this the types of cells shown in examples (a)–(d) are classified as *primary sense cells*, while those exemplified by (e) are called *secondary sense cells*. It should be clearly understood that the differentiation between the two types hinges on the presence or absence of a transmission apparatus (axon). As we shall note shortly, aside from the morphological differences between the two basic types there are highly significant functional and operational differences as well.

1. The Primary Sensory Cell

This structure has the appearance of a classic neuron with three fairly well defined substructures. The first, the receptive apparatus, is the analog of the dendritic region. This segment is physiologically defined as that portion of the neuron where stimulus transduction actually takes place. This transduction in general implies the absorption of appropriate physical stimulus by the cell and a local process that culminates in the generation of a receptor current. This current is an ionic flow across the cell membrane, and it is controlled by the absorbed stimulus. The potential drop across the cell membrane that is generated by the ionic current is designated as the *generator potential*. This potential is conducted by electrotonus to the portion of the sense cell that is electrically excitable and where the generator potential creates a sufficient local deplorization of the cell membrane to initiate all-or-none spike activity. The region in which this process takes place is designated as the initial segment of the neuron. It is clearly the demarcation between receptive region and transmission apparatus. It is worth emphasizing at this point that the receptive region is *not* electrically excitable; in other words, in this segment of the neuron no spike activity is originated. This segment can be excited only by an appropriate type of physical stimulus to which the receptive region is specialized.

Once the spikes are originated in the initial segment, they travel centripetally on the axon of the sense cell. When the impulses arrive at the presynaptic region they liberate chemical transmitter agents that activate adjacent neurons in a process of synaptic transmission. This process involves the arrival of neural spikes from the axon to the distribution zone, the activation of chemical transmitter substances that are stored at the distribution zone in characteristic packets (vesicles), the diffusion of these chemicals through the synaptic gap, and their absorption by the dendritic region of the adjacent neuron. The distribution apparatus possesses a number of characteristic morphological features that can be used to identify the "sending end" of a synaptic junction. Most characteristic of these is the appearance of a large number of vesicles in a concentrated region and the presence of certain identifiable presynaptic structures such as synaptic bars, synaptic ribbons, and differentiated cell membranes. The actual synaptic cleft is a space between two adjacent neurons; its typical width is 150–250 Å. The gap is contiguous with the intercellular substance. Such chemically operated synapses predominate in the vertebrate nervous system and these are the only types that have been identified in mammals (Mountcastle and Baldessarini, 1968). It is now clear that chemical synaptic transmission is not the only possible way for a synapse to function. Electrical synapses have also been identified (Furshpan and Potter, 1959) in which the transfer of information is achieved by electrical current flow through the synapse instead of by chemical transmission. The flow of current in electrical synapses is unidirectional, and thus both chemical and electrical synapses transmit information in one way only. The two basic synaptic types are distinguished not only by their functioning but also by their morphology. As we have mentioned the chemical synapse is typically a gap about 150–250 Å wide and it is characterized by typical presynaptic structures. In contrast, the electrical synapse shows a greatly reduced separation (or no separation at all) between two neighboring cells; these tight junctions are thought to provide a low-resistance current path.

Let us now summarize the salient features of the primary sensory cell. This cell possesses, both functionally and structurally, all three elements of the typical neuron: receptive region, transmission apparatus, and presynaptic region. The cell maintains *two types* of electrical activity. (a) A graded generator potential is set up as a consequence of the transduction process, and (b) this potential initiates all-or-none responses in the axonal segment. The two potentials thus coexist within the same cell even though at different locations of the cell. This implies that the cell membrane has different properties in different regions; it is electrically inexcitable in the receptive region, while it is electrically excitable in the transmission region. At this time we have no clear-cut information on the morphological features that render certain portions of the cell membrane inexcitable and others electrogenic.

2. The Secondary Receptor Cell

In the vertebrate special sense organs (with the exception of the olfactory epithelium) the sensory structure is more complex than the previously described primary sense cell. Here a specialized receptor cell, of epithelial origin, receives the external stimulus, converts it to a form that is compatible with the receptive properties of adjacent cells, and activates these surrounding cells. The distinctive structural features of the receptor cell are that it does not possess an axonal segment and, hand in hand with this, it does not transmit pulsatile information. All-or-none signal transmission was developed in the nervous system to make "long-distance" communication possible. In secondary sensory receptor systems the sense cell is in intimate contact with the succeeding neuron, and thus there is no need for pulsatile transmission. Since the receptive pole of the neighboring neurons is generally chemically excitable, the output of a sense cell is in the form of secretion of chemical transmitter substances. Between the sensory cell and the following neuron the information transfer takes place via the already discussed synaptic mechanism.

Grundfest (1961) very strongly emphasizes the secretory function of the sense cell. He states that the cell is probably not electrically excitable, and it may or may not generate an electrical potential upon absorption of stimulation. If a potential does appear it might be either depolarizing, hyperpolarizing, or both, depending on stimulus parameters. In any case, if the potential does appear it might be only a secondary process, essentially an electrical sign of secretory activity of the cell. If an electrical potential does appear in the sensory cell that does not sustain pulsatile activity, this potential should not be confused with the generator potential of the simple sensory cell. Davis (1961a) proposed a very useful distinction according to which the term *generator potential* denotes the graded electrical activity that is directly responsible for the initiation of all-or-none neural responses, while the term *receptor potential* describes the graded electrical activity that occurs in the sensory receptor cell as a direct consequence of the absorption of stimulus. Of course, in simple sensory receptor cells the distinction between the two potentials is meaningless since they are the same in that case. Thus whatever graded potentials are recordable from the vertebrate special sense organs are properly described as receptor potentials. Such potentials have been obtained intracellularly from taste buds (Beidler, 1961), from retinal cones (Tomita, 1965), and from hair cells of the lateral line organ (Harris *et al.*, 1970), among others. The slow potentials recordable from the olfactory epithelium are true generator potentials, since the cells there are primary receptors. The microphonic and summating potentials of the cochlea are thought to be an aggregate external manifestation of receptor potentials originating in the hair cells (Davis, 1961a, 1965).

Let us summarize the scheme of operation of the secondary receptor system. In this structure the sensory cell has lost its axonal segment and thus it has only two of the three main portions of a generalized neuron: the receptive region and the distribution apparatus. The former is specialized to absorb a specific type of stimulus and to perform a transduction process on this stimulus. The latter is a presynaptic region, and it is specialized in liberating chemical transmitter agents. Between the sense cell and the following neuron there is a (generally) chemically functioning synapse. The neuron that is in contact with the synapse functions as a classical neuron and has the three basic functional components:* receptive region, transmission apparatus, and presynaptic region. A distinction is made between two types of potential in the secondary receptor system. The first, receptor potential, is set up in the sense cell as a direct consequence of the transduction process. The second, generator potential, is a postsynaptic potential and its distinguishing function is to initiate all-or-none responses in the axon of the secondary neuron.

3. Special Features of the Receptive Region

Since this segment of the sensory receptor system, primary as well as secondary, is of utmost importance in determining the functioning of the structure, it is appropriate to dwell in somewhat more detail on the specific properties and morphological features that can be commonly associated with this segment of the receptor.

A small class of all receptors possesses receptor segments whose structure is modality specific, in other words, segments in which particular architectural features are uniquely correlated with the specific type of stimulus that they are specialized to transduce. The most conspicuous modality-specific receptor segment is associated with photoreceptors in which the terminal segment of the sense cell possesses a folded membrane structure. This folded membrane yields an extension of the active surface area (in which the photosensitive pigments are incorporated) of up to hundredfold increase compared to the surface area of the enveloping structure without the invaginations. The folded membrane structure is so typical of photoreceptors that one can identify from this morphological feature the light-sensitive nature of the cell with near certainty. The only other modality-specific morphological feature

---

* The retina is an exception because there the rods and cones (sensory cells) first make contact with intermediate neurons (horizontal and bipolar cells) and only through these do they connect with the true second-order neurons (ganglion cells).

that has been identified is the presence of microtubules in certain primitive mechanoreceptors. Aside from these two types all other receptive regions must be classified as modality unspecific. This means that one cannot infer from the microstructure of the receptive region of most sense cells to the particular physical stimulus the cell is specialized to receive. In spite of our inability to identify stimulus specificity from microstructure, we can recognize certain features that characterize receptive regions in general. Such features are the presence of large numbers of mitochondria and in many cases the presence of ciliary structures.

Mitochondria are known to mediate oxidative energy metabolism in cellular structures. Their presence in large numbers in the receptive region of sense cells clearly indicates that there is a high level of energy consumption in this vicinity. It is highly probable that the mitochondria provide the energy supply of the transducer process and more specifically that they supply the metabolic energy needs for the receptor current. In analogy with axonal processes, one is probably justified in assuming that the ionic membrane current that comprises the receptor current is dependent on ion pump mechanisms, which in turn are known to be dependent on oxidative metabolism. It has been shown for photoreceptors (Hagins, 1965) and for the cochlea (von Békésy, 1950) that these receptors do operate as power amplifiers in the sense that the energy content manifested in the receptor currents is greater than that of the absorbed stimulus. The excess energy is presumably derived from the local metabolic processes and the mitochondria are most likely to be, at least in part, instrumental in supplying the local energy pool.

One of the most fascinating observations concerning the receptor segments of many sensory cells is that they contain structures that closely resemble modified forms of motile cilia. These structures have the type of cytoarchitecture that has been closely associated with motile cilia, as typified by the epithelial cells in the trachea. The characteristic components are a basal body from which the cilium erupts and the ciliary shaft. The cross section of the structure at any point reveals a characteristic, highly organized structure that is easy to recognize from its nine longitudinal outer filaments and the two additional inner filaments confined to the shaft region. In many receptor cells there is a geographical separation between the stimulus-specific receptor segment and the energy-supplying (mitochondria-rich) region. In these the connection between the two segments is made by what appears to be a modified cilium. In these structures the cilia act as connecting links between two segments of the receptive region that have developed to their ultimate degree of specialization. Receptors of this type are known to subserve many sense modalities, and it is conspicuous that very similar ciliary structures are in evidence in all. In these receptors the ciliary portion resembles the basal part of motor cilia, while the mobile ciliary shaft has given way to the specialized receptor segment. It is then the basal body portion of the cilia that apparently developed to perform an important function in sensory cells. It is assumed that in ciliated sensory cells the basal body is the site of actual transduction. The basal body develops from the centriole, which is the center of morphogenesis in cell development.

The mechanoreceptor sensory cells of the vertebrate vestibular apparatus are ciliated structures of the type discussed above. These cells are equipped with two types of cilium: a number of stiff stereocilia and one flexible kinocilium. It is the kinocilium that is analogous to motile and sensory cilia. A great deal of diligent effort has failed to uncover any sign of kinocilia in the organ of Corti. The cochlear hair cells of course possess stereocilia, about 100 on each outer hair cell and about 50 on each inner hair cell. The kinocilium, however, is absent. In some species throughout life, and in others only during early development, a basal body is present in both inner and outer hair cells. In guinea pig these structures can be observed at any age of the animal (Flock *et al.*, 1962; Engström *et al.*, 1962), while they can be found in only very young kittens and they disappear later in life (Spoendlin, 1966). Realizing the great importance of modified kinocilia in sensory receptors of many types, Engström *et al.* (1962) suggested that the basal body of the cochlear hair cell is the fundamental excitable structure. They considered the stiff stereocilia to act as microlevers in "rocking" the cuticular plate of the hair cells. The basal body is inserted in a small opening of the cuticular plate, and thus as the entire plate is moved by the mechanical stimulus that is passively transmitted to it by the hairs, the basal body becomes deformed. The mechanical deformation of the basal body is considered by Engström *et al.* to be the crucial step in the excitatory process of the hair cell. As we have noted above, Spoendlin (1966) discovered that basal bodies are not present in all species and on that basis he discounts the basal body as the seat of excitation. It appears to us that Spoendlin's argument is most persuasive in that it is unlikely that the basal body per se would be of great functional significance. It should be noted, however, that at the position of the basal body (whether this structure is present or not) the cuticular plate is discontinuous and at this region the cell makes its most intimate contact with the endolymph. It is quite possible that this region of the cell is very significant as the site of excitation. At this point we shall review in some detail the structure of the cuticular plate–reticular lamina–stereocilia region in order to better speculate on the probable process of hair cell excitation.

The cochlear hair cells are capped by the cuticular plate, a structure of irregular depth and shape. It is always thicker toward the modiolus and becomes thinner toward the other side, where it actually disappears over a roughly oval-shape opening. The stereocilia are anchored in the cuticular plate. When a section is made through the plate the picture shown in Fig.

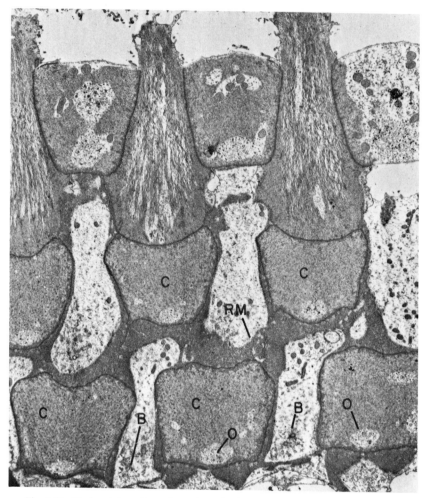

Fig. 5.61. Horizontal section through cuticular plates (C) of outer hair cells and reticular membrane (RM). Basal bodies (B) are seen only in the supporting cells and not in the openings (O) of the cuticular plate. (From Spoendlin, 1970, p. 9.)

5.61 (from Spoendlin, 1970) emerges. The plates are imbedded into a matrix formed by processes of supporting cells; this matrix is known as the reticular lamina. Both cuticular plate and reticular lamina appear to be extremely dense, rigid structures, and the contact between the lamina and the cuticular plates appears to be quite intimate. These observations strongly suggest that there is very little relative motion (if any) possible between the cuticular plates and the surrounding framework and also that deformation of any individual cuticular plate is probably very minimal (if any). The stereocilia are clublike structures, 2.5–5 μ in length, and their diameter is up to 0.35 μ on inner hair cells and up to 0.15 μ on outer hair cells (Engström *et al.*, 1962). An electron micrograph of some stereocilia is shown in Fig. 5.62. Engström and colleagues give the following description of the structure and attachment of the hairs:

> The outer surface of the hair is a direct continuation of the cuticular plasma membrane which forms an uninterrupted sheath around the hair. Inside this membrane and at a distance of about 70 Å, another membrane can be seen having direct continuity with the root portion of the hair. Thus, each hair is surrounded by two membranes of different origin and attachment. The root continues almost through or perhaps straight through the entire cuticle of the hair cell. It tapers downward forming a tubelike structure with a rather opaque wall. In the center of the tube a dark but extremely delicate filament can sometimes be observed. The tube also extends upwards into the lower part of the hair proper, forming a hollow-appearing central core. (Engström *et al.*, 1962, p. 1360.)

According to Spoendlin (1966) between the rootlet that extends upward into the hair and the hair membrane there is only material of low density. Only the rootlet itself is composed of high-density material. The organization of the hair substance is longitudinal; apparently elongated molecules form an orderly arrangement in constituting the basic building material of the hair (Iurato, 1961).

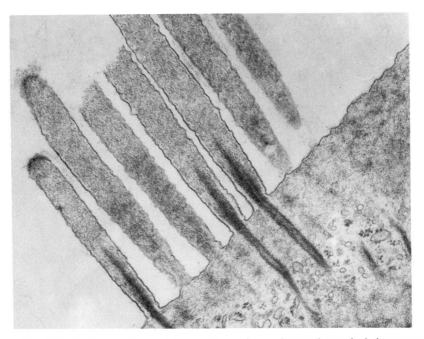

Fig. 5.62. Basal end of several hairs with rootlets and central core in hair proper. Central part of core and rootlet is less dense than outer layer. (Courtesy of Dr. H. Engström.)

   The necessity for ruling out the basal body as the site of excitation, or the site of actual receptor function, places the stereocilia themselves in the role of front contender for this honor. As we noted earlier in this chapter there have been some suggestions for the mechanism of CM production involving the cilia to a greater extent than mere mechanical linkages. Examples are Dohlman's (1959, 1960), Christiansen's (1963), and to some extent Naftalin's (1965) schemes. The more classic theories of Wever (1949) and Davis (1965) treat the hairs as connective structures that transmit mechanical deformation to the cell body or to the cuticular plate. The deformation of the cell body or of the cuticular plate by action of the stereocilia is a somewhat tenuous mechanism, as we have noted above, because of the great rigidity and density of the cuticular plates and because of the strong coupling between them and the reticular lamina. The small cuticle-free region in which the basal body is located (or from which it disappears during maturation) and which protrudes above the cuticular plate is the only place where direct ionic exchange between the cell body and the endolymph could take place. This is because the cuticular plate is too dense to permit the passage of ions. Communication between the cell body and the endolymph might have important functional significance in allowing the endolymph to supply at least partial nutrition to the cell.
   One of the most attractive propositions is that the cilia themselves are the transducers, not passive types serving merely as capacitive couplers as envisioned by Dohlman, Christiansen, and Naftalin, but active receptor structures that can convert minute deformations to electrical currents. One of the simplest ways to envision this operation is to compare the cilium, more specifically its inner tube or filament, to a strain gage. Such a device consists of some resistive material which when subjected to mechanical stress changes its resistivity. As a result, when a potential is applied to the strain gage it signals the presence of stress (commonly an elongation of the resistive filament) by a change of current. The resistance change of a strain gage can be expressed in terms of its change of length as $\Delta R/R = S\Delta L/L$, where S is the so-called gage factor, dependent on the material used to construct the device. The gage factor can range from less than unity to several hundred. Large values are associated with semiconductor materials, small values with simple wire gages. Semiconductors are of course characterized by their orderly crystalline structure (as well as by the peculiar energy levels of their valence electrons); highly organized molecular structure in living material can suggest organic semiconductor function. It is thus conceivable that the fine, longitudinally organized central structure of the cilium that passes from the body of the hair into the cuticular plate, forming the rootlet, does function as a semiconductor strain gage. In this situation a relatively high gage factor could be expected, with the result that the structure could function essentially "isometrically"; that is, it could provide relatively sizable

resistance change with extremely minute displacement. It can be assumed that the stress would be provided by the bending of the cilia under the shearing force that is exerted on it by the differential displacement of the tectorial membrane and the cuticular plate–reticular lamina matrix. This scheme of course is still a "resistance-modulation" model; the endocochlear potential and the intracellular negativity of the hair cells are assumed to act as the polarizing voltages for the strain gage formed by the internal structure of the stereocilia. As the gage resistance changes, the current driven through the resistive structure (here the hairs) also changes. This current is funneled through the hair cells and can thus serve as receptor current. The distinguishing feature of the scheme is that it associates the variable resistor with the hairs as opposed to the apical pole of the hair cells. It also provides for possibly greater sensitivity due to the semiconductor action of the strain gage. This "amplification" is not available in the scheme in which the hair cell is simply construed as a variable resistor.

A second possibility that ought to be considered is that the hair membrane, or some portion of it, or perhaps the inner membrane acts as an active receptor structure upon deformation. The deformation could occur in the form of stress due to bending of the hairs or due to pressure (or impact) on the tip of the hairs by the tectorial membrane. The receptor action would consist of the change of the resting permeability of the membrane due to absorption of stimulus energy (deformation). In the active membrane region where the permeability is altered, movement of ions can occur through the membrane. The current path is from endolymph, through the active membrane segment, through the ciliary shaft into the cytoplasm of the hair cell. Inactive regions of the cell membrane also sustain a current flow, balancing that occurring across the active segment. The voltage drop generated by the flow through the inactive regions (portions of hair membrane and the cell membrane) *is* the receptor potential. In this scheme the primary energy source for the active ionic current flow is the intracellular polarization of the hair cells. The positive endocochlear potential is relegated to a secondary role; it hyperpolarizes the cell (and hair) membrane and effectively boosts the ionic current.

This scheme, envisioning an active permeability change at the site of excitation, is in complete analogy to most other receptor mechanisms that have been described thus far. It is generally agreed (Mellon, 1968) that the first step upon absorption of stimulus energy at a receptor site is a local change in membrane permeability. In primary receptors (i.e., those possessing axonal segments) the resulting potential change is by necessity always depolarizing, so that it is capable for initiating nerve impulses. In secondary receptor systems, that is, in specialized sensory cells, the potential change need not be depolarizing. In this case the output of the cell is secretion of chemical transmitters, and this function can be accomplished by both depolarizing and hyperpolarizing receptor potentials (Grundfest, 1964). Both depolarizing and hyperpolarizing receptor potentials have been observed experimentally.

Aside from the two mechanisms of passive resistance change and permeability change, one should consider a third possibility as well: that the transduction effect results from the alteration of membrane capacitance as a result of deformation. As in the resistance-modulation scheme, here the critical membrane could be associated with either the cuticle-free region at the apex of the hair cell or the unit membrane of the cilia themselves. As the appropriate membrane is deformed it can change its capacitance and, since there is a dc polarizing voltage across it, a capacitive current can result. This current would be different from that envisioned in the resistance-modulation scheme in that no actual ion transport would take place in the capacitive circuit. This is an attractive feature of the capacitive modulation process, since it is somewhat difficult to conceive how ion flow could be effectively modulated at the upper frequency range of CM production. There is no experimental evidence available today with which one could conclusively discriminate among the three possible mechanisms of current modulation that are based on resistance changes, permeability changes, or capacitance changes. Clearly it is very important that such discrimination be obtained.

4. A Summary of Cochlear Receptor Function

Probably the easiest way to summarize the operation of the organ of Corti as a sensory receptor organ is with the aid of the three-part schematic in Fig. 5.63. On the left a sketch of a hair cell is shown together with a portion of the tectorial membrane and a few attached afferent nerve endings and fibers. The block diagram in the center of the figure depicts the distinct structural regions of interest, while the block diagram on the right shows a functional classification of the different regions. The stimulus is filtered and then distributed to the cells by the accessory structure, only a small portion of which is shown here. The accessory structure of the cochlea certainly includes the entire basilar membrane–organ of Corti complex. Here only a segment of the tectorial membrane and the reticular lamina are shown. The sensory input structures in this case include the tectorial membrane, the stereocilia, and probably the reticular membrane–cuticular plate structure. The function of the sensory input structures is to transmit the stimulus to the receptive region of the sense cell. The most common assumption is that the stimulus is the bending of the cilia brought about by the relative sliding motion between the tectorial membrane and the reticular lamina. The receptive region is specialized to absorb the stimulus and to generate a local electric response, the receptor current, whose outward manifestation is the receptor potential. It has been assumed by most authorities that the receptive region is the uppermost portion of the cell, probably only the cuticle-free region where the basal body can be found in some species. As we noted above, it is quite probable that the ciliary membrane, or the central ciliary

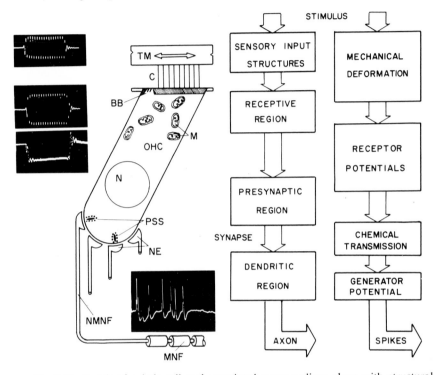

Fig. 5.63. Sketch of a hair cell and associated nerve endings along with structural (center) and functional (right) block diagrams of the system. The inserts demonstrate the waveforms of the various quantities that are indicated in the functional block diagram, namely, stimulus, CM, DIF SP, and neural discharges. Abbreviations: TM, tectorial membrane; C, cilia; OHC, outer hair cell body; N, cell nucleus; M, mitochondria; PSS, presynaptic structures; NE, afferent nerve endings; NMNF, nonmyelinated segment of nerve fiber; MNF, myelinated segment of nerve fiber; BB, basal body. (Adapted from Dallos, 1972, p. 30.)

core, might function as the actual sensory receptor structure that is specialized to respond to stimuli. On the far left of the figure some sample waveforms are shown for the various processes described in the block diagram at the right. The stimulus is assumed to be a brief sinusoidal burst. Here the actual sound pressure change is shown, but it is highly probable that the time course of the effective stimulation, that is, of the bending pattern of the cilia, is quite similar. Two receptor potentials are shown, the CM and the DIF SP. These are presumably generated or controlled at the cell's receptive region.

The lowermost portion of the cell body is the presynaptic region. It is distinguished by the presence of characteristic structures such as synaptic bars and accumulation of vesicles, all of which are typical at the sending end of a chemical synapse. It is presumed that the receptor potentials act on these presynaptic structures and initiate the release of packets of chemical transmitter substances (as yet unidentified). The transmitters diffuse through the synaptic clefts formed between the bottom of the cell and surrounding endings of afferent nerve fibers. The initial nonmyelinated segment of the fibers of the 8th nerve form the dendritic region. The chemical transmitters arriving at the nerve endings alter the local membrane permeability and thus set up a local depolarization of the membrane. This potential change is the generator potential. We cannot show a picture of the time course of this potential because thus far none is available. The generator potential is decrementally conducted in the nonmyelinated fibers to the so-called initial segment of the nerve axon, where it is instrumental in setting up all-or-none action potentials. The distinguishing feature of the initial segment is that it is electrically excitable as opposed to the dendritic region, which can conduct electricity only in a passive manner. It is widely assumed that the initial segment of the 8th nerve axons is at the habenula perforata, where the fibers gain their myelin sheath, and where in passing through the habenulae they are severely constricted in diameter. It is a common notion that such radical structural changes as, for example, diameter shifts are the appropriate conditions for a fiber to become electrogenic, that is, for it to be electrically excitable. In the myelinated segment of the nerve fiber the information travels in the form of an impulse train, an example of which is given in the insert of Fig. 5.63.

It might be worthwhile to stop at this point and dwell a little on the question of the location of the initial segment. As we have just mentioned, the habenula is most commonly assumed to mark this region. This location appears to be the logical choice for several reasons. First, distinct structural changes in the fibers, such as the beginning of myelination and changes in diameter, are seen here. Second, the extensive adrenergic plexus innervating the cochlea terminates largely in this region, and controlling function by this innervation is most likely to take place in the region of impulse initiation (Spoendlin, 1970). The only problem with associating the initial segment with the habenula perforata is that the majority of fibers that innervate outer hair cells have to travel considerable distances before they reach this site. It is estimated that the average dendrite from an outer hair cell is 700 μ long and that a sizable number might reach lengths in excess of 1 or 2 mm. These dendrites, if they are dendrites, would conduct generator potentials with decrement. The attenuation of these potentials would be excessive for the longer fibers, and it can be legitimately questioned whether the greatly diminished generator potential would be capable of initiating nerve impulses in an effective manner. It can be estimated that the decrement for fibers with diameters of 0.3–0.5 μ (the diameter of the cochlear dendrites) over a length of 1 mm might be of the order of 10,000-fold. A very conservative estimate (taking a space constant $\lambda = 0.2$ mm) would still yield an approximate attenuation of 150-fold.

While this consideration of attenuation of graded electrical signals on long dendrites is not sufficient to rule out the habenula perforata as the initial segment for outer hair cell fibers, it certainly indicates that one must entertain the possibility that the initial segment for these fibers is at a more peripheral location. It is conceivable that the "major" initial segment is at the habenula, that is, where fibers innervating the inner hair cells would begin all-or-none conduction. This would be the more dominant place of impulse initiation because, first, afferent axons to the inner hair cells are about ten times as numerous as those to the outer hair cells (Spoendlin, 1966) and, second, in this scheme the initial segment to the outer hair cell fibers would be more diffuse, probably in the region of arborization of the dendrites. Of course, if the initial segment is more peripheral for some fibers one would expect neural impulses within the organ of Corti. These have never been detected. It must be noted, however, that the extracellular potential field of very thin fibers running in sparse bundles would be very small, and the customary recording electrode, the high-noise-level pipette, would probably be incapable of detecting it. Thus the fact that spikes have not been seen within the organ of Corti might be simply a consequence of the adverse recording conditions and not an indication of their absence.

B. THE ROLE AND SIGNIFICANCE OF COCHLEAR POTENTIALS

As our extensive discussions above indicate, the receptor potentials in a sense organ are the first electrical signs of the stimulus transduction process. In a secondary receptor system (such as the cochlea) the receptor potentials arise in the specialized sensory cell. The actual function of these potentials has never been established with certainty. Two possibilities exist. The first and more attractive possibility is that the receptor potential (or receptor current) is a direct mediator of the release of chemical transmitters at the presynaptic zone. This scheme assumes that the receptor current is set up as a direct consequence of absorption of stimulus energy by the cell and that this receptor current serves as the intermediary link between the stimulus and the cell output, the chemical transmitters. One of the most important considerations in support of this scheme is that the receptive pole of the cell and its presynaptic region are as a rule on two opposite ends of the cell structure. In other words, these two regions are physically separated. It is very clear that the transmitter substance is stored in the synaptic vesicles that are concentrated in the presynaptic region. The excitable structure of the cell, its receptive region, is many tens or hundreds of microns away from this concentration of transmitters. Thus the excitatory process in the cell must be communicated to the presynaptic region, and the most likely assumption is that the communication between these regions takes place via the receptor potential. The scheme then is as follows. Upon excitation a receptor current is set up in the input region of the cell. The current generates a potential drop (receptor potential), which is passively conducted in the cell structure to the presynaptic region. There the receptor potential initiates the liberation of chemical transmitters. It should be noted that either depolarizing or hyperpolarizing receptor potentials could function as effective agents of the liberation of transmitter substances.

The second possibility is to assume that the receptor potentials are merely incidental by-products of the transducer process. In other words, whatever physical process subserves the absorption of stimulus energy by the cell, and the subsequent liberation of transmitters, has a by-product: the receptor potential. In this case the receptor potential is a *sign* of the functioning of the cell instead of being the essential result of that functioning. In this case the receptor potential is designated as an *epiphenomenon*. The main argument in favor of this scheme is that the function of the sense cell is secretory. Whether a potential accompanies this operation is incidental even the presence of the potential is not required. This scheme is certainly more direct than that which requires an intermediary process between stimulus absorption and chemical transmission. There does not seem to be, however, a clear mechanism described that would tie together the physically separated input and output processes in the cell. It is quite possible that such a mechanism is not really necessary, and that it is only our incomplete understanding of cellular and receptor function that forces us to seek and feel more comfortable with such an intermediary process.

In the following, bits and pieces of evidence are collected that might have a bearing on this rather fundamental problem. It should be said at the outset that information concerning this problem is fragmentary and indirect. The best one can do at this juncture is to speculate on this basis and at least be aware of the problem. It is commonly assumed that CM and SP are the receptor potentials of the cochlea. Thus our basic problem can be stated simply by asking whether the CM and SP (or certain components of the SP) are epiphenomena or if they serve an essential intermediary role between stimulation and the release of chemical transmitters from the presynaptic region of the hair cells. An even more general question is whether these potentials actively (causally) participate in the initiation of neural responses in the auditory nerve. The history of this questioning is as old as the history of cochlear potentials itself. Immediately upon the discovery of the CM two camps formed, those who thought that the new potential was significant in auditory information transfer and those who assumed it to be an epiphenomenon. The arguments have swayed back and forth, and their details are not very illuminating. At present, most authorities assume that the CM is probably an important intermediary step (Wever, 1966; Davis, 1968). The SP was also considered everything from important physiological process to simple artifact during its two-decade history. At present, many people discount its importance, probably because this potential is more difficult to obtain consistently than the CM, and because certain misconceptions tend to be accepted (for example, that the SP is significantly smaller than the CM or that it is present only at high frequencies or at high stimulus levels).

The most important idea that one must accept when inquiring into the role of CM and SP is that *all* information currently available is on the aggregate, gross CM and SP. We have already spent considerable time in this chapter discussing the fundamental differences between the recorded gross potential and the outputs of individual generators. It should be clear at this point that one treads on thin ice when attempting to make one-to-one tie-ins between these. The crucial point is the *we have no direct intracellular recording of either CM or SP from cochlear hair cells.* One might say that the aggregate response as we see it with the gross electrodes almost certainly has no direct relation to the initiation of neural responses. The individual hair cell potential that is represented by the gross response only to a certain extent might or might not be a crucial causative factor. In the following we shall treat some properties of the aggregate response. Most of the items that will be brought out are negative in the sense that they indicate a lack of correlation between the gross response and neural components, and they tend to indicate that the gross responses are epiphenomena. It must be kept in mind that this might not be the case, that the lack of correlation might simply reflect the poor correspondence between gross response and unit response from a single cell.

One of the most uncompromising proponents of the CM and opponents of the SP as significant receptor potentials is Wever (1966). In his later writings Davis (1968) also argues for the CM and against the SP, which he now considers as a simple nonlinear distortion component of the CM. Wever's primary arguments in favor of the CM are worth summarizing here. He notes that the CM is ". . . invariably present when the ear is functional. When . . . absent, as in albinotic cats and certain strains of guinea pigs, dogs, and mice, the animals are wholly unresponsive to sounds." He further notes that "When the ear is exposed to sounds of extreme intensity the cochlear potentials show reductions in magnitude . . . when the ear is later studied histologically only the hair cells show changes as an alteration of staining properties." Further, "A correlation of 0.91 was found . . . between the magnitudes of cochlear potentials and the number of hair cells present. . . ." Finally, "There is a reasonable degree of correspondence between the forms of the sensitivity curves for various species of animals as shown in their cochlear potentials and in the behavioral threshold curves" (Wever, 1966, p. 120). It appears to me that the first three points prove that CM and hair cells are intimately related, but do not necessarily provide information on the relation between CM and hearing. In other words, there is no hearing without hair cells, and there is no CM without hair cells. These two points however, do not yield the conclusion that there is no hearing without CM.

Let us review some evidence against the CM as an excitatory agent. Hawkins (1959) noted that one effect of certain ototoxic drugs (kanamycin and streptomycin) when administered in relatively mild doses is to depress the CM while hardly affecting the AP. Hawkins' oscilloscope traces show AP responses with very little CM preceding them when obtained from a kanamycin-treated cat while, in other traces corresponding to responses from a normal animal, the CM is seen as a prominent response preceding the AP. The CM is easy to identify, for it reverses polarity when the polarity of the stimulus click is reversed. No absolute calibration is available; the stimulus level is such that it is 50 dB above the required click intensity to elicit an AP. One can guess that for a round-window recording that level is about 100 dB SPL. This means that the AP response is from the high-intensity second segment of the input–output function. It is remembered that we tentatively identified this segment with primary innervation from inner hair cells. It is known that the ototoxic drugs first destroy the basal outer hair cell population. We shall come back to this result after reviewing some of our own relevant data.

We have already discussed in the section on compound action potential (Section V) some results on sound-damaged cochleae (Dallos and Bredberg, 1970). It was noted that AP sensitivity is well correlated with outer hair cell population but that almost normal maximum AP can be achieved with severe reduction of the outer hair cell (OHC) population provided that the inner hair cells (IHC) are normal. Our results have also indicated that CM and all components of SP are very well correlated with OHC population and rather poorly with IHC population. It was stated that if IHC's do produce CM, their output is about 30–50 dB down from that of the OHC's. Similar relations probably exist for SP also. Davis *et al.* (1958b) also concluded that CM originates in outer hair cells but they assigned SP to inner hair cells. I believe on the basis of more complete evidence that all gross receptor potentials (CM and SP) are produced primarily by OHC's. If this assessment is correct then we are clearly confronted with a seeming contradiction. On the one hand the receptor potentials are apparently correlated with one hair cell group (OHC), and on the other hand the majority of auditory nerve fibers (90–95%) innervate the *other* hair cell group (IHC). It is also apparent from the work of Hawkins (1959) and from ours (Dallos and Bredberg, 1970) that at high intensities compound AP can be normal in the presence of severe destruction of the OHC group. These facts appear to strike a severe blow at the hypothesis that CM and SP are important excitatory agents. Clearly, situations do exist in which very good or normal compound AP can be seen together with severely diminished CM and SP.

Another line of evidence indicating possible lack of correlation between neural responses and CM can be obtained from studies of the distortion component $2f_1 - f_2$. Considerable detail on this cochlear distortion product is presented in the following chapter; the reader is referred to it for specifics. Here I merely wish to call attention to the fact that the distortion component $2f_1 - f_2$ has some peculiar characteristics, detectable by psychoacoustic methods (Zwicker, 1955; Plomp, 1965; Goldstein, 1967), which can be confirmed in measurements of single-unit discharge patterns in the cat auditory nerve (Goldstein and Kiang, 1968). In contrast none of the unique properties of $2f_1 - f_2$ appears to be present when measurements are made in the CM (Dallos, 1969b). In other words, it appears that whatever cochlear process is responsible for the generation of the nonlinear component $2f_1 - f_2$ does not generate a CM. Since the component is clearly audible and since indications are that it is present in the discharge pattern of the 8th nerve, one can conclude that CM is not a prerequisite to neural responses and thus to hearing sensation.

It is important to emphasize again in closing that our contentions relate to *gross* CM. It is this overall, aggregate response of probably thousands of hair cells that is clearly poorly correlated with neural components. The possibility cannot be ruled out at this time that this lack of correlation reflects primarily the inability of the gross CM to represent the elementary hair cell process. Nevertheless, the discrepancies between CM and neural responses are striking in certain cases, sufficiently so to alert us to the continuing need for careful study of receptor potentials and their function.

The final considerations in this chapter are addressed to the interrelationships among the various cochlear potentials, specifically between resting potentials and receptor potentials and between CM and SP. Much has been said about these issues in this chapter; here primarily a concise summary is in order. There is considerable experimental evidence that both CM and SP (specifically the high-level DIF SP⁻ that was studied by all investigators) are dependent on the endocochlear potential. Studies that tend to show this include those in which by appropriate maneuvering of the cochlear blood supply the EP was reduced or eliminated (cf. Davis *et al.*, 1958b; Konishi *et al.*, 1961; Butler, 1965) and studies in which the dc potential gradient was altered by electrical polarization of the cochlear partition (Tasaki and Fernández, 1952; Konishi and Yasuno, 1963; Honrubia and Ward, 1969b). It appears that whenever the dc potential gradient is altered, a concomitant change in SP and CM occurs. The characteristics and the time course of the alteration of the CM do not appear to correlate well with changes in EP alone. It was demonstrated by Butler (1965), however, that the decrease of CM over time has the same time course as the decrease of the potential gradient across the reticular lamina. This observation was made by monitoring both EP and the organ of Corti potential together with CM in anoxic guinea pigs. The EP and the organ of Corti potential were assumed to add in providing the effective dc voltage drop across the cuticular plate. The organ of Corti potential is presumably a manifestation of the intracellular resting potential of the hair cells. Thus it is appropriate to state that the correlation between CM and the dc potential gradient formed by the sum of the EP and the intracellular negativity is quite good. This observation strongly suggests that the CM is derived from the resting potentials and that both resting potentials are intimately involved as energy sources. This consideration forms the basis of Davis' resistance-modulation hypothesis. Further evidence is supplied by experiments in which the dc potential gradient is altered by pumping current across the organ of Corti. The most sophisticated and successful such experiment is the one by Honrubia and Ward (1969b). As we have seen, these authors noted that in anoxic cochleae even with moderate external currents one is capable of actually reversing the potential gradient. Upon doing this, they noted that when the dc gradient did reverse polarity, so did the SP and the CM. Their experiments provide an indication of the dependence of these receptor potentials on the resting potentials.

The SP (specifically the high-level DIF SP$^-$) has been considered by many to be a manifestation of nonlinear distortion of the CM (Whitfield and Ross, 1965; Engebretson and Eldredge, 1968). Some good theoretical arguments have been advanced to support this notion. If this is indeed the case then one can expect the SP to depend on the CM to a very close degree. Experimental evidence on this subject has not been provided as yet.

Some interrelationships among cochlear potentials can be highlighted by examining their dependence on biochemical manipulations of the inner ear. When the perilymph is replaced by Na$^+$-free solutions (technically the NaCl is replaced with either choline chloride or sucrose) there is virtually no observable effect on either CM or EP (Konishi and Kelsey, 1968a). It is notable that choline chloride is an electrolyte and thus its substitution for perilymph should not effect electrical conductivity, while sucrose is not an electrolyte and consequently it should have an effect on conductivity. When compensation is made for the apparent resistance changes one sees no differential effect on CM or EP by either substitution. While CM and EP are unaffected (and apparently so is the organ of Corti potential) by the removal of Na^+ from the perilymph, the AP is significantly influenced by the manipulation. In Fig. 5.59 AP input–output functions are shown for before and after perfusion with sucrose Locke's solution of the perilymphatic space. It is probably highly significant that the low-intensity segment of the function shows the greatest detriment; the maximum AP changes by only 10–30%. The fact that AP is diminished clearly indicates that the perfusate could freely diffuse through the basilar membrane and that the removal of Na^+ from the surrounding of the 8th nerve dendrites has a profound effect on impulse generation. It is worth speculating that since the more sensitive segment of the AP input–output function is generally associated with fibers connected to the outer hair cells, and since this is the segment that is affected by the removal of Na^+, the effect is primarily on the tunnel fibers or on the bare cell bodies of the outer hair cells. It is interesting to note in contrast that the CM, which we associate primarily with the outer hair cells, is unaffected. This seems to imply that Na^+ is *not* an important ion species in the production of CM.

When the composition of endolymph is altered, that is, when perfusates that are low in K^+ ion content are introduced into the scala media, the result is a slow decline of the EP and a faster decrease of CM and AP (Konishi et al., 1966). The decrease in the EP is relatively unspectacular; 30 minutes after the start of perfusion it declines by about 50%. In contrast about 10 minutes after perfusion the CM reaches the postmortem level. The negative organ of Corti potential is only slightly affected by the removal of K^+ from the scala media, which probably signifies that the reticular lamina is an effective barrier to diffusion. The fact that a dearth of K^+ in the cochlear duct affects the CM quite significantly tends to indicate that the flow of these ions from scala media into the hair cells might mediate the CM production process.

The third appropriate change in ionic composition entails not only the removal of Na^+ ions from the perilymph, but their replacement with K^+ ions. This procedure was performed by Tasaki and Fernández (1952). The maneuver results in the rapid depression of AP, CM, and the organ of Corti potential. At the same time there is a moderate increase in EP. Since there is apparently good diffusion through the basilar membrane, the results tend to indicate that potassium in the fluid spaces of the organ of Corti has a devastating effect on all potentials. This effect is clearly the result of the removal of the K^+ concentration gradient from across the hair cell and dendrite membranes and thus the effective depolarization of these structures.

The paradoxical increase in EP is likely to be the result of increased K^+ concentration in perilymph, and the consequent reduction in the K^+ diffusion potential.

The final change in fluid composition is the removal of calcium from the perilymph. This process causes a slowly developing, nonreversible depression of the CM and at the same time a rapid decrease of AP. Significantly, it is again the low-level portion of the AP input–output function that is affected; the high-level response is barely altered (Konishi and Kelsey, 1970). The usual effect of Ca lack in extracellular fluid is the depolarization of nerve fibers and the reduction in the generator potentials. These effects are produced through a mechanism of change in permeability of excitable membranes due to the absence of Ca^{2+}. Similar processes apparently are at play in the organ of Corti when Ca^{2+} is removed from the perilymph.

The metabolic poison tetrodotoxin has the effect of eliminating the inward (Na) current through a cell membrane during active permeability changes. Consequently its effect is to suppress action potentials without a significant influence on either resting membrane potential or graded generator potentials. When introduced either into scala tympani or media, tetrodotoxin has no effect on EP, and thus active Na current is probably not necessary for the maintenance of this resting potential. In line with the general insensitivity of membrane potentials to tetrodotoxin, the organ of Corti potential (i.e., the intracellular negativity) is unaffected by the administration of this drug. The CM is also unaffected by it, when introduced into either scala media or scala tympani. In marked contrast, when the drug is introduced into scala tympani the AP is very rapidly decreased. Again, the major effect is seen in the lower segment of the input–output function, even though there is a sizable reduction in the high-intensity AP response as well. Interestingly, when tetrodotoxin is introduced into scala media, it does not influence normal AP production. This indicates that this agent cannot diffuse through the reticular membrane (Konishi and Kelsey, 1968b).

Procaine has the general effect of decreasing membrane permeability and thus it decreases the resting membrane potential. When this drug is introduced into the organ of Corti, its effect on cochlear potentials is very similar to that of tetrodotoxin (Konishi and Kelsey, 1968b). When introduced into scala tympani, it radically decreases AP (primarily the low-level response). It apparently has no effect on the organ of Corti negativity, but it does create a mild depression of CM. Like tetrodotoxin, procaine does not diffuse through the reticular lamina, as attested by a lack of influence on the AP when introduced into scala media. The endocochlear potential increases somewhat after the infusion of procaine into any of the cochlear scalae. This is apparently a result of increased membrane resistance and consequently a lesser load on the generator of EP.

The various bits of evidence reviewed above can now be summarized. It appears that diffusion through the reticular lamina is quite minimal, but in contrast the basilar membrane does not present a diffusion barrier to the ions and substances that have been used in the experiments. This contention is well in line with the electron microscope observation that the reticular lamina and the imbedded cuticular plates appear to be dense, impermeable structures. The stria vascularis is clearly responsible for the development of the EP and also for supplying the metabolic energy that is required to maintain the K^+ concentration of the endolymph. It appears that while K^+ and Na^+ can diffuse into the scala media space through the basilar and

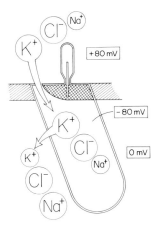

Fig. 5.64. Schematic of ionic concentration and primary ion flow around and through the membrane of the outer hair cell. It is assumed here that the major flow of K^+ ions from endolymph into the cell is through the cuticle-free apical pole. This flow could also take place through the unit membrane of the cilia. The excess K^+ ions move down their concentration gradient across the extensive, cortilymph-surrounded cell membrane around the body of the cell.

Reissner's membranes, there is an active transport process in the stria that selectively removes Na^+ from the endolymph and into the bloodstream. The most important observation probably pertains to the very strong dependence of CM on the K^+ content of endolymph and the imperviousness of this response with manipulations of the Na^+ content of perilymph. It appears that CM should be construed as a result of flow of K^+ ions from endolymph into the hair cells. Figure 5.64 shows a schematic of this process. First note that there is virtually no concentration gradient for K^+ across the cuticular plates since both the endolymph and the inside of the hair cells are rich in potassium. However, there is an electrical gradient maintained by the combined effect of the EP and the intracellular negativity. The electrical gradient can produce a steady K^+ flow into the hair cell (either through the small cuticle-free region or through the ciliary membranes). The flow can be modulated by resistance changes to yield the CM. The excess K^+ is removed from the cell body by diffusion down its concentration gradient into the organ of Corti fluid space, which is low in potassium content. The initiation and maintenance of action potentials apparently follow well established rules. Thus removal of Na^+ from the extracellular spaces has a profound effect on AP and so does any interference with sodium currents such as produced by tetrodotoxin. Similarly, the removal of calcium from the surrounding of the nerve fibers interferes with spike production and consequently diminishes the AP. The fact that most manipulations have their primary effect on the low-intensity AP seems to go hand in hand with our previous observation that it is fibers innervating the outer hair cells that are responsible for this segment of the AP input–output function. The dendritic processes of these fibers are much more accessible to the fluids in the spaces of the organ of Corti, for they are at least partially bare, and the cells that they innervate are completely surrounded by the fluid. Thus these fibers should be highly susceptible to any alteration in the ionic content of their environment. In contrast, the inner hair cells and the fibers that innervate them are all tightly packed within a matrix of supporting cells and consequently could be protected, at least on a short-term basis, from changes in the cortilymph.

CHAPTER 6

Nonlinear Distortion

I. Description of Nonlinear Systems

One of the most frequently studied and yet least understood aspects of the ear's operation is its production of distortion. Some manifestations of distortion were noted as early as 1744 (Sorge; cf. Jones, 1935), but even today the mechanism of distortion generation is a subject of considerable disagreement. That there is confusion about this topic is not at all surprising. The classic development of mathematics, physics, and engineering, let alone quantitative biology, followed the treatment of linear or linearizable systems. Not until relatively recently did the basic premise begin to permeate our corporate thinking that *life is very nonlinear*. Consequently it is a relatively recent development that engineers purposely design nonlinearities into their systems rather than take the classic approach of linearizing at any cost. Along with the increased awareness of the nonlinearity of nature, more and more use is made of available but hitherto ignored mathematical techniques, and the quest is on for the development of more general and adequate methods for the analytic treatment of nonlinear systems. The difficulties attendant on treating and understanding nonlinear behavior are some of the prime causes for inadequate and often confused treatment of such phenomena.

Another, probably more important reason for much of the controversy and misunderstanding that surround the topic of nonlinear behavior is the basic property of all nonlinear systems that they resist simple descriptions which purport to be all encompassing. To explain, a nonlinear system might behave in a particular fashion for a certain combination of the parameters of the input stimuli, while another combination could bring about a seemingly unrelated and apparently opposing behavior. Clearly a simple description of the operation in one range cannot serve a similar function in the other range. Quantitative, but even qualitative, descriptions of a nonlinear system must contain information about the range of applicability of the mathematical or conceptual model. An example will illuminate the importance of adequate specification of experimental conditions. Certain systems exhibit a phenomenon called jump resonance. In such a system the amplitude of the output signal depends not only on the amplitude of the input and the frequency of the input (which is the familiar linear case) but also on the *direction* in which a particular frequency is approached. Figure 6.1 illustrates the situation in depicting a nonlinear resonance curve that gives the relationship between output magnitude and input frequency when the input amplitude is held constant. Note that above f_1 and below f_2 the amplitude is uniquely defined but that between these two frequencies the output can be any of three different values. If this region is approached from the low-frequency side then the system output follows the upper portion of the curve. If, however, the frequency is decreasing from above f_1 then the lower portion of the curve is of importance. (The dashed portion of the curve describes unstable behavior, that is, values that cannot be observed over a prolonged duration.)

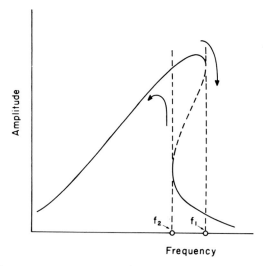

Fig. 6.1. Frequency response curve of a system exhibiting the phenomenon of jump resonance.

It is conceivable that hypothetical experimenters could create considerable controversy about the operation of such a system if one experimenter used only frequencies below f_1 while the other used only frequencies above f_2, and if both generalized from their findings for all frequencies.

Another possible contributing factor to some of the disagreements over nonlinear behavior is the extreme susceptibility of the measurement of such behavior to instrumental artifacts. It is now generally appreciated that in order to describe the nonlinear behavior of the auditory system one must use a nondistorted test stimulus. Clearly if the input signal contains distortion components then it is extremely difficult, if not impossible, to separate such distortion products in the output that arise in the system itself from those that are merely transduced from the input. While there is growing awareness of the necessity of using pure input signals, experimenters still too commonly do not use adequate precautions to avoid distorted stimuli or, even when they are careful, they rarely report exact figures. The reporting of quantitative information on the purity of the test signal is extremely important. It is also imperative that tests for lack of distortion in the signal be conducted under circumstances that closely mimic actual experimental conditions. The reader's attention is again called to the potentially large discrepancies that can exist between signal distortion measured in a rigid-walled coupler and that measured in front of the eardrum. This problem was discussed at length in the second chapter, but its relevance here cannot be sufficiently emphasized.

Finally, much confusion has arisen in the past because of simple semantic difficulties. Beats, a simple linear phenomenon, are often confused with difference tones, which can arise in nonlinear systems only. Apparent distortion of complex signals, which occurs in any linear system that is not purely dissipative (that is, a system that possesses some filter characteristics), can be easily confused with amplitude distortion.

In order to provide a clear understanding of the distinction between linear and nonlinear systems, it is now proper to provide a formal definition of a linear system. Assume that a rule H describes the operation that is performed by a system upon an input. Such a rule might be as follows. Add 5 to the input, or multiply the input by 2, or square the input. If input signals are denoted by the functions $f(t)$, $g(t)$, ..., $z(t)$ while a, b, ..., x are constants, then the operator H is said to be linear if the following equality is satisfied:

$$H[af(t) + bg(t) + \ldots + xz(t)] = aH[f(t)] + bH[g(t)] + \ldots + xH[z(t)] \quad (6.1)$$

This condition can also be written in a somewhat simpler form as two simultaneous conditions:

$$H[f(t) + g(t) + \ldots + z(t)] = H[f(t)] + H[g(t)] + \ldots + H[z(t)]$$

and

$$H[af(t)] = aH[f(t)] \quad (6.2)$$

The first condition is that the additive property or superposition be satisfied. The second condition is that of homogeneity. The first condition requires that the output of a linear system in response to a number of independent inputs be expressible as the sum of the outputs that would have been obtained if each input were present alone. The second property requires that the outputs of a linear system to inputs of different magnitudes differ only by a constant of proportionality. Systems that do not satisfy these requirements are classified as nonlinear. Two simple examples will illuminate how these rules operate. Assume first that the operator H assigns the following rule. Multiply the input by 2 in order to obtain the output. Our two input functions are $f(t) = 5 \cos t$ and $g(t) = 7 \cos 3t$. The rule of homogeneity requires that

$$2[5 \cos t] = 5 \cdot 2[\cos t] = 10 \cos t; \qquad 2[7 \cos 3t] = 7 \cdot 2[\cos 3t] = 14 \cos 3t$$

Clearly this condition is fulfilled. The requirement of superposition is expressed as

$$2[\cos t + \cos 3t] = 2[\cos t] + 2[\cos 3t]$$

This requirement is again clearly fulfilled. Thus the operation of multiplying by 2 is shown to be linear. Next let us assume that the operator H requires that the input be squared in order to obtain the output. Using the same functions and constants as before, let us examine the two rules. First the rule of homogeneity.

$$[5 \cos t]^2 = 5^2 \cos^2 t = 25 \cos^2 t \neq 5[\cos t]^2 = 5 \cos^2 t$$

This requirement is not satisfied. The additive property is expressed as

$$[\cos 2t + \cos 3t]^2 = \cos^2 2t + 2 \cos 2t \cos 3t + \cos^2 3t \neq [\cos 2t]^2 + [\cos 3t]^2$$
$$= \cos^2 2t + \cos^2 3t$$

The second requirement is likewise unsatisfied. Thus, clearly, the squaring operation must be considered nonlinear.

In connection with the second example we can see a property of nonlinear systems that is probably most important for our purposes. The term $2 \cos 2t \cos 3t$ can be rewritten as $\cos 5t + \cos t$. Thus in this case the input consists of the functions $\cos 2t$ and $\cos 3t$, but after the squaring operation functions at other frequencies also appear, such as $\cos 5t$ and $\cos t$. One can state that the output of a linear system *never* contains frequency components that were not present in the input signal, whereas the output of a nonlinear system can contain frequencies introduced by the system itself, not originally present in the input. These newly created frequencies have traditionally been the focal points of any treatment of auditory nonlinearities. Thus in auditory physiology one customarily discusses the subject of harmonic generation, to mention the simplest case, as a seemingly independent entity. Other *manifestations* of nonlinear behavior are treated in their own right. This style of attack on nonlinear problems in hearing is a rather natural consequence of our customary reliance on pure tones as input stimuli to the auditory system. In physical terms such an input (pure tone) constitutes harmonic forcing of a nonlinear system. The most common behavior of a nonlinear system when driven by a sinusoidal force is to generate new frequency components. Thus it is not surprising that almost the entire literature on the nonlinear behavior of the ear revolves around the description of the properties of such new products. Only recently have attempts been made to suggest models that could account for several attributes of the nonlinear operation of the hearing organ.

In this chapter the traditional approach will be followed in that nonlinear behavior will be discussed in terms of new frequencies generated in the peripheral auditory system. When the stimulus consists of a single pure tone three new frequency components can appear under appropriate circumstances. These are harmonics (or overtones), subharmonics (or undertones), and dc. The latter, direct-current or zero-frequency component, has actually been treated in Chapter 5 in great detail. I am referring to the summating potential of course, which, as we have already mentioned, is a distortion component, being a dc response to an ac stimulus. When two or more pure tones are simultaneously present, so-called intermodulation components (combination tones) can be observed. All these nonlinear distortion products will be separately discussed below. In addition a few other relevant topics will be treated, such as interference and squelch.

II. Distortion Components in Cochlear Potentials

A. HARMONICS

When a pure tone is fed through a system whose behavior is nonlinear, the output waveform is seen to depart from the simple sinusoidal time course of the input. The tops of the sinusoid might be clipped off or the shape might become more peaked. The change in waveform depends directly on the properties of the nonlinearity. These properties (if known) can be described either analytically, that is, by providing a mathematical relationship between input and output, or by graphical means, that is, by showing a plot that depicts the dependence of the output on the input. A simple example of the former is the statement that $y = ax^2$, where x is the input, y is the output, and a is a constant. This mathematical description indicates a so-called quadratic nonlinearity where the output is proportional to the square of the input. One of the simplest graphical relationships giving a nonlinear characteristic is that which shows saturation (Fig. 6.2). Here the system is linear below a certain value of the input (x_0) but the output does not increase in proportion to the input once the value of x_0 is surpassed. Incidentally, such a simple graphical representation can also be given analytically by a set of equalities or inequalities. In the present case, for instance, the following description provides an adequate representation of the system's behavior:

$$y = \quad bx \qquad \text{for} \qquad -x_0 \leqslant x \leqslant x_0$$
$$y = +bx_0 \qquad \text{for} \qquad x > x_0$$
$$y = -bx_0 \qquad \text{for} \qquad -x_0 > x$$

It should also be mentioned that any such simple, single-valued, characteristic function can also be approximated to any desired degree of accuracy by a polynomial in the form $y = a_0 + a_1 x + a_2 x^2 + \ldots + a_n x^n$. In this polynomial series the value and sign of the coefficients $(a_0, a_1, \ldots, a_n)$ depend on the

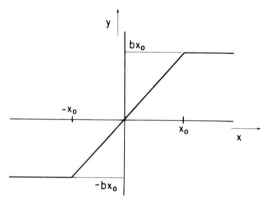

Fig. 6.2. Input–output characteristic of a system showing saturation at high input levels.

exact form of the function to be approximated, while the number of terms determines the accuracy of approximation. In general if the graphic function is symmetrical around the origin (such as the example is) then the polynomial approximation contains only odd terms, that is, $a_1 x + a_3 x^3 + \ldots + a_{2k-1} x^{2k-1}$. When the function is symmetrical around the ordinate the series is composed of even terms, $a_0 + a_2 x^2 + \ldots + a_{2k} x^{2k}$.

Functions that can be described in terms of a polynomial approximation represent nonlinearities whose effect on the input signal is the same no matter what the frequency of that signal might be. Such nonlinearities are often called frequency independent or memoryless. The latter designation arises from the observation that this type of nonlinearity by itself does not allow energy storage; namely, the output from it follows the input instantaneously.

In this respect these simple nonlinearities behave as purely dissipative (resistive) elements; they modify the amplitude of a sinusoid but not its phase. The characteristic function of a memoryless nonlinearity is easy to recognize, for the output and input magnitudes of the signals are related by a single-valued function. Such a function is characterized by the rule that to any given input magnitude only one uniquely related output magnitude corresponds. Multivalued characteristic functions signify a nonlinearity with memory, or in other words one that possesses energy storage capability and thus alters not only the amplitude but also the phase of an input sinusoid. Multivalued nonlinear functions cannot in general be approximated by a simple polynomial series, and consequently the treatment of their behavior is greatly complicated. One of the most common multivalued nonlinearities is hysteresis. Hysteresis implies directional sensitivity in that increasing and decreasing input signals do not generate the same output even if of equal magnitude. Such a nonlinearity creates frequency-dependent effects. Thus far all attempts to model the nonlinear behavior of the peripheral auditory system (Newman *et al.*, 1937; Engebretson and Eldredge, 1968; Nieder and Nieder, 1968; Pong and Marcaccio, 1963), based on physiological data, have employed single-valued nonlinear characteristic functions.

The distortion of the waveform of the sinusoidal input signal by the nonlinearity is customarily expressed in terms of the harmonic distortion components that are generated in the process. Even after considerable distortion of the input, the output signal remains periodic with the same repetition rate as the undistorted input. According to the theorem of Fourier any periodic function can be expressed as the sum of harmonically related sinusoids. That is, if $f(\omega t)$ is an arbitrary periodic function with period $T = 2\pi/\omega$, then

$$f(\omega t) = a_0 + a_1 \cos \omega t + a_2 \cos 2\omega t + \ldots + a_n \cos n\omega t + \ldots$$
$$+ b_1 \sin \omega t + b_2 \sin 2\omega t + \ldots + b_n \sin n\omega t + \ldots \quad (6.3)$$

This series expressing the function in terms of sine and cosine functions is called a Fourier series, while the process of describing a periodic function in these terms is called Fourier analysis. The rule for obtaining the coefficients in the series is expressed by the following equations:

$$a_0 = \frac{1}{2\pi} \int_0^{2\pi} f(\omega t) d\omega t \qquad a_n = \frac{1}{\pi} \int_0^{2\pi} f(\omega t) \cos n\omega t \, d\omega t$$

$$b_n = \frac{1}{\pi} \int_0^{2\pi} f(\omega t) \sin n\omega t \, d\omega t \qquad (6.4)$$

In general the evaluation of the coefficients of a Fourier series can be quite laborious. Fortunately some savings in effort, and incidentally some deeper insight into the process of distortion, can be gained if the periodic function to be analyzed exhibits some form of symmetry. We can distinguish two types of symmetry. A sine function is symmetrical to the zero point; this symmetry can be expressed by the relationship $f(\omega t) = -f(-\omega t)$. Such functions are called *odd*. The Fourier series of an odd function contains only odd terms or, stating it in another way, the series consists of only sine functions. Conversely, a cosine function is symmetrical about the vertical coordinate axis. Such functions are called *even* and they can be classified by the relationship $f(t) = f(-t)$. The Fourier series of an even function contains only cosine terms.

One more important simplifying idea has to be introduced. The first term in the series, a_0, is also called the dc component. This term expresses the average value of the periodic function. If there is no dc component (when the areas under the function above and below the time axis are equal) the a_0 term vanishes. This condition always prevails for odd functions, but for even functions the dc term may or may not be zero. Of course, to describe a general periodic function that does not show any symmetry one would have to have a series containing both even and odd terms. In general the coefficients a_n and b_n decrease in magnitude with increasing n. Stated in different terms, the tendency is for progressively smaller high-frequency terms. If a series describes its periodic function quite accurately with only a few terms it is described as rapidly convergent. A slowly convergent series is one in which the coefficients decrease to negligible proportion after only a large number of terms.

The concept of the Fourier series was introduced in the previous paragraphs not only because this elegant technique allows one to mathematically specify a complex repetitive wave in terms of simple and familiar sinusoids, but, more importantly, because a complex repetitive wave is actually *composed* of this series of sinusoids, and the individual components can in reality be measured with suitable instrumentation. The appropriate instrument for the measurement of the harmonic content of a signal is some sort of spectrum or wave analyzer. Such an instrument is capable of providing a measure of the magnitude of the individual spectral components. If a system contains a nonlinearity which distorts the waveform of a pure sinusoidal input signal then the distortion can be quantified by measuring the individual harmonic components in the system's output. This approach has been used frequently, and almost exclusively, in treating the distortion of a pure tone by the peripheral auditory system.

The first systematic study of the harmonic content of the CM potential was reported by Stevens and Newman (1936) and by Newman et al. (1937). Cochlear microphonic input–output functions were measured for several fundamentals and for harmonics up to the fifth order. Both cats and guinea pigs were studied. All measurements were made with round-window electrodes, and thus the reader should keep the limitations of this type of recording in mind when evaluating these experimental results. Incidentally, with very few exceptions CM distortion has been measured in the past with the round-window method, and thus much of the published information describes fairly limited behavior. Somewhat similar to the Newman *et al.* (1937) investigation was the experimental series of Wever and colleagues (Wever and Bray, 1938; Wever *et al.*, 1940b; Wever and Lawrence, 1954). These investigators also utilized the round-window technique, and again the guinea pig was the experimental animal. The results of the above experiments, which to date are among the most detailed on cochlear distortion, are summarized below.

Input–output functions of harmonic components were seen to have the same general shape as the familiar CM magnitude versus sound intensity function, which we discussed in detail in Chapter 5. When plotted in a log–log coordinate system the harmonic functions show a straight-line segment at moderate intensities, which at higher levels is followed by satura-tion, maximum, and a bend-over portion. The first distortion component that becomes measurable at the lowest sound level is invariably the second harmonic. This component can first be detected 30–40 dB above the level at which the fundamental becomes measurable. The second harmonic is followed by the higher overtones in an orderly fashion. It was immediately noticed that the slope of the harmonic functions is steeper than that of the fundamental. Wever and Bray (1938) state that the slopes become increasingly steeper with the order of the harmonic. Their second- and third-harmonic plots have slopes very close to 2 and 3, respectively. In theory the slopes of the harmonic input–output functions should be proportional to their order, that is, 2 for a second harmonic, 3 for a third harmonic, and so forth. Wever and Bray's experience, as well as ours, is that the functions tend to conform to the theoretical expectation at the lowest orders only. When one attempts to ascertain the slope of harmonic functions of fourth and higher orders, the task is usually made difficult by the very narrow range over which these functions exhibit straight-line segments in the logarithmic coordinate system. The reason for this is that progressively higher-order components become measurable at progressively higher sound intensities, but they tend to have input–output functions that saturate at approximately the same level. As a consequence the measurable straight-line segments become truncated. It seems that the slopes seldom become steeper than 30 dB/10 dB.

Stevens and Davis (1938) made a distinction between the shapes of the harmonic input–output functions depending on the order of the harmonics that these represented. Apparently the input–output functions belonging to odd harmonics had a smooth appearance, not unlike the fundamental functions: a straight-line segment followed by saturation, but no bend-over portion. In contrast, the even functions all exhibited pronounced bend-over segments. The input–output functions shown by Wever and Bray (1938) are also of different character for the even and odd harmonics. The input–output functions of the odd-harmonic components all show straight-line segments, followed by saturation, maximum, and bend-over. All maxima occur at the same SPL for a given fundamental frequency. The even-harmonic functions have their maxima at a lower SPL, and this maximum is followed by a dip, after which the function rises again. Our experience is that the odd harmonics *tend* to have simpler input–output functions and that the even harmonics *tend* to show local minima and generally more complex behavior. It is fair to say, however, that not all cases conform to the patterns shown by Stevens and Davis and by Wever and Lawrence. When recordings are made from the first turn of the guinea pig cochlea, and the input–output functions are classified as to whether or not they possess a local minimum, one notes that all fundamental functions and the vast majority of the third-harmonic functions are of the simple variety; that is they have no local minima. At low frequencies the simple functions predominate among the second-harmonic input–output plots also, but above 5 kHz more and more of these become complex.

Some examples of the shapes of the various harmonic order input–output functions are shown in Fig. 6.3. These plots are obtained with an automatic tracing method whereby the signal intensity is increased at a rate of 2 dB/ second. Both CM and SPL are automatically plotted on logarithmic scales. These functions show all phenomena that have been mentioned before, such as steepening slopes at higher orders, difference between even- and odd-order functions, and the interesting notches in the even functions. In addition, this method of tracing (as opposed to discrete measurements) reveals the sharpness and actual depth of the notches. The presence of two segments in the even functions strongly suggests that there are two distinct processes that produce the even-harmonic distortion in the auditory system. Since there is a notch between the segments, indicating partial cancellation of the CM at a given intensity, the microphonic potentials produced by these processes are out of phase. It is quite possible that the high-level process is generated in the middle ear. As we shall see, the low-level process is most likely cochlear in origin. The suggestion that the middle ear is the sight of the even-harmonic-producing high-level process must be weighed against the finding of Guinan and Peake (1967) that the middle ear is quite linear (see Chapter 3). It should be remembered, however, that the stroboscopic method used by Guinan and Peake is not sensitive to even-harmonic distortion, and thus it could have gone undetected.

To study the spatial distribution of CM harmonic components we recorded these at various locations in the guinea pig cochlea with the differential-electrode technique. Of primary interest was to determine whether a given harmonic component would have a spatial pattern corresponding to that of a pure tone of identical frequency or maybe to that of the eliciting fundamental. Several approaches were used to determine these spatial patterns. Input–output functions for fundamentals, harmonics, and for pure tones having the same frequency as the harmonics were obtained simultaneously from more than one cochlear location; the magnitudes of fundamental and harmonic CM components were measured at constant sound pressure level over several

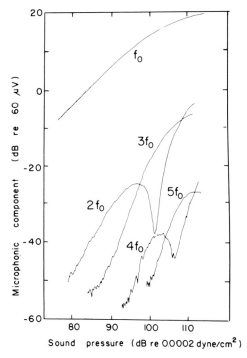

Fig. 6.3. Input–output functions of CM fundamental, second, third, fourth, and fifth harmonics. Recording is from the first turn of a guinea pig cochlea with differential electrodes; stimulus frequency is 6000 Hz. (From Niswander, 1970.)

fundamental frequencies; finally, cancellation of the harmonic CM components was attempted by introducing a controllable signal of the same frequency with bone conduction.

In Fig. 6.4 CM input–output functions are shown from both first and third cochlear turns, for a fundamental of 650 Hz, its third harmonic, and for a pure tone having the same frequency as the third harmonic (1950 Hz). The plots for the 650-Hz fundamental show the expected unity slope at lesser sound pressure levels, then gradual saturation and bend-over. Because of the different sensitivity of the two turns, in the linear region the output of the third turn is about 20 dB higher than that of the first turn. Nonlinearity, however, occurs in the third turn at a much lower level than in the first, with the consequence that above approximately 80 dB SPL, the first-turn CM becomes greater. Since the first turn is considerably more sensitive to a frequency of 1950 Hz, the CM response from it to such a pure tone stimulus is greater at all intensities than the third-turn potential.

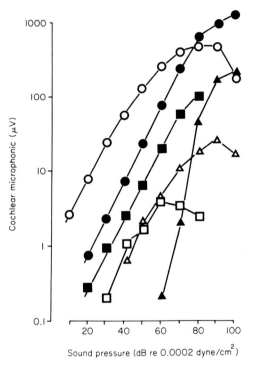

Fig. 6.4. Cochlear microphonic input–output functions from first and third turns of the guinea pig cochlea for a 650-Hz pure tone (●, turn 1; ○, turn 3), its third-harmonic component (1950 Hz; ▲, turn 1; △, turn 3), and for a 1950-Hz pure tone (■, turn 1, □, turn 3). (From Dallos and Sweetman, 1969, p. 41.)

The third-harmonic (1950-Hz) component rises steeper than pure tones at low intensities. At low intensities, the harmonics are considerably more prominent in the third turn than in the basal turn. With increasing primary intensity, the third-turn response shows saturation before the basal-turn response, and thus the latter becomes larger at high sound pressure levels. It is immediately clear from these plots that the relationship between responses from the two turns is much closer between fundamental and harmonic than between harmonics and pure tones mimicking them in frequency. This means that the relative magnitudes of harmonic components from turn to turn correspond to the relative magnitudes of their eliciting fundamentals, rather than to those of pure tones of identical frequency. Thus, the indication is that the spatial distribution of a given harmonic in the cochlea does not depend on the frequency of the harmonic component in question, but rather on the frequency of its fundamental.

To investigate this suggestion further, plots of fundamental and harmonic components in the CM were obtained at various fundamental frequencies, but at a constant sound pressure level of the eliciting stimulus. Such plots are essentially the tuning curves for a given cochlear location. In Fig. 6.5 such curves are shown in the fundamental frequency range of 300–3000 Hz, from an electrode pair located in the third turn of the guinea pig cochlea. The

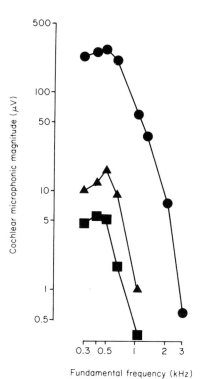

Fig. 6.5. Cochlear microphonic potentials as the function of frequency from turn 3 in response to 60-dB-SPL fundamentals. Fundamental (●), second- (▲) and third-harmonic (■) CM components are all plotted at the frequency of the fundamental. (From Dallos and Sweetman, 1969, p. 42.)

sound pressure of the fundamental was 60 dB. In this plot, the CM response to the 60-dB fundamental and the CM components at the second- and third-harmonic frequencies are shown, with the ordinate expressed in units of microvolts. All components are plotted at the frequency of their fundamental; thus, for example, both second and third harmonics of a 300-Hz fundamental are plotted at the abscissa point corresponding to 300 Hz. It is clear that the third-turn electrodes seem to be maximally sensitive in this animal to about 500 Hz. Below this frequency, there is a gradual decrease in response and, above this frequency, there is a rather precipitous drop. The shape of the second- and third-harmonic functions is quite similar. The most significant observation is the most obvious one. All three functions show maximum sensitivity for the same frequency region. It it is recalled that the harmonic functions are *not* plotted according to the actual harmonic frequency, but rather according to the fundamental frequency, it would appear at face value that the maximum sensitivity of the third turn occurs at different frequencies, depending on the harmonic order of the signal in question. To explain, it would appear that when the signal is a fundamental the third turn is most sensitive to 500 Hz; when the signal is a second-harmonic component, however, maximum response at this same point occurs at 1000 Hz. Since the frequency sensitivity of the electrode location is clearly described by the curve for the fundamental component, the fact that harmonic curves follow the pattern of their fundamentals, and not their own frequencies, must indicate that harmonic components are not distributed in the cochlea as one would expect them to be according to their frequencies and the place principle. Instead, any harmonic component is localized in the region that is most sensitive to its eliciting fundamental. Consequently, it is unlikely that harmonic components are mediated by traveling waves.

In an extensive series of experiments with von Békésy type of models, Tonndorf (1958a) sought to describe hydrodynamic distortion processes inherent in the cochlea. He concluded that harmonic distortion is closely tied in with the formation of eddies in the perilymphatic fluid. He demonstrated that eddies occur only at relatively high driving levels, while particle and membrane motion is clearly visible at much lesser intensities. With the appearance of the eddies, the particle orbits become distorted, i.e., flattened and asymmetrical. The distorted particle motion evidently found a coupling mechanism with the membranous partition, for Tonndorf was able to demonstrate that each harmonic formed its own maximum on the membrane at the same place where an externally applied tone of the same frequency would have. We see that these results seem to contradict our findings in that the harmonic components in Tonndorf's model were "well behaved" in their distribution; they were accompanied by their own traveling waves. The following explanation is offered. The eddies, which Tonndorf so closely associates with distortion, are a high-intensity phenomenon. We do not know exactly what intensity is required for reaching eddy threshold in a given species, say in guinea pigs, but a reasonable assumption is that sound pressure levels of the order of 80–90 dB might be needed. Now let us assume that the eddies are required, as a type of feedback mechanism, to couple the fluid-borne distortion to wide segments of the membrane and to initiate traveling waves. Without eddies, then, one would not expect localized distortion, if present, to be redistributed according to the place principle. There is no reason, however, why such localized distortion could not cause limited excitation.

Tonndorf (1958b) followed up his model experiments with electrophysiological studies of harmonics in the CM of guinea pig cochleae. In those experiments, he reaffirmed the conclusions that were obtained in the model study, namely, that each harmonic forms a traveling wave pattern of its own. His most conclusive evidence is presented in his Fig. 9, which depicts the same type of information as our Fig. 6.5. In his figure, the magnitude of a fundamental, and its second and third harmonic, are plotted as the function of frequency at a constant sound pressure level. In that figure, he shows that the two harmonics are distributed as one would expect on the basis of their frequency if they had been externally introduced pure tones, rather than internally generated harmonics. The reader will recall that this is directly contrary to the data presented in our Fig. 6.5. Here we must invoke the intensity differences between the two sets of data. Our curves were obtained at 60 dB SPL measured at the eardrum, while Tonndorf's functions were generated at 90 dB SPL measured in a coupler. It is very likely that the sound pressures at the animals' drum membranes would have been considerably higher than the coupler figures indicate. Thus, there is at least a 30-dB intensity difference between the two experiments. In our case, probably no eddies were present in the cochlea; thus, we measured localized distortion (hydraulic or electrical). In Tonndorf's case, the eddies were operative in carrying distortion components to different regions of the cochlea. We would now like to amplify these contentions. First, examination of the second-harmonic function of the Tonndorf article (1958b, Fig. 9) clearly shows two peaks 1 octave apart. One of these peaks (the larger) appears at a frequency that would be expected if traveling waves were present; the other appears at a frequency that would be expected if the harmonic were distributed as its fundamental (as it was in our Fig. 6.5). To us, this second peak in Tonndorf's function clearly signifies the presence of two processes, one localized and one distributed, according to the traveling wave mechanism.

Let us now turn back to our own data for higher intensity levels. We did collect CM versus frequency functions like those in Fig. 6.5 with more intense sound stimuli. While the functions of Fig. 6.5 are clear-cut, the high-intensity plots that one can obtain do not appear to show any clear tendency to favor either localized distortion processes or distributed ones. In fact, functions for 80–90 dB appear to depict a transitory stage during which two processes might coexist and neither can dominate the other.

B. INTERMODULATION COMPONENTS

When the input to a nonlinear system contains two or more frequency components then in general a host of frequencies appear in the output of the system that are not present in the input signal. These frequencies are called intermodulation distortion components or, in acoustics (sometimes quite inaptly), combination tones. When two frequency components are present in the input, f_1 and f_2, the output can contain all frequencies that are obtained as $|if_1 \pm jf_2|$, where i and j are any integers. It is clear that this series of frequencies contains the complete harmonic series of the two primary input frequencies for the special case when i or j is zero. It is fairly common to designate those components that result from taking the difference between if_1, and jf_2 as difference tones, and conversely to designate the sum as summation tones. When the nonlinearity that is responsible for the generation of the intermodulation component is the polynomial type, that is, when an analytic expression for the relationship between input and output can be formulated as a power series, then the number and type of intermodulation components generated depend on the order of the power series that represents the nonlinearity. In general, if the highest power that appears in the series is n, then the distortion components can be expected to satisfy the inequality $i,j \leqslant n$. We gave an example earlier in this chapter in which the nonlinearity was represented by a simple squaring operation. We had $y = x^2$ with $x = \cos 2t + \cos 3t$, and thus we had $y = \cos^2 2t + 2 \cos 2t \cos 3t + \cos^2 3t$. With the use of simple trigonometric identities one can rewrite the last expression and obtain $y = 1 + \cos t + \frac{1}{2} \cos 4t + \cos 5t + \frac{1}{2} \cos 6t$.

Clearly the resulting expression contains a dc term, frequencies of 4 and 6 (twice the input frequencies), and 1 and 5 (difference and sum of input frequencies). Simple inspection reveals that in this case all resulting frequency components are predicted by but do not exhaust the possibilities included in $|i \cdot 2 \pm j \cdot 3|$ with $i,j = 0, 1, 2 \leqslant n = 2$. The example clearly indicates that the number of frequency components and their order are dependent on the type of nonlinearity that is responsible for their generation.

When cochlear microphonic potential is recorded at gradually increasing intensity levels one observes that the CM response to simple sinusoidal input (pure tone sound stimulation) becomes more and more distorted, that is, less and less sinusoidal. The change in waveform according to Fourier's theorem implies that the CM must contain harmonics of the stimulus frequency. With suitable means these harmonics can actually be measured. Similarly, when the sound stimulus consists of two or more sinusoidal signals at relatively high sound levels, the resulting CM contains intermodulation distortion components that can be measured with relative ease. The first such measurements were accomplished by Newman *et al.* (1937) and Wever *et al.* (1940a,b,c). Cats and guinea pigs and the round-window recording technique were used in these measurements. These early measurements provided a storehouse of useful information on the nature of cochlear distortion, aside from their contribution that proved that distortion components actually exist in the ear as physically real, objective phenomena. We have to consider the early data in light of our present knowledge on the limitations of round-window recording and in light of the realization of the extreme'importance of using sources of high-purity sound. Discounting these problems, the following phenomenological aspects of combination tone generation in the cochlea emerge from the Newman *et al.* and the Wever *et al.* investigations.

Intermodulation CM components apparently do not have real thresholds; the lowest SPL at which they are measurable depends strictly on the instrumentation used. This observation is in harmony with that made for the fundamental CM component itself or for harmonics. The magnitude versus stimulus intensity behavior of the distortion components, that is, their input–output function, is also very similar to that of the fundamental component. When plotted in a double logarithmic coordinate system the input-output functions have the now-familiar straight-line segment at low stimulus levels, followed by saturation and actual bend-over. The main distinction between input–output functions for primary components (f_1 and f_2) and those for the intermodulation products ($|if_1 \pm jf_2|$) is manifested in the slope of the initial straight-line segments of the functions. While the slope of a primary function is always equal to unity, the slopes of the combination tone functions are determined by their order. A simple empirical rule is that the slope is equal to $i + j$. The rule must be explained through the use of a few examples. Let us assume that we measure the simple difference or summation tone ($i = j = 1$) *and* we change the intensity of both primaries equally. Under this condition the slope of the component at $f_1 \pm f_2$ is 2. If, however, only one of the primary intensities is changed while the other primary is kept at a constant intensity, the resulting slope is 1. In the case of a combination tone $2f_1 \pm 3f_2$, the resulting slope is 2 when the intensity of f_1 is changed and that of f_2 is constant; it is 3 when the intensity of f_2 is changed while that of f_1 is constant, and finally it is 5 when the strengths of both primaries are changed equally. In practice this formula holds quite well for low-order combination tones, specifically when the variable $i + j \leqslant 3$. For the higher-order situations the straight-line segments of the functions become exceedingly short, the accurate measurement of slopes is difficult, and the slopes do not appear to become systematically steeper.

Engebretson and Eldredge (1968) provided some simple computations to put the above observations on more quantitative bases. They assumed that the nonlinearity can be expressed as a polynomial; that is, the relation between input (x) and output (y) was taken as $y = a_1 x + a_2 x^2 + a_3 x^3 + \ldots + a_n x^n$. When the magnitudes of the two input components of frequency f_1 and f_2 were taken as A_1 and A_2, the analytical expression for the input–output function of the combination tone $if_1 \pm jf_2$ was shown to be in the form $A_{i \pm j}(A_1, A_2) = A_1^i A_2^j$ ($b_{i,j}$ + terms involving the powers of A_1^2 and A_2^2), where $b_{i,j} = 2(\frac{1}{2})^{i+j}[(i+j)!/i!j!]a_{i+j}$. The important concept that emerges from this formulation is that if A_1 and A_2 are small all terms that contain their square will be negligible compared to the first-order term. This means that under such circumstances the magnitude of the $A_{i \pm j}$ combination tone can be approximated as

$$A_{i \pm j}(A_1, A_2) = A_1^i A_2^j b_{i,j} \tag{6.5}$$

The result implies that, when A_1 is variable and A_2 is constant, the slope of the $A_{i \pm j}(A_1)$ function is equal to i, and when A_2 is variable and A_1 is constant the resulting slope is j, whereas the slope of the $A_{i \pm j}(A_1, A_2)$ function is $i + j$ when both A_1 and A_2 vary together. These results are of course identical to the empirical formulation of Wever et al. When neither A_1 or A_2 can be considered small the higher-order terms can no longer be neglected, and as a consequence the slope of the combination tone input–output function does not conform to the simple formula given above, but it becomes very complex. Empirical evidence obtained with round-window recording bears this contention out as well.

One can obtain further correlations between CM data and the Engebretson–Eldredge formulation of combination tone behavior. At low levels of stimulation, that is, when A_1 and A_2 are small, the magnitude of the $A_{i \pm j}$ component decreases with increasing $i + j$ (assuming that $b_{i,j}$ is convergent in i and j). This implies that the lower-order combination tones are more prominent than the higher-order tones. In practice the simple difference and summation components $f_1 \pm f_2$ appear at the lowest intensity, followed by the $2f_1 \pm f_2$ and $f_1 \pm 2f_2$ components, then the $2f_1 \pm 2f_2$ products, and so on. An illustration of the order of appearance of the various combination frequencies of a given pair of primaries is given in Fig. 6.6. Here the two fundamental frequencies are 1000 and 1120 Hz, always presented at equal intensity levels. Only the intermodulation components that are obtained as $(n+1)f_1 - nf_2$ are measured, and these components form the series 880, 760, ..., 160, and 40 Hz as n changes from 1 to 8. Notice that in this series $i + j$ changes from 3 to 17; in other words, the series of frequencies encom-

passes low and very high orders of combination tones. It is apparent that all
input–output functions are highly similar in the location of their maxima.
Their initial slopes tend to become somewhat steeper with increasing $i + j$,
but this increase is very moderate, certainly nowhere near in line with the
prediction of slope by the formula, slope $= i + j$. Both the sensitivity and the
maximum are clearly ordered according to $i + j$; the lower the number the
lesser the SPL required to elicit a measurable combination tone and the
greater the maximum CM corresponding to this tone. One interesting
observation is that the high-order functions tend to bunch up; they seem to
converge to a common minimal function.

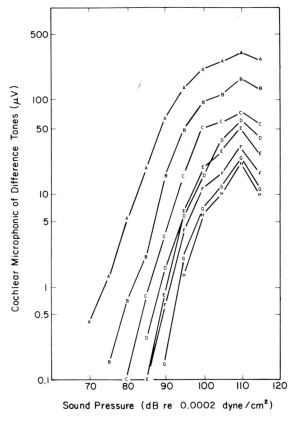

Fig. 6.6. Cochlear microphonic input–output functions for the series of combination
components $(n+1)f_1 - nf_2$; $f_1 = 1000$ Hz, $f_2 = 1120$ Hz. Recording is from the first turn
of a guinea pig cochlea. Legend: A, $2f_1 - f_2 = 0.88$ kHz; B, $3f_1 - 2f_2 = 0.76$ kHz; C,
$4f_1 - 3f_2 = 0.64$ kHz; D, $5f_1 - 4f_2 = 0.52$ kHz; E, $6f_1 - 5f_2 = 0.40$ kHz; F, $7f_1 - 6f_2 = 0.28$
kHz; G, $8f_1 - 7f_2 = 0.16$ kHz; H, $9f_1 - 8f_2 = 0.04$ kHz. (Modified from Dallos, 1969b,
p. 1441.)

One often tends to use primary frequencies that have a relatively large common divisor. Under such circumstances more than one of the possible combinations of $if_1 \pm jf_2$ would yield the same frequency intermodulation component. For example, if $f_1 = 1000$ and $f_2 = 1100$ Hz, then $f_2 - f_1 = 10f_1 - 9f_2 = 100$ Hz, or $2f_2 - 2f_1 = 9f_1 - 8f_2 = 200$ Hz. In these cases the resulting input–output functions tend to have more complex shapes than the single-maximum plots given in Fig. 6.6. Examples are given in Fig. 6.7 where the primaries $f_1 = 1000, f_2 = 1100$ Hz change together and the resulting combination frequencies $(n + 1)f_1 - nf_2$ are shown for $1 \leqslant n \leqslant 9$. All plots are labeled

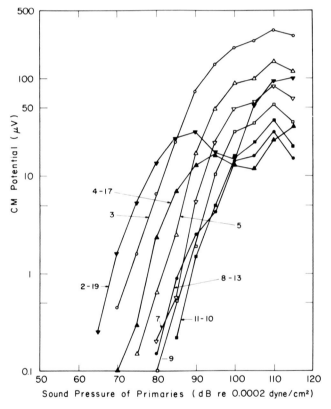

Fig. 6.7. Cochlear microphonic input–output functions for the series of combination components $if_1 - jf_2$; $f_1 = 1000$ Hz, $f_2 = 1100$ Hz. Recording is from the first turn of a guinea pig cochlea. The numbers indicate the combination of $i + j$ that yielded a given function. For example, the curve 2–19 is the response curve at 100 Hz, and it can be construed as either $f_2 - f_1(i + j = 2)$ or $10f_1 - 9f_2(i + j = 19)$. Similarly, the curve 7 reflects the measurement at 700 Hz; this component could be produced only by $4f_1 - 3f_2(i + j = 7)$. Note that all functions that are described by one index only are simple (open symbols), whereas the functions that correspond to two indices are more complex in shape (closed symbols).

with their corresponding order as expressed by $i + j$. The interesting idea that we are attempting to show here is that many of the functions correspond to two orders. The above numerical examples pertain to 100 Hz, whose order $(i + j)$ is both 2 and 19, and to 200 Hz, whose order is both 4 and 17.

Notice that all input–output functions that have multiple labels are complex in appearance. The lowest SPL at which a given component appears is determined by the lowest order that can be associated with it. Thus there is a clear progression in sensitivity from $i + j = 2$ on toward higher orders. The functions that can arise from two combinations of $if_1 \pm jf_2$ have two maxima with a trough in between. Such a shape strongly suggests that two components of differing strength and phase in different intensity regions interact to produce the resultant input–output function. It can be conjectured that in the low-intensity region the lower-order component dominates the resultant response, while at higher levels the high-order component becomes increasingly more important. This possibility can actually be proven correct by the simple method of detuning one of the primaries a slight amount so that the two primaries no longer have a common divisor. This way the two components that have had equal frequencies are now split. For example, if in the above case f_1 is increased by 5 Hz, from 1000 to 1005 Hz, then $f_2 - f_1$ becomes 95 instead of 100 Hz, while $10f_1 - 9f_2$ becomes 150 instead of 100 Hz. Measurements show that at low sound levels only the 95-Hz component is present, while at high intensities both the 95- and 150-Hz intermodulation distortion products can be detected. This means that at low levels the simple difference tone $f_2 - f_1$ dominates, while both $f_2 - f_1$ and $10f_1 - 9f_2$ coexist at high levels.

It is a common finding that, when the two primaries are nominally set so that they have a large common divisor and produce distortion components of different order but nominally identical frequency, then in certain intensity regions the distortion component exhibits very strong beats. This finding can be easily explained by noting that a slight discrepancy in the frequencies of the primaries would split the nominally coincident frequencies and that beats would ensue between closely spaced products. An example can easily illuminate this situation. In the above case we nominally had 1000- and 1100-Hz primaries. If the actual frequencies are 1000.1 and 1100 Hz then the $f_2 - f_1$ component is 99.9 Hz, while the $10f_1 - f_2$ component is 101 Hz. In the intensity band where these two components coexist a 1.1/second beat results.

Probably one of the best-controlled and most extensive studies of the input–output properties of CM combination tones was done by Worthington (1970). He measured such functions with six pairs of primary tones and over a wide range of primary intensities. Two features distinguish his measurements. First, the differential-electrode recording technique was used and, second, equipment distortion was rigidly controlled by estimating the actual amount of CM that was due to distortion in the sound system. The method used to accomplish this estimation was described in Chapter 2. Worthington measured only first-order difference tones, $f_2 - f_1$. Previous experiments (Wever and Lawrence, 1954; Sweetman and Dallos, 1969) indicated that the behavior of the simple summation tone $f_1 + f_2$ and of higher-order combination tones is largely predictable when the difference tone is known. Four of Worthington's primary pairs contained the same higher-frequency primary, 4500 Hz. With this he had primaries of 4000, 1530, 500, and 210 Hz, resulting in difference tones of 500, 2970, 4000, and 4290 Hz. His other combinations were 760- and 500-Hz primaries with a 260-Hz difference tone and 1530- and 1740-Hz primaries with a 210-Hz difference tone. Notice that this array of primaries is so chosen that in four cases one primary generates its maximal activity in the first cochlear turn while its companions are best localized in the first, second, third, and fourth turns of the guinea pig cochlea. Three combinations are so arranged that both primaries are very close to one another in frequency and their best locations are in the first, second, and third turns.

In Fig. 6.8 the magnitude of the difference tone is shown in all four cochlear turns as the function of the frequency difference between the primaries when the higher-frequency primary is 4500 Hz. The parameter in

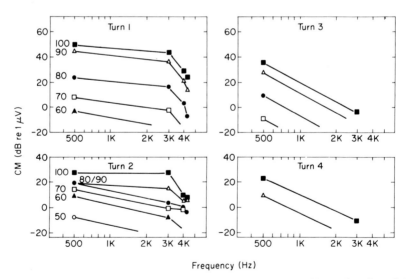

Fig. 6.8. The magnitude of the first-order difference tone ($f_2 - f_1$) as a function of the frequency interval between the primary tones (the primary frequency f_2 is kept constant at 4500 Hz). The parameter is stimulus intensity in decibels SPL. Median values are shown. (From Worthington, 1970, p. 155.)

the graphs is the common SPL of the two primary signals. In all situations shown the difference tone decreases with increasing separation between the primaries. The decrease is very gradual when the separation is moderate, but it becomes significant when the lower-frequency primary generates its maximal excitation in the apical region of the cochlea. In general one can state that combination tones are the biggest when their eliciting primaries are closely spaced in frequency.

Worthington classified his input–output functions into three categories according to their shape. Category A consisted of functions having the classically described appearance of approximately 40 dB/decade slope at the low sound levels followed by saturation, maximum, and bend-over portion. Category B contained functions that started out with a slope of 2 (40 dB/decade) but that had an intermediate minimum at relatively moderate SPL's, followed by another steep segment having a slope of approximately 2 and then the usual saturation and bend-over. Category C consisted of functions whose initial slope was less than 1.5 but which at an intermediate intensity assumed steeper slopes, followed by saturation and bend-over. It was found that a particular type of input–output function tended to occur with given primary pairs. Thus for example in the first turn type A functions predominated with $f_1 = 4500, f_2 = 210$ Hz, while type C functions were seen with $f_1 = 760, f_2 = 500$ Hz. In general, the closer together the primaries were, the better was the likelihood that type C functions would result.

In Table 6.1 the distribution of the various types of input–output functions is given for all experimental conditions. It is notable that in turn 1 the above-mentioned trend is very clear but that in the higher turns the situation is not as easy to define. This can be attributed, first, to smaller number of functions available for a given condition from the higher turns* and, second, to the fact that in higher turns the straight-line segments of the functions on which the slopes and classification are based are of very limited extent. This necessitated the use of yet a fourth category, U, for unclassifiable. It is quite fascinating to observe that in the three cases where the primaries are far apart, no type C function is ever generated. On the other hand, in the three cases with closely spaced primaries such functions are in the majority. In fact with $f_2 = 500, f_1 = 760$ Hz only type C functions were seen in the first turn.

Typical first-turn input–output functions are shown in Fig. 6.9. Panel (a) of the figure contains examples of the types of functions that were seen with the primary frequencies far apart (4500, 500 Hz) while in panel (b)

---

* The experiments were conducted with two pairs of electrodes in any given cochlea. Of these one pair was always in the first turn, while the second pair was in either second, third, or fourth turn. Altogether 15 animals were tested; thus the first turn is represented with an N of 15, while the higher turns are represented with an N of 5.

TABLE 6.1

SUMMARY OF THE NUMBER OF ANIMALS DEMONSTRATING VARIOUS TYPES
OF INPUT–OUTPUT FUNCTIONS[a]

Distortion product (Hz)	Primaries (Hz)	Turn 1	Turn 2	Turn 3	Turn 4
$DT_1 = 4290$	$f_1 = 210$	A, 12	A, 1	U, 5	U, 5
	$f_2 = 4500$	B, 3	B, 1	U, 5	
			U, 3		
$DT_1 = 4000$	$f_1 = 500$	A, 11	A, 3	U, 5	U, 5
	$f_2 = 4500$	B, 4	B, 1		
			U, 1		
$DT_1 = 2970$	$f_1 = 1530$	A, 12	A, 1	A, 1	
	$f_2 = 4500$	B, 3	B, 2	U, 4	U, 5
			U, 2		
$DT_1 = 500$	$f_1 = 4000$	A, 3	A, 1	A, 2	
	$f_2 = 4500$	B, 4	B, 4	C, 2	A, 3
		C, 8		U, 1	B, 1
$DT_1 = 260$	$f_1 = 500$	C, 15	B, 2	A, 4	C, 1
	$f_2 = 760$		C, 2	B, 1	A, 2
			U, 1		B, 2
$DT_1 = 210$	$f_1 = 1530$	A, 5	A, 3	A, 2	C, 1
	$f_2 = 1740$	C, 10	B, 1	B, 1	B, 3
			C, 1	C, 1	U, 2
				U, 1	

[a] From Worthington (1970, p. 137).

examples are shown for the functions that were generated by closely spaced
primary pairs (4500, 4000 Hz). In both panels, aside from the actual CM
distortion component, input–output functions are given for the corresponding
estimated distortion that in any case would have been due to nonlinearities
in the sound system. Dashed lines indicate slopes of 1 and 2 so that the reader
can readily compare the various segments of the input–output functions. In
general, with wider frequency separation between the primaries, a greater
SPL is required to produce a measurable difference tone, and a lower maximal
CM is achieved. With the primaries far apart in frequency, only type A and
B functions are produced. Irrespective of the type, both sensitivity and maximum are about the same in a given condition. When type B functions are
generated the transition region occurs in the vicinity of 80 dB SPL.

In panel (b), examples are shown for input–output functions in which
the primaries are relatively closely spaced in frequency. Here all three
function types are represented, but keep in mind that for the combination
760, 500 Hz only type C functions were produced. Considerable uniformity

is seen in the high-intensity pattern of the various functions, and thus all three functions, types A, B, and C, are virtually identical above 80 dB SPL. The sensitivities of the type A and B functions do not appear to differ much, but the sensitivity of the type C function is generally greater. In Table 6.2

TABLE 6.2

MEDIAN SPL LEVEL OF THE PRIMARIES WHERE $DT_1 = 1 \mu V$ IN TURN 1 AND MEDIAN SLOPE OF THE LOW-LEVEL PORTIONS OF THE DISTORTION PRODUCT[a]

Distortion product (Hz)	Primaries (Hz)	Type of curve	Median SPL of primaries to achieve $DT_1 = 1 \mu V$ (dB)	Median slope of low-level distortion[b]
$DT_1 = 500$	$f_1 = 4000$	A	68.5	2.2
	$f_2 = 4500$	B	62.25	1.9
		C	57.25	0.87
$DT_1 = 260$	$f_1 = 500$	C	74	0.6
	$f_2 = 760$			
$DT_1 = 210$	$f_1 = 1530$	A	69	1.9
	$f_2 = 1740$	C	58.5	0.8

[a] From Worthington (1970, p. 139).
[b] Below approximately 70 dB.

some comparisons are made among the three types of function for the primary combinations where all three could be obtained. A measure of sensitivity (SPL required to elicit 1-μV CM) and the slopes of the functions are given. It is notable that for any given primary pair the type C function appears at the lowest SPL; in fact the median sensitivity difference between type A and C patterns is about 10 dB. The low-level median slopes for type A and B functions are very close to 2, while that for type C is less than unity.

Input–output functions with distinctly different segments, such as types B and C, might indicate that they are produced by the interaction of more than one process that dominates in differing intensity regions. In this context the observation of the type C function might be a significant advance in the quest for the delineation of the underlying properties of cochlear distortion production. It is commonly assumed (Wever, 1966) that the type of decelerated function that is represented by the low-intensity segment in a type C pattern is produced by high noise level in the recording system. In other words, if the noise level at the frequency of interest is commensurable with the measured signal then the growth of the signal appears to be slowed until

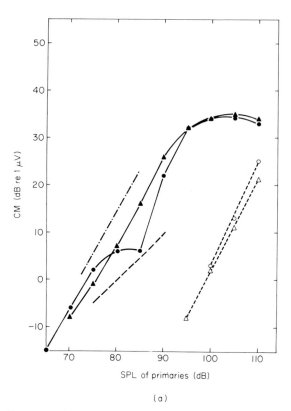

CM (dB re 1 μV)

SPL of primaries (dB)

(a)

Fig. 6.9. Representative cochlear microphonic input–output functions obtained from turn 1 for two distortion components: (a) $4500 - 500 = 4000$ Hz and (b) $4500 - 4000 = 500$ Hz. Functions are given in each panel from different animals. In addition, curves estimating the amount of distortion that one would anticipate in the CM as a result of distortion in the sound are also given (open symbols). For illustration, two straight-line segments have been added, one with a slope of 1 and the other with a slope of 2. (From Worthington, 1970, pp. 121, 122.)

it clearly emerges from the noise floor. It appears that in the case of the type C input–output functions such a simple explanation is not sufficient. The CM responses to pure tones at the frequency of the distortion component can be measured in proportion to the stimulus intensity in magnitudes at or below the point at which the shallow segment of the type C function begins. All examples of such pure tone input–output functions show unity slopes and there is no sign of interaction with noise at very low CM levels. While the simple difference tone often exhibits the type C behavior when the primaries are closely spaced, other combination tones elicited by the same f_1 and f_2 do not have input–output functions with shallow initial slopes. In Fig. 6.10

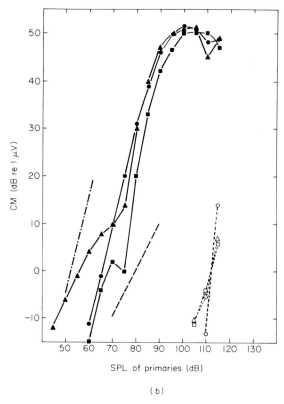

Fig. 6.9(b).

the distortion products $f_2 - f_1$ and $f_2 + f_1$ are compared when recorded from the first cochlear turn with primaries of 500 and 760 Hz. The two components are highly similar in course and magnitude above approximately 60 dB SPL, but below this there is a significant departure. The difference tone grows as a type C function, while there is no apparent slope change in the function that describes the growth pattern of the summation tone. They are not shown in the figure, but other combination tones such as $2f_1 - f_2$ and $2f_2 - f_1$ behave very similarly to the summation tone in that they also fail to exhibit the characteristic shallow initial slope of the type C function. It is notable in connection with the type C functions that these are recordable from cochlear regions that are *not* maximally sensitive to the primary tones. For example, in the situation where the primary pair 500, 760 Hz was used by Worthington, all input–output functions were type C from turn 1, but none were such from turn 3, which is the best location for the two primaries.

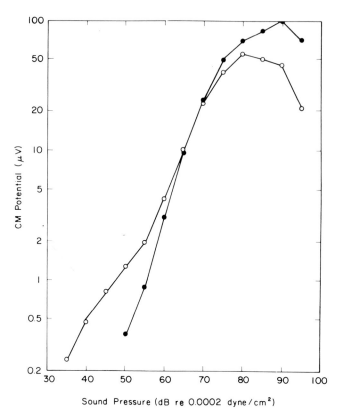

Fig. 6.10. Comparison of the CM input–output functions of a first summation component ($f_1 + f_2$, ●) and a first difference component ($f_2 - f_1$, ○) obtained from the same guinea pig. Recording is with differential electrodes from the first turn; $f_1 = 500$ Hz, $f_2 = 760$ Hz. The noise level within the 3-Hz bandwidth of the measuring instrument is 0.2 μV at 260 Hz, less at 1260 Hz.

From the input–output data of all 15 of his guinea pigs, Worthington obtained spatial distribution patterns of difference tones, primaries, and pure tones having the same frequency as the difference tone. Since in any given animal only two pairs of electrodes were used, the construction of spatial plots necessitated the combination of data from several animals. This was accomplished by taking the median CM from all animals from a given electrode location for a given experimental condition. Some of the results are presented below (Worthington, 1970; Worthington and Dallos, 1971).

Figure 6.11 shows the four distribution patterns that are obtained with primaries $f_1 = 4000$, $f_2 = 4500$ Hz. In each panel the families of graphs depict the CM magnitude as the function of electrode location with SPL as the

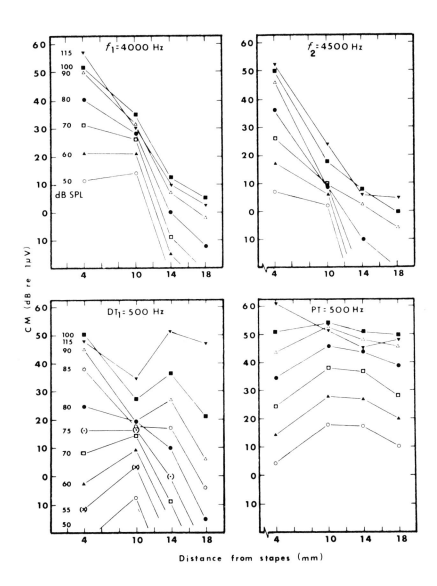

Fig. 6.11. Spatial distribution pattern for primaries (f_1, f_2), difference tones (DT = $f_2 - f_1$), and pure tones (PT = $f_2 - f_1$). Data points are medians. The parameter is the primary or pure tone intensity in decibels SPL, $f_1 = 4000$, $f_2 = 4500$, DT = PT = 500 Hz. (From Worthington and Dallos, 1971, p. 1825.)

parameter. The CM magnitudes that correspond to f_1 and f_2 are given in the top panels, while that of $f_2 - f_1$ and the pure tone $f = f_2 - f_1$ is shown on the bottom. When the CM of either f_1 or f_2 was measured, it was done in the presence of the other primary in equal intensity. The spatial pattern of the pure tone, $f = f_2 - f_1$, was obtained without a secondary tone being present. For the four cases in which the higher primary (f_2) was 4500 Hz, at the lowest intensity levels the spatial pattern of $f_2 - f_1$ is virtually unchanged. It is remembered that this invariability in the location of the first appearance of CM combination tone production comes about in spite of a change in the lower-frequency primary from 210 to 4000 Hz. The cochlear site where measurable $f_2 - f_1$ can be seen at the lowest level of the primaries is in the second turn of the cochlea in all four cases. It is notable that the higher-frequency primary CM (4500 Hz) is most prominent in the first turn. These observations suggest that the distortion components are first generated at a site somewhat apical from the location of the maximum of the higher-frequency primary, irrespective of the frequency of the lower primary. When the primary intensities are increased above the level at which distortion first appears, first subtle and then quite obvious changes in the CM patterns of $f_2 - f_1$ can be seen. At the highest levels the spatial pattern of the difference tone is quite similar to that of the pure tone having the same frequency. These results suggest a redistribution of CM distortion along the cochlea with increasing stimulus strength. The intensity shift can be seen with great clarity in Fig. 6.11. From the low-level second-turn location the distortion component maximum gradually shifts to the third turn. The shift is accompanied by an apparent suppression of the difference tone in the location where it originally appeared. This suppression results in two maxima at the higher levels with a trough in between. The probable cause of this suppression will be discussed in a subsequent section on the interference phenomenon. It is sufficient to mention here that apparently interference (the suppression of the CM response to a tone in the presence of another tone) is a nonlinear phenomenon that probably originates in the same mechanism as CM combination tone generation (Engebretson and Eldredge, 1968) and thus would be most prominent in the region where the distortion components are greatest. Thus interference has its maximal effect in the region where the difference tone first appears and it produces the reduction in the high-level $f_2 - f_1$ in that very region.

Both the input–output functions and the spatial patterns of cochlear distortion components can be explained with the greatest ease if one assumes that CM distortion production is not a unitary process. There appear to be at least two major components that predominate in different intensity regions in producing the overall CM pattern. The first of these components is most apparent at the lowest intensity levels. It produces maximal CM somewhat apically from the location of the higher-frequency primary, and its growth pattern might not conform to what one would expect on the basis of a polynomial nonlinearity (recall the type C input–output function). This low-level distortion component is fairly well localized in the cochlea; it does not spread as widely as a pure tone would. Above approximately 80 dB SPL of the primaries a second process assumes dominance over the CM response to distortion components. The spatial pattern of this constituent is very much like that of the CM responses to pure tones. Thus with increasing stimulus intensity an apparent redistribution of the CM takes place in the cochlea. This redistribution is very apparent from the above-cited results, which were foreshadowed by the earlier findings of de Boer and Six (1960) and Sweetman and Dallos (1969), as well as some of Tonndorf's model experiments (1959).

C. Origin of Distortion Components

The site and mechanism of origin of intermodulation distortion have been the subjects of a century-old debate. Von Helmholtz (1863; see von Helmholtz, 1954) was the first to relate the presence of audible combination frequencies with nonlinear distortion in the auditory system, but he assigned the site of this nonlinearity to the middle ear, specifically to the asymmetrical vibration of the eardrum. Von Békésy (1934) thought that combination tones arose in nonlinear vibrations of the stapes, while the extensive animal experiments of Wever *et al.* (1940b) showed that they originate even more centrally, namely in the cochlea. The latter view is now widely accepted. It is fully realized that *all* constituents of the auditory periphery are nonlinear; they simply differ in their degree of nonlinearity. In this sense, then, the cochlea is more nonlinear than the middle ear, with the result that at a given sound pressure level most of the distortion components have their origin in the inner ear. The experiments of Wever *et al.* were deceptively simple. They measured the CM harmonic and combination tone pattern (input–output functions) in normal guinea pigs when the stimuli were delivered via the usual air-conduction route. Then they amputated the middle ear except for the stapes and subsequently delivered the stimuli directly to the stapes in the form of mechanical vibrations and remeasured the CM response. They noted that both the combination tone and harmonic patterns in the CM were very similar in both experimental situations, yielding the conclusion that the major portion of the distortion content of the CM originates beyond the stapes.

It is fairly clear that the cochlea is the site of the controlling nonlinearity; the question still remains, however, as to which cochlear process possesses the type of nonlinear response that can produce the observed CM behavior. There are at least three possible cochlear mechanisms that can be implicated. The first of these is the basic hydrodynamic process of which Tonndorf

(1970b) is the strongest advocate. The second possibility is tied to the actual motion pattern of the basilar membrane; while no detailed theory for combination tone and harmonic generation from this process has been put forth, it is implied in the work of Johnstone and Johnstone (1966), who proposed this mechanism to explain summating potential production. The third possibility is that the dominant nonlinearity is in electrical processes, either in the functioning of the hair cell or in the gross CM-producing process. Wever and Lawrence (1954) believe that the transduction process in the hair cell is the most nonlinear link. We have shown in the previous chapter that the resistance-modulation process of CM generation is itself inherently nonlinear and can be responsible for some of the harmonic content of the CM. The same process can contribute to combination tone generation as well.

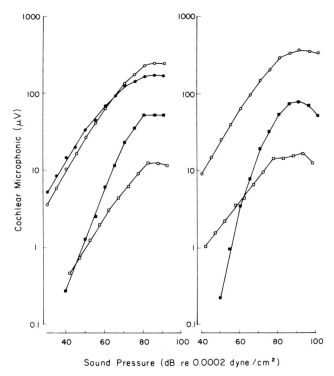

Fig. 6.12. Demonstration of the fact that a CM distortion component can be larger than a pure tone response of the same frequency. Recordings with differential electrodes from the third turn of the cochlea. Left panel: input–output functions for primaries $f_1 = 750$ Hz ($\bigcirc$), $f_2 = 1000$ Hz ($\bullet$), summation component ST $= 1750$ Hz ($\blacksquare$), and pure tone PT $= 1750$ Hz ($\square$). Right panel: input–output function for fundamental $f_0 = 750$ Hz ($\bigcirc$), second-harmonic CM component $2f_0 = 1500$ Hz ($\blacksquare$), and pure tone PT $= 1500$ Hz ($\square$).

In the previous pages we have already provided considerable evidence on the basis of which one can zero in on the most plausible source of CM distortion. It is remembered that at low intensities the distortion components have spatial distributions in the cochlea that are markedly different from that of pure tone responses at similar frequencies. We would now like to emphasize this point with the aid of Fig. 6.12. The two panels of the figure depict a family of input–output functions, recorded with differential electrodes from the third cochlear turn of a guinea pig. In the left-hand panel the CM magnitude functions are given for primaries of 750 and 1000 Hz, for the first summation tone elicited by these primaries, and for a pure tone whose frequency is the same as that of the summation tone, that is, 1750 Hz. In the right-hand panel the CM function is given for a 750-Hz fundamental, for the second-harmonic component generated by the fundamental, and for a pure tone that has the same frequency as the second harmonic: 1500 Hz. There is only one important idea that we wish to illustrate, namely, that in both situations chosen here the distortion components reach magnitudes that corresponding pure tone responses cannot attain at *any* sound pressure level. This means that at a favorable recording location the CM distortion components are in exces of the microphonic that can be generated by a stimulating pure tone. If this is the case then the spatial patterns of the distortion component and the pure tone response cannot be the same. This indicates that at least at low levels the intermodulation and harmonic products do not arise from traveling waves, that their source and distribution are fairly well localized to the region in which the primaries generate their major disturbance.

These facts strongly suggest that hydrodynamic nonlinearities that could result in the generation of traveling waves are unlikely to be responsible for the CM distortion at low and moderate sound levels. There is of course the possibility that a peculiar hydrodynamic process, localized and not coupled to the basilar membrane, could be the source or, more likely, that the nonlinearity is in the fine motion pattern of the organ of Corti or in the electrical processes. It is remembered that our evidence further indicated that at high intensities the CM distortion components behave just as pure tone responses of like frequency; in other words, their spatial pattern strongly suggests that these components are mediated by traveling waves of the von Békésy type. This observation in turn results in the conclusion that the high-level distortion is intimately tied to nonlinearities that reside in the basic fluid dynamics of the cochlea. Nonlinear pressure waves are expected to be resolved into their Fourier components by the spectral filtering characteristics of the cochlear partition that we have discussed at length in Chapter 4. It is equally clear that electrical nonlinearities could not possibly result in traveling waves and that it is unlikely that nonlinearities in the motion pattern of the organ of Corti could either. The latter contention is based on our previous observations that the major path of energy flow in the cochlea is from the fluid to the membrane and not from one membrane segment to an adjacent one. Thus the high-level distortion constitutes a fairly clear-cut case. The only question in connection with it is to determine the type of hydrodynamic process that is responsible for its generation. The low-level process requires more thorough scrutiny.

Tonndorf (1970b) summarized his thinking on cochlear distortion, primarily on the basis of his extensive studies on mechanical cochlear models. It is his contention that there are two nonlinear hydrodynamic processes that can explain his observations on the nonlinear behavior of the models. These processes, an amplitude-independent and an amplitude-dependent process, roughly correspond with what we have identified as the low- and high-level distortion. In Tonndorf's view fluid motion in the cochlea is very much like shallow-water surface waves where the restoring force is provided by capillary action between the fluid and the cochlear partition. In the boundary layer of fluid next to the vibrating partition a vorticity of the particle motion can be observed in that the closed particle orbits (generally ellipses) are not parallel with the major axis of the model in the region of maximal partition displacement. The vorticity apparently results in asymmetrical particle orbits in scalae tympani and vestibuli. The elliptical particle orbits are displaced with respect to one another in the two scalae and they result in an out-of-phase, push–pull movement that produces an asymmetrical partition displacement and consequently an asymmetrical traveling wave envelope. It should be emphasized that this asymmetrical envelope belongs to a traveling wave that corresponds to the difference tone (what Tonndorf calls the "beat response"). This process is a demodulation or amplitude detection phenomenon. Apparently its existence in the cochlear models depends on the appropriate choice of primary frequencies. It is not at all clear whether the process generates any other combination frequencies besides the dc component (the basic asymmetry) and the simple difference tone (the amplitude detection component). While such a nonlinear process is clearly present in the mechanical cochlear model it does not seem to correspond to distortion seen in the CM. The vorticity component is apparently resolved in a traveling wave that corresponds to the difference frequency. Such a traveling wave is absent in the low-level response, as can be determined from the CM. In addition, the simple difference and summation tone components are of equal strength in the CM, as are other combination frequencies of equal order. It does not appear that these components are also present in the model's response.

While this hydrodynamic nonlinearity does not appear to correlate well with CM responses, the other phenomenon described by Tonndorf, the amplitude-dependent event, does. At relatively high signal levels, at the peak of the traveling wave, eddies appear in the cochlear fluids in both perilymphatic scalae (von Békésy, 1928). The lower the signal frequency the greater the spatial extent of the eddy. When eddies first appear they have a fairly smooth, elliptical shape. As intensity increases the eddies flatten out as if the vertical vector (perpendicular to the partition) would saturate. Concomitant with this peak clipping of the eddies, smaller eddies also appear inside the main loop. These small eddies correspond in location to the place of the harmonics of the driving frequency. Tonndorf does not mention it, but presumably with dual frequency drive similar side eddies would also correspond to at least some of the combination frequencies. The eddies are intimately related to traveling waves, specifically to the maximum amplitude region. Thus the high-level distortion process that produces eddy motion in the cochlear fluids is a mechanism that distributes individual frequency components according to their own frequency by traveling waves. It is probably the mechanism that generates the high-level combination frequencies seen in CM.

Wever and Lawrence (1954) concluded that cochlear distortion arises in the final transducer process, that is, in the CM-generating mechanism. They measured the relative distortion (rms sum of distortion components divided by the rms sum of the fundamentals) in the CM and in the sound radiated by the round window. They argued that if the distortion is hydromechanical in origin then the relative distortion in the CM should be equal to or less than that in the sound produced by the nonlinearly vibrating round-window membrane. In other words, they assumed that the round-window vibratory pattern would reflect distortions that have mechanical sources. They found that the relative distortion content of the CM was greatly in excess of that of the sound field in front of the round window. From this they arrived at the conclusion that we have stated above, namely, that the distortion originates in the hair cell transducer. As we shall demonstrate below, this deduction is quite correct for the low-level distortion, but there is some question as to whether the data actually permitted the drawing of this conclusion by Wever and Lawrence. One problem is that, as Tonndorf has pointed out (1958b, 1970b), the horizontal component of the eddy is not distorted; it is only the vertical component that saturates. The round-window vibration reflects the horizontal vector, and thus even if hydrodynamic distortion were present it would not necessarily set the round window in nonlinear vibration. Another problem is that one cannot be certain if the sealing of the round window by the measuring probe tube microphone was good enough to assure that some leakage of the primary components of the stimulating sound did not occur. The basis of the original argument of Wever and Lawrence is that whatever the probe microphone measures is due to the sound generated by the vibration of the round-window membrane, and thus the relative distortion figure is representative of its motion pattern. If considerable leakage from the sound source occurs, the relative distortion of the round-window-generated sound becomes artificially lowered because of the inflated denominator in the fraction that represents the relative distortion. Now we do not know whether such inflation actually occurred but, knowing the difficulties of sealing a probe tube around the round window, we cannot rule out its presence.

Fairly conclusive evidence supporting the final conclusions of Wever and Lawrence was obtained by Dallos *et al.* (1969a). It was hypothesized that if the distortion originates in electrical hair cell processes then the changing of the electrical bias of the cell should significantly alter its distortion-producing

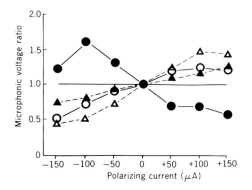

Fig. 6.13. Ratio of magnitude of microphonic potential with and without polarization. Measurements made at various current levels and at two sound pressures of the primary tones. The two primaries (4000 and 4500 Hz) were presented at equal sound levels. The distortion component of interest is the 500-Hz difference tone. Legend: ▲, primary at 67 dB; △, primary at 97 dB; ●, difference tone at 67 dB; ○, difference tone at 97 dB SPL of the primaries. (From Dallos *et al.*, 1969a, p. 450.)

properties. Conversely if the distortion occurs prior to the deformation-to-CM transduction then the electrical biasing of the transducer would have the same effect on a distortion component as on the response to a fundamental or to any pure tone. Electrical biasing was accomplished by direct-current polarization of the cochlear partition patterned after the procedure of Tasaki and Fernández (1952). The results were striking. At low stimulus levels the polarizing current had exactly the opposite effect on the distortion components as on pure tones or on the primaries. At high levels the effects were the same. As Fig. 6.13 demonstrates, the relative change in the CM response to a primary tone and the first difference tone is essentially the same as the function of polarizing current at high stimulus level. In other words, there is a proportional increase in all CM components when the scala vestibuli is made positive relative to the scala tympani and the current strength is increased.

In contrast, at a low stimulus level, while the CM of the primary changes exactly as at high levels, the difference tone component decreases with increasing scala vestibuli positivity. This dramatic difference between high- and low-level response demonstrates that different nonlinear processes dominate at different intensity levels in consonance with our findings from CM spatial patterns. In addition, the results strongly suggest that the low-level distortion is clearly tied to the CM-generating mechanoelectrical process.

For the sake of completeness it should be mentioned that in the transition zone between the low- and high-level response segments the effect of dc bias on the distortion components can be quite spectacular. As Fig. 6.14 demon-

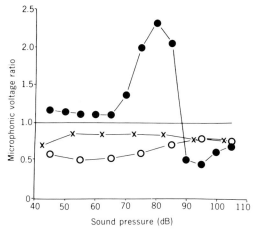

Fig. 6.14. Ratio of magnitude of microphonic potential with and without polarization. The primary frequencies are 4000 and 4500 Hz presented at equal sound intensity, and the distortion component is the 500-Hz difference tone. The effect of polarization on a 500-Hz pure tone is also shown. The polarizing current is 100 μA; scala vestibuli is negative with respect to scala tympani. Legend: $\bigcirc$, 4000-Hz primary; X, 500-Hz pure tone; $\bullet$, 500-Hz difference tone. (From Dallos *et al.*, 1969a, p. 450.)

strates, the relative change in the CM distortion component can be several hundred percent in this region. The figure depicts the relative change in one of the primaries, in a pure tone response whose frequency was the same as the difference tone, and in the difference tone with a change in sound pressure when the biasing current was maintained at the same strength. Note that at low SPL's the pure tone responses and the distortion component are affected in an opposite manner, while at the highest levels all effects converge. In the transition zone the distortion component undergoes large and bizarre changes as dominance apparently shifts from one constituent process to

another. Similar results have been obtained on harmonics by Legouix and
Chocholle (1957) and in more detail by Durrant and Dallos (1971).

Before summarizing the current status of thought concerning cochlear
distortion we must discuss one final possibility for the generation of the
nonlinear components. We clearly demonstrated in Chapter 5 that the

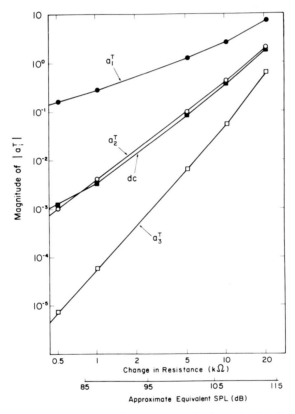

Fig. 6.15. Magnitude of Fourier components in the series that describes the harmonic
content of the CM in scala tympani where the distortion is due to the circuit nonlinearity
of the cochlear electroanatomy. Computation is based on Eq. (6.12). Abscissa gives both
the change in hair cell resistance and the approximate equivalent SPL.

resistance-modulation scheme of CM production is an essentially nonlinear
process. It is remembered that the CM magnitude versus resistance change
functions are decidedly nonlinear and that the computed CM waveforms are
distorted. In the following a brief formal analysis of such a distorted waveform is presented in order to inquire into the properties of the Fourier
components of the response and their relationship to observed CM distortion

components. In Chapter 5 the following formulas were derived for voltages in the two cochlear scalae, vestibuli (E_V), and tympani (E_T):

$$E_V = \frac{A + B \cos \phi}{C + D \cos \phi}$$

$$E_T = \frac{E}{C + D \cos \phi} \tag{6.6}$$

In these formulas $A = 7.7232$, $B = 0.384R$, $C = 2213.32$, $D = 61.4R$, $E = 21.6756$, where R is the magnitude of the change in the hair cell resistance due to stimulation, and $\phi = 2\pi ft$. The Fourier expansion of a function $f(\phi)$ can be written as

$$f(\phi) = a_0/2 + a_1 \cos \phi + a_2 \cos 2\phi + ...$$

$$+ b_1 \sin \phi + b_2 \sin 2\phi + ... \tag{6.7}$$

where

$$a_n = 1/\pi \int_0^{2\pi} f(\phi) \cos n\phi \, d\phi \quad \text{and} \quad b_n = 1/\pi \int_0^{2\pi} f(\phi) \sin n\phi \, d\phi \tag{6.8}$$

It is apparent that both E_T and E_V are even functions of ϕ; in other words, for both the equality $f(\phi) = f(-\phi)$ is satisfied. This implies that all b_n values are uniformly zero. Consequently we can make the following substitutions:

For E_T,
$$a_n^T = \frac{E}{\pi C} \int_0^{2\pi} \frac{\cos n\phi}{1 + [(D/C)\cos \phi]} \, d\phi \tag{6.9}$$

For E_V,
$$a_n^V = \frac{1}{\pi} \int_0^{2\pi} \frac{A + B \cos \phi}{C + D \cos \phi} \cos n\phi \, d\phi = \frac{A}{\pi} \int_0^{2\pi} \frac{\cos n\phi}{C + D \cos \phi} \, d\phi$$

$$+ \frac{B}{\pi} \int_0^{2\pi} \frac{\cos \phi \cos n\phi}{C + D \cos \phi} \, d\phi = \frac{A}{\pi} \int_0^{2\pi} \frac{\cos n\phi}{C + D \cos \phi} d\phi$$

$$+ \frac{B}{2\pi} \int_0^{2\pi} \frac{\cos(n+1)\phi + \cos(n-1)\phi}{C + D \cos \phi} \, d\phi$$

$$= \frac{A}{E} a_n^T + \frac{B}{2E} a_{n+1}^T + \frac{B}{2E} a_{n-1}^T \tag{6.10}$$

It is seen that a_n^V can be expressed with a recursion formula from the various values of a_n^T. The task is then to complete the integration in the expression for a_n^T. This can be accomplished by noting that

$$\int_0^{2\pi} \frac{\cos n\phi}{1 + K \cos \phi} \, d\phi = \frac{2}{(1 - K^2)^{1/2}} \left[\frac{(1 - K^2)^{1/2} - 1}{K} \right]^n \tag{6.11}$$

Thus

$$a_n^T = \frac{2E}{C[1-(D/C)^2]^{1/2}} \left\{ \frac{[1-(D/C)^2]^{1/2}-1}{D/C} \right\}^n$$

$$= \frac{0.007872}{(1-0.0007695R^2)^{1/2}} \left[\frac{(1-0.0007695R^2)^{1/2}-1}{0.02774R} \right]^n \qquad (6.12)$$

The values of a_0^T, a_1^T, a_2^T, and a_3^T as the function of R are plotted in Fig. 6.15. In this log–log plot all functions appear as approximately straight lines. The slope of the line depicting the growth of the fundamental component (a_1^T) is unity, that of the second harmonic (a_2^T) and the dc component (a_0^T) is 2, while that of the third harmonic (a_3^T) is 3. One of the most interesting findings is that the magnitudes of the second harmonic and the dc component are virtually equal. Very similar plots can be obtained for the spectral content of the scala vestibuli potential; they differ in magnitude but not in character. The percent distortion is the same in the scala vestibuli and scala tympani potentials; the value is approximately 15% at $R = 10$ kΩ. The latter probably is the maximal change in the hair cell resistance within the physiologically important range. At an R value of 2.2 kΩ [which was the change in resistance that Johnstone *et al.* (1966) noted at a sound pressure level of 95 dB] the harmonic distortion predicted by our Fourier analysis of the CM is of the order of 2.7%. The corresponding value that one can glean from actual CM distortion measurements is about 20%. This discrepancy tends to indicate that the nonlinearity that arises from the basic electrical circuit properties of the resistance-modulation process is not the dominant factor in controlling the distortion content of CM; at least it is not at moderate intensity levels. At very high SPL's the actual distortion content of the CM and that predicted by Fourier analysis are commensurable, but at these levels other nonlinearities are probably also active and significant.

One can catalog the plausible sources of nonlinearity that are manifested in the harmonic or combination tone content of the CM. Some of these sources are intimately related to the actual CM-generating process, and others exist independent from that mechanism. In the former category we can consider the essential nonlinearity of the network that converts resistance variations to potential changes and also the possible nonlinearity of the hair cell transducer itself. In the latter category are hydrodynamic processes, nonlinearities in the fine motion patterns of the structures of the basilar membrane and organ of Corti, and at very high SPL's possibly even middle ear nonlinearities. All experimental evidence seems to substantiate the notion that at high sound levels the behavior of distortion components, as discerned from CM or in cochlear scale models, is not materially different from that of pure tone responses at corresponding frequencies. The most important

corollary of this observation is that these distortion components are correlated with traveling waves of their own. Consequently these components must
arise in nonlinearities of either the middle ear or of cochlear hydrodynamics.
Various experiments indicate (Wever and Lawrence, 1954; Guinan and
Peake, 1967) that the middle ear is less nonlinear than the cochlea, and thus
we must conclude that hydrodynamic nonlinearities produce the dominant
distortion at high sound intensities. In contrast with the high-intensity
behavior, for low sound levels our experiments firmly support the hypothesis
that distortion originates in transducer processes. Thus, at low levels, it is
not localized hydrodynamic or mechanical processes that dominate the
nonlinear response (even though these processes are undoubtedly nonlinear
to some extent), but electrical processes. Of the two clear possibilities,
nonlinearity of the transducer and nonlinearity of the CM-producing circuit,
the former appears to be the more significant. Lest some confusion arise
as to the difference between these two electrical processes, it should be noted
that what we call a circuit nonlinearity arises from the simple property of the
network that describes the production of CM via the resistance-modulation
process, and voltage changes that result from *linear* resistance changes are
nonlinear. Thus in this scheme, even though the basic tranducer (the variable
resistance) is linear, the resulting potential variation is not. In contrast, when
the transducer is nonlinear then (if the resistance-modulation scheme is
assumed to operate) the resistance change itself is not proportional to the
stimulus. In this situation of course the nonlinearity of the transducer
(resistance change) and of the network can be compounded to produce a
response that is more distorted than could be expected from either nonlinearity alone. Our results and computations seem to indicate that it is the
actual transducer nonlinearity that dominates the distortion process at low
and moderate sound pressure levels.

D. THE INTERFERENCE PHENOMENON

Soon after the discovery of cochlear microphonic potentials it was noted
by Black and Covell (1936) and in more detail by Wever *et al.* (1940d) that
the CM corresponding to a given tone can be diminished by the addition of
a second tone to the stimulus. Normally a single stimulating tone is presented
and its resultant CM is measured. A second tone is then introduced and its
intensity is gradually increased. At low levels of the second tone the CM
corresponding to the first tone is unaltered, but at higher levels it begins to
decrease. Concomitant with the decrease in the CM, the input–output function of the primary tone becomes more linear as a result of the interference
process. Above the level at which interference becomes noticeable, it is an
approximately linear function of the intensity of the interfering tone; in other

words, the CM of the primary tone is decreased by about 10 dB for every 10-dB increase in the magnitude of the interfering tone.

The interference phenomenon, particularly its linearizing effect on the input–output function of the primary CM, remained somewhat mysterious until 1968, when Engebretson and Eldredge demonstrated that many aspects of tonal interference can be accounted for by a relatively simple nonlinear model. They assumed that the controlling nonlinearity can be represented by asymmetrical saturation and constructed a simple network to simulate such behavior. The network consists of a resistive mixer for the addition of

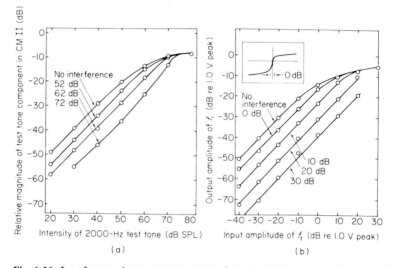

Fig. 6.16. Interference input–output curves for the cochlea (a) and the nonlinear network (b) showing the linearization effect. A wave analyzer with a 10-Hz narrow-band filter was used to measure the magnitude of the fundamental components of the distorted waveforms. In the presence of the interfering tone a higher test-tone intensity is reached before the curves become nonlinear. Also, the curves are linear for larger output magnitudes of the test-tone fundamental. Parameter in (a) is intensity of 3300-Hz interfering tone in decibels SPL. Parameter in (b) is amplitude of interfering f_2 in decibels re 1.0-V peak. (From Engebretson and Eldredge, 1968, p. 551.)

the primary and interfering sinusoids, a set of diodes to simulate the asymmetrical peak limiting, and a low-pass filter to simulate the Whitfield and Ross (1965) spatial filtering effect. The two sets of input–output functions shown in Fig. 6.16 are from actual CM data and from recordings made from the network output. It is clear that the two families of curves are highly similar. In both the essential features of the interference effect are discernible. These are the proportional decrease in the primary response with the increase of the interfering signal, and the linearization of the primary input–output function.

Engebretson and Eldredge assumed that the transfer function (output–input relation) of the nonlinearity could be approximated as a power series: $Y = a_0 + a_1 X + a_2 X^2 + a_3 X^3 + \ldots + a_n X^n + \ldots$, where X is the input and Y is the output. If the input consists of two sinusoids, that is, if $X = A_1 \sin 2\pi f_1 t + A_2 \sin 2\pi f_2 t$, then the magnitude of the component at frequency f_1 is

$$M_1(A_1;A_2) = A_1[a_1 + (3/4)a_3(A_1^2 + 2A_2^2) + (5/8)a_5(A_1^4 + 6A_1^2 A_2^2 + 3A_2^4)$$

$$+ (35/64)a_7(A_1^6 + 12A_1^4 A_2^2 + 18A_1^2 A_2^4 + 4A_2^6) + \ldots] \qquad (6.13)$$

Assume now that the primary frequency (f_1) is present with a much greater amplitude than the secondary, i.e., $A_1 \gg A_2$. Under such circumstances the expression for $M_1(A_1;A_2)$ is reduced to what would correspond to the input–output function for a single sinusoid of frequency f_1 and magnitude A_1. In other words, in this case

$$M_1(A_1;A_2) \simeq M_1(A_1) = A_1[a_1 + (3/4)a_3 A_1^2 + (5/8)a_5 A_1^4$$

$$+ (35/64)a_7 A_1^6 + \ldots] \qquad (6.14)$$

This situation of course corresponds to the case in which the interfering tone is relatively small and its effect on the primary is negligible. The converse situation can be assessed when the magnitude A_2 is greater than A_1, that is, when the interfering signal is greater than the primary. Under such conditions the magnitude of the frequency component f_1 can be written as

$$M_1(A_1;A_2) \simeq A_1[a_1 + (3/2)a_3 A_2^2 + (15/8)a_5 A_2^4 + (35/16)a_7 A_2^6 + \ldots] \qquad (6.15)$$

This expression can be written in the form

$$M_1(A_1;A_2) = A_1 F(A_2) \qquad (6.16)$$

Note that this expression is linear in A_1. In other words, the input–output function for the component f_1 becomes linear in the presence of a substantial interfering signal. This is exactly the behavior that can be seen in CM. Thus the simple nonlinear model of Engebretson and Eldredge can explain the linearizing effect of interference. This same simple model can also produce intermodulation distortion components and a dc component that could explain at least some aspects of summating potential production. Engebretson and Eldredge made no attempt to correlate their saturating, asymmetrical nonlinearity with a particular cochlear process. We can attempt to do this by briefly reviewing some additional data on interference and combination tone generation.

In his study of cochlear difference tones, Worthington (1970) also obtained significant data on the interference effect. He noted that interference first appears at the same cochlear location where difference tones are first measurable in the CM. Thus for example the first sign of interference upon an approximately 4000-Hz CM response appears in the second turn of the cochlea, *irrespective* of the frequency of the interfering tone. It is remembered that the first difference tone, elicited by an approximately 4000-Hz tone and another arbitrary frequency primary, is always localized to the second turn. As the intensity of the interfering tone increases, the maximal amount of interference shifts from the location that is just apical from the best site for the primary to a location that corresponds to the interfering tone. An example of this shift is shown in Fig. 6.17, where the interference on a

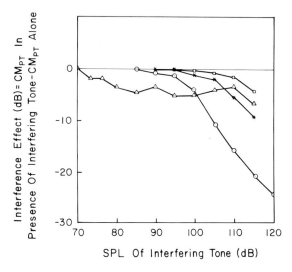

Fig. 6.17. Median effect of interference in cochlear turns 1 (circles), 2 (triangles), 3 (squares), and 4 (stars), caused by one tone acting on another. Ordinate shows the effect in decibels, that is, the ratio of the CM of the tone in the presence of the interfering tone and alone. Abscissa is the SPL of the interfering tone. The pure tone in this case is 2970 Hz, while the interfering tone is 4500 Hz. (From Worthington, 1970, p. 167.)

2970-Hz primary by a 4500-Hz secondary input is shown. Below 90 dB SPL of the interfering tone the only effect is in the second turn (the same site at which a difference tone between a 2970-Hz and a lower-frequency primary would be localized). This effect is relatively constant with the change of the interfering tone level. At higher intensities the maximal decrease in the 2970-Hz CM occurs in the first turn, which is of course the best location for the 4500-Hz interfering tone. The interference in the first turn above 90 dB SPL is exactly proportional to the magnitude of the interfering tone. These observations strongly suggest that the interference phenomenon is also a two-stage distortion process, and based on the considerations of Engebretson and Eldredge it is eminently reasonable to assume that the two stages of interference originate in precisely the same processes that give rise to the two stages of harmonic and intermodulation distortion generation. Thus at low levels a transducer nonlinearity produces harmonics, intermodulation products, *and* tonal interference, while at high levels hydraulic nonlinearities produce similar effects. The only requisite, that the nonlinearity can be expressed in a power series, is extremely liberal and it does not represent a significant constraint. There are of course some differences in the results of the two stages of distortion such as the growth of the effects, the location in the cochlea where they occur, and probably others. The important conclusion can be drawn, however, that no matter what their origin might be the manifestations of the various distortion processes are interrelated.

One additional interesting facet of tonal interference is worth discussing. Since interference and combination tone production are apparently very closely related it is worth inquiring how interference takes place on a combination tone. The following discussion (from Dallos, 1969b) relates to this problem. In both panels of Fig. 6.18, the magnitude of a CM component at

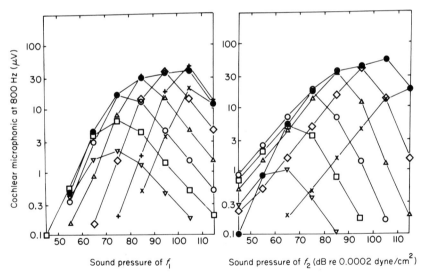

Fig. 6.18. Microphonic input–output functions recorded from the third turn of the cochlea of a guinea pig for the combination tone $2f_1 - f_2$ ($f_1 = 1000$ Hz, $f_2 = 1200$ Hz). Left panel: Intensity of f_1 is variable, and that of f_2 is the parameter. Right panel: Intensity of f_2 is variable, and that of f_1 is the parameter. Closed symbols indicate the function that was obtained when both intensities were identical. Sound pressure is given in decibels re 0.0002 dyne/cm². Parameter is fixed SPL: $\triangledown$, 55; $\square$, 65; $\bigcirc$, 75; $\triangle$, 85; $\diamondsuit$, 95; +, 105; and X, 115 dB. (From Dallos, 1969b, p. 1441.)

$2f_1 - f_2$ is given. On the left, functions are shown with the intensity of f_1 as the variable and that of f_2 as the parameter, while in the right-hand panel the intensity of f_2 is varied with the strength of f_1 held constant at a variety of values. These functions present a very systematic picture; they all peak at or near the point where the intensities of both primaries are equal. On the low-intensity side of the peak, the functions grow with either approximately unity or approximately double slopes as expected; that is, those functions in which f_1 is the variable have initial slopes of 2, while the functions generated by a variable f_2 grow at a unity rate. In direct contrast, the declining slopes are reversed. Specifically, the high-intensity slopes of the functions of a variable f_1 decline at an approximate rate of -1, while the variable f_2 functions decline with the approximate slope of -2. The implications of these observations are fairly straightforward. The cause of the proportional decline in the distortion components at the high-intensity end of the functions must be sought in the interference phenomenon. These results demonstrate that at levels where the variable-intensity tone exceeds the magnitude of the fixed-intensity tone, the combination tone generated by these declines. The very important consideration emerges that interference takes place by the variable-intensity tone interfering on the fixed-intensity tone and not on the combination tone itself. To explain, if the high-intensity decline in the combination tone magnitude that is so clearly evident in the plots of Fig. 6.18 were due to interference by the primary on the combination tone, then one would expect to see a decrease that was independent of which primary did the interfering (i.e., which primary was the variable). In contrast, we see that when f_1 is the variable the decreasing slope is -1, which means that f_1 depresses f_2. This depression is linearly proportional to the intensity of f_1 but, since the combination tone magnitude is also linearly related to the magnitude of f_2, a -1 slope results. In contrast, when f_2 is the variable, it linearly depresses the response to f_1, but a unity depression in f_1 causes a doubled depression in the combination tone; thus, a -2 slope clearly results in this situation.

E. SUMMATING POTENTIALS

We devoted a sizable fraction of Chapter 5 to the discussion of the stimulus-related dc response of the cochlea, the summating potential (SP). At this point it is necessary to return, very briefly, to this phenomenon and to discuss it in the context of the nonlinear behavior of the cochlea. It should be stated at the outset that the SP, being a dc response to an ac stimulus—the sound, is an *inherently nonlinear response*. In other words, there is no linear process that could result in the production of an SP-like phenomenon in response to the ac sound stimulation. When mention is made in the literature that the SP is a nonlinear distortion component (Whitfield and Ross, 1965; Davis, 1968; Engebretson and Eldredge, 1968) the meaning is usually that this dc component arises in the nonlinearity of the CM-producing process. To state this premise in different terms, the tacit assumption is that there is some nonlinearity that results in a distorted CM waveform, expressible as the sum of a fundamental, a dc, and harmonic components. The dc component in this Fourier expansion is taken to be the SP.

There have been few specific suggestions for the mechanisms of SP generation. Davis (1958) and Davis and Eldredge (1959) assumed that the SP resulted from a unidirectional longitudinal shear of the cilia between the reticular lamina and the tectorial membrane. They consequently assumed at that time that the nonlinearity was tied to the relative motion patterns of the basilar membrane and the fine structures of the organ of Corti. Tonndorf (1970b) attributed a significant role in SP generation to hydrodynamic dc modulation processes. Johnstone and Johnstone (1966) developed a formal model based on functional asymmetry in the mechanical displacement of cilia. Their model provided for both SP^- and SP^+. The basic idea of a morphologically polarized hair cell (i.e., asymmetrical hair arrangement and asymmetrical location of basal body) itself suggests a possible nonlinear mode of functioning. Indeed, in the lateral line organ such basic structural asymmetries yield a highly distorted gross microphonic potential, one whose major energy content is at the second-harmonic frequency of the stimulus (Flock and Wersäll, 1962). The relatively low harmonic content of the CM as compared to the lateral line microphonic mediates against very close comparisons, even though the theory of Whitfield and Ross (1965) purports to remove this difficulty by showing that the cochlea as a mechanoelectrical network discriminates against high frequencies, i.e., against harmonics. As we have already mentioned their argument is valid for harmonics associated with traveling waves but not for distortion generated in hair cell processes, such as that called for by the morphological asymmetry of the transducers. Finally, we have demonstrated that even if all mechanical and hydraulic components of the cochlea function in a linear manner, if the CM is produced by modulation of the resting current through the hair cells by the (linear) resistance change of the hair cells, even in this case the potential variations in the cochlear scalae are nonlinear as the consequence of the properties of the electrical network of the inner ear. We have shown by Fourier analysis that a sizable dc component results from this nonlinear network function.

Clearly there is a multitude of potentially possible sources of nonlinearity, all capable of generating dc demodulation components. We must couple with the abundance of theoretically feasible means of production the apparent multiplicity of SP components. A brief review of the section on SP of Chapter 5 indicates that there are at least four possible dc components that make up the composite response and that there might be more. The obvious four are the DIF$^-$ and DIF$^+$, the AVE$^-$ and the AVE$^+$ components. At present, it is somewhat hazardous to attempt to assign mechanisms of origin to the various components; work to establish the correlations is now under way.

Aside from our Fourier analysis that showed dc potential components in the response of the cochlear network, another formal analysis of SP production was offered by Johnstone and Johnstone (1966). These authors derived a geometrical model of ciliary motion, on the basis of which they contend that the external hair cells produce SP$^-$ and the internal hair cells SP$^+$. If α is the angle of movement of the basilar membrane due to stimulation, ϕ_0 is the angle of the hairs when the membrane is at rest, and ϕ is the hair angle associated with the membrane angle of α, then the following relationship can be derived:

$$\cot \phi = k\alpha + \cot \phi_0 \tag{6.17}$$

where k is a constant depending on anatomical dimensions. As a result of this functional relationship, symmetrical changes in α (i.e., linear vibrations) result in asymmetrical hair bending around any resting angle ϕ_0 (except at $\phi_0 = 90°$, where the change in ϕ is also symmetrical). In other words, due to the geometry, a linear angular motion of the basilar membrane is converted to a nonlinear angular motion of the hairs. Thus linear basilar membrane vibration can result in nonlinear cochlear potentials. The nonlinear potential would consist of a fundamental ac component (CM), its harmonics, and a dc component (SP). Now it is the basic property of this theory that the sign of the produced dc component is directly related to the initial hair angle ϕ_0. If $\phi_0 < 90°$ then the dc component is positive, while if $\phi_0 > 90°$ then it is negative. Johnstone and Johnstone assume that the hair angle of the internal hair cells is less than 90°, while that of the external hair cells is greater than 90°. Thus their theory associates SP$^+$ with the former and SP$^-$ with the latter. All anatomical data (for example, Spoendlin, 1967; Engström et al., 1965) clearly indicate that, while these assumptions are correct for the basic orientation of cell bodies, the hairs themselves are *always* perpendicular to the reticular lamina, irrespective of their origin, be it external or internal hair cells. Thus the anatomical evidence refutes the differential bending of the hairs between the two groups of cells and thus takes a great deal away from the arguments. It is interesting that qualitative agreement is obtained fom this model for many properties of the SP, such as input–output functions from the model that are similar to those obtained from the cochlea, at least for some stimulus conditions. The behavior under conditions of pressure in either cochlear scala is also correctly predicted. Unfortunately, to provide the appropriate qualitative behavior, the model requires excessive angular movements.

It appears that, for the small angular hair displacements that can be computed on the basis of either the Johnstone and Johnstone (1966) or the Rhode and Geisler (1967) geometrical models with the aid of either the von Békésy (1960) or the Johnstone and Boyle (1967) basilar membrane displacement data, the nonlinearity originating in the basilar membrane to hair cell angle transformation is too small to account for a significant portion of the recorded SP. More likely sources of this potential are sought in basic nonlinearities of the hair cell transducer, in cochlear hydrodynamics, and possibly in nonlinear network properties of the inner ear.

F. INTERMODULATION COMPONENTS AT $(n+1)f_1 - nf_2$

In discussing intermodulation distortion in CM potentials we have treated all orders of distortion products as if their order were not of importance in their overall description and in their mode of production. This was done for the simple reason that there is no indication whatsoever to the contrary on the basis of CM data. Our discussion of cochlear nonlinearities would not be complete, however, if some mention were not made of a class of observations (psychoacoustic as well as electrophysiological) that strongly indicate that there is a distinct difference in some properties and in the mode of production of the intermodulation distortion components $(n+1)f_1 - nf_2$ and all other orders. Zwicker (1955), Plomp (1965), and Goldstein (1967) investigated this class of combination tone by psychoacoustic means. A brief description of some pertinent observations made by Goldstein is presented in the following.

Goldstein used a pitch cancellation method to assess the quantitative features of the subjective difference tone $2f_1 - f_2$. In other words, he presented his subject with the two primaries (f_1 and f_2) that produced the difference tones of interest. He then introduced a cancellation tone at frequency $2f_1 - f_2$ that was generated from a common source with f_1 and f_2. (In other words, it was phase coherent with the primaries and with a distortion component at $2f_1 - f_2$ that was generated in the auditory system.) The phase and amplitude of the cancellation tone were adjustable. During experiments the parameters of the cancellation tone were adjusted until the pitch of the difference tone disappeared from the complex sensory experience of the subject. This method provides clear quantitative information on the subjective difference tone. For the sake of comparison Goldstein studied both the simple difference tone $f_2 - f_1$ and $2f_1 - f_2$ (other difference tones were also examined in lesser detail). He observed that $2f_1 - f_2$ is audible at a much lower intensity level than the simple difference tone. A second important difference concerns the dependence of the difference tones on frequency separation of the primaries. All the $(n+1)f_1 - nf_2$ components decrease with

f_2/f_1 at a rate of approximately 100 dB/octave, while $f_2 - f_1$ is largely insensitive to frequency separation. A third important consideration relates to the growth of the difference tones with increasing primary intensity. This growth, as reflected in the amplitude of the canceling tone, is quadratic for $f_2 - f_1$; that is, when both f_2 and f_1 are increased equally, for each 10-dB increase in the primary level the cancellation tone must be increased by 20 dB. In contrast, $2f_1 - f_2$ appears to grow at the same rate as the primaries, 10 dB for each 10 dB. There is apparently a great asymmetry between the higher- and lower-frequency components that are complementary in the combination tone series. Thus $2f_1 - f_2$ is very prominent, but $2f_2 - f_1$ is almost negligible. All these peculiar psychoacoustic observations point to the conclusion that the series $(n + 1)f_1 - nf_2$ does not originate in a saturating-type, polynomial nonlinearity. Goldstein concluded that because of the very sharp frequency dependence of these components they must be cochlear in origin. Further, since cancellation can be accomplished they are most likely present as traveling waves in the inner ear and thus they appear to have hydromechanical origins.

Goldstein and Kiang (1968) continued the investigation of $2f_1 - f_2$ by physiological methods. They studied the discharge patterns in single units of the cat's auditory nerve with bitonal stimulation and compared firing patterns that were synchronized to f_1, f_2, and $2f_1 - f_2$. Their main finding was that unit responses that were time locked to $2f_1 - f_2$ behaved as if this frequency were actually present in the sound stimulus. In other words, the distortion component $2f_1 - f_2$ that is generated in the inner ear is transduced into neural impulses in the same manner as ordinary external stimuli. They obtained PST (poststimulus time) histograms in response to continuous pure tones of f_1 and f_2, and f_1 and f_2 together. The frequencies were so chosen that the fiber's best (characteristic) frequency would correspond to $2f_1 - f_2$. It is impressive that the fiber did not respond to either f_1 or f_2 alone to any degree, but a well-developed response, with periodicity corresponding to $2f_1 - f_2$, was present when the two tones were sounded simultaneously.

An even more interesting demonstration is seen in Fig. 6.19. Here the responses from three different fibers are shown with the same stimuli. The experiments were designed to duplicate the cancellation procedure used by Goldstein in the psychoacoustic experiments. Thus provisions were made to present to the animals, in addition to tones f_1 and f_2, a tone having a frequency of $2f_1 - f_2$ whose amplitude and phase could be controlled by the experimenter. It was possible to cancel the time-locked responses at $2f_1 - f_2$ by the addition of this secondary tone. Note that in the figure the top row depicts the PST histograms obtained when f_1 and f_2 were presented. In all cases the dominant periodicity is at the frequency $2f_1 - f_2$. The second row shows the responses to a pure tone of frequency $2f_1 - f_2$ when the parameters of

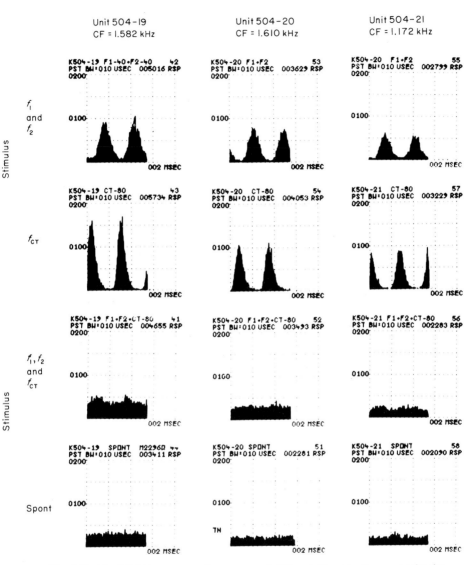

Fig. 6.19. The PST histograms of responses of different fibers to the same stimulus. All histograms are synchronized to $2f_1 - f_2$. Stimulus frequencies: $f_1 = 2.10$ kHz, $f_2 = 2.72$ kHz, $f_{CT} = 2f_1 - f_2 = 1.48$ kHz. Stimulus levels re 200 V peak-to-peak into earphone: $L_1 = -54$ dB, $L_2 = -54$ dB, $L_{CT} = -74$ dB. The top row of histograms shows the response when the two primaries are the stimulus. Note the strong synchronization to $2f_1 - f_2$. The second row shows the responses to the canceling tone alone when it is adjusted for optimal cancellation. Note the 180° phase difference between the histograms of the first and second rows. In the third row the primaries and the cancellation tone are simultaneously present. (From Goldstein, 1970, p. 241.)

this tone were so chosen that it could cancel the combination tone response in the first fiber. Notice that the peaks in the PST histogram in the second row are exactly 180° apart from those in the first row. The third row shows the histograms when both the primaries and the cancellation tone are presented together. It is noteworthy that the time-locked activity so apparent for both the combination tone (first row) and the canceling tone (second row) is now eliminated and the fiber responses do not significantly exceed the spontaneous level. In other words, the combination tone and the canceling tone eliminated one another in destructive interference prior to the spike-generating process.

The experiments of Goldstein and Kiang appear to demonstrate that a very prominent class of distortion components having frequencies $(n + 1) f_1 - n f_2$ is generated in the cochlea from mechanohydraulic nonlinearities. These distortion components have certain characteristic properties that set them apart from other more "classical" combination tones. Not the least of these is their relative strength; psychoacoustically the relative level of $2f_1 - f_2$ can be as high as 20% in contrast with 0.2% for $f_2 - f_1$. Consequently this class of combination tones can have a very important role in pitch perception (Greenwood, 1971; Smoorenburg, 1970).

As must clearly be apparent to the reader after studying Section II,B, combination tone components in CM do not show similar dichotomy between a group of classically behaving components and the $(n + 1)f_1 - n f_2$ series. To underscore this, some results on the CM components $f_2 - f_1$ and $2f_1 - f_2$ are contrasted below. The discussion is based on the author's 1969 report (Dallos, 1969b).

Experiments were performed by fixing f_1 and changing f_2 so that the ratio f_2/f_1 varied between 1.05 and 1.8. Microphonic potentials at the frequencies $2f_1 - f_2$ and $f_2 - f_1$ were recorded from both the first and third cochlear turns for constant, and equal, sound pressure levels of the primaries. Some of our results are shown in Fig. 6.20. Here the lower primary was 1000 Hz, while the higher primary ranged from 1050 to 1800 Hz. Presentations were made at constant 60, 80, and 100 dB SPL. In the left-hand panel, the potentials measured from the first turn are shown, while the third-turn data are given in the right-hand panel. Inspection of the left panel reveals that neither distortion component ($2f_1 - f_2$ or $f_2 - f_1$) was radically influenced by the frequency separation of the primaries. The microphonic potentials do not change more than about 10 dB for any one condition, and the fluctuations appear to be random. There is no discernible difference between the behavior of the two types of difference tone. In the third turn, both types of difference tone, at all three intensity levels, are strongly influenced by the primary frequency ratio. Above the f_2/f_1 ratio of 1.2, the microphonic response for both distortion components falls at an approximate rate of

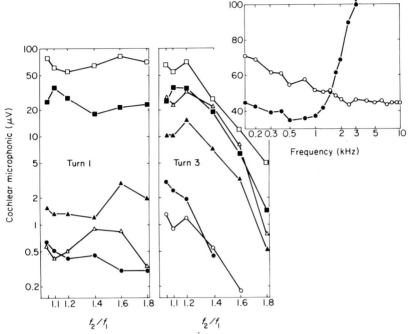

Fig. 6.20. Magnitude of combination tones $2f_1 - f_2$ (open symbols) and $f_2 - f_1$ (closed symbols) as the function of f_2/f_1 at 60 (circles), 80 (triangles), and 100 (squares) dB SPL of the primaries. Left panel: Recording from turn 1. Right panel: Recording from turn 3. The insert shows the 3-μV isopotential curves of this animal from both turn 1 (open circles) and turn 3 (closed circles). Note that the rapid decrease of both combination components from the third turn corresponds to the decrease in sensitivity of this recording location to the higher-frequency primary, f_2. (From Dallos, 1969b, p. 1438.)

32 dB/octave. I wish to emphasize that *both* difference tones behave in like manner.

The difference between the flat curves obtained from the basal turn and the rather precipitous drop in microphonic from the third turn are easily explained by noting the relative sensitivity of the two electrode locations to the primary frequencies. To facilitate the comparison, the insert in Fig. 6.20 shows the 3-μV isopotential curves (i.e., the sound pressure required to elicit a 3-μV CM response at the various test frequencies) for both electrode pairs for this particular animal. Note that the basal-turn electrodes are almost equally sensitive to all frequencies between 1000 and 1800 Hz, which is the range of the primaries in Fig. 6.20. In contrast the third-turn electrode pair is about 30 dB less sensitive to 1800 than to 1000 Hz. Since the low-level isopotential curve for the third-turn electrode location presumably is indicative of the degree of excitation at various frequencies in that region of the cochlea, one can conclude that the apparent diminution of both distortion components with increasing f_2/f_1 is simply due to a decrease in the magnitude of excitation by the higher-frequency primary. It should be emphasized that the decrease in difference-tone magnitude is not a consequence of declining sensitivity of the cochlear location to the difference tone itself. Note that the $2f_1-f_2$ component varies in frequency between 250 and 900 Hz, while the f_2-f_1 component ranges from 50 to 800 Hz. The third-turn sensitivity decreases at the lowest frequencies at an approximate rate of 6 dB/octave, but the total change between 250 and 900 Hz is only 3 dB. Thus one can state that it is the sensitivity of a particular cochlear location to the primary frequencies that determines the magnitude of a distortion component and not its sensitivity to the frequency of the distortion component itself. This observation is in complete harmony with some of our previous results (Sweetman and Dallos, 1969; Dallos and Sweetman, 1969; Dallos 1969b). The decrease in distortion magnitude is not analogous to the decrease of $2f_1-f_2$ in Goldstein's experiments. In the cochlear region that is most sensitive to the two primaries, the CM distortion-component magnitude remains unchanged with increased frequency separation of f_1 and f_2. Thus, we have considerable data showing flat responses from the basal turn with $f_1 = 4000$ Hz and f_2 varying from 4200 to 7200 Hz, and also from the third turn with $f_1 = 500$ Hz and f_2 varying between 550 and 900 Hz.

   The intensity dependence of the magnitude of the combination tone $2f_1-f_2$ was approximated by Goldstein (1967) by the function $L = a^2b/(a+b)^2$, where a and b are the intensity of the two primaries. This description indicates that if both a and b are changed equally then the relative distortion stays constant, while if only b changes then the relative distortion achieves a maximum value for $a = b$ and decreases for $b < a$ and for $b > a$. If only the intensity of the lower-frequency primary a changes then, according to the formulation, the combination tone magnitude should asymptotically approach the magnitude of b with increasing a. This latter situation was not tested by Goldstein.

   According to a polynomial nonlinearity the magnitude of the distortion component $2f_1-f_2$ should increase linearly if the intensity of f_1 is held constant while f_2 is changed. Furthermore, the increase should be proportional to the square of the magnitude of f_1 if this primary is variable while the other is held constant. Finally, if both primaries are increased equally and simultaneously the distortion product should rise as the cube of the intensity.

   In Fig. 6.21 representative CM magnitude versus SPL (input–output) functions are plotted. Three different functions are shown. In the first case, the intensity of f_1 is held constant while f_2 is varied; in the second, the converse is true; in the third, both primary intensities are changed equally. In conformity with results for other CM combination tones, the initial slope of these functions is determined by whichever of the primaries is the variable.

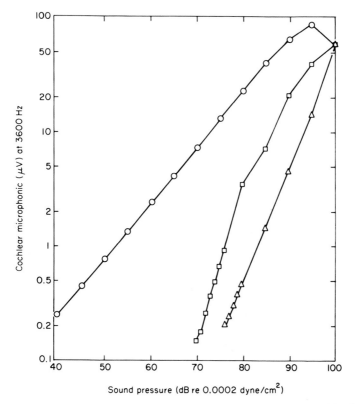

Fig. 6.21. Cochlear microphonic input–output functions for the combination $2f_1 - f_2$ ($f_1 = 4000$ Hz, $f_2 = 4400$ Hz). In one function ($\square$), the intensities of both primaries are the same; in another ($\bigcirc$), the intensity of f_1 is a constant 100 dB SPL; and in the third ($\triangle$), the intensity of f_2 is a constant 100 dB SPL. Recording is from the basal turn of the guinea pig cochlea. (From Dallos, 1969b, p. 1440).

Clearly defined unity slopes (tenfold change in CM for 20-dB change in SPL) were seen in the cases examined by us when the intensity of f_1 was held constant and f_2 was the variable. Similarly the initial slope of the $2f_1 - f_2$ microphonic function is double (hundredfold change in CM per 20-dB change in SPL) with little or no variability when the magnitude of f_2 is constant and the sound pressure of f_1 is the variable. When both primaries change together the initial slopes of the CM functions are seen to vary between 1.5 and 3.0. It will be remembered that, on the basis of polynomial distortion, one would expect to obtain a slope of 3 (thousandfold change in CM per 20-dB change in SPL) in this situation. Since the slopes of the CM distortion functions, when only one of the primaries varies, conform to this polynomial pattern, an explanation is in order for the frequent departures from the cubic slope in those cases where both primaries are changing. It appears that the steeper the initial slope of a CM function, the narrower the intensity range covered by a pure power-function segment (i.e., a straight line in the log–log coordinate system). As a consequence, one is often unable to measure a straight-line segment between the noise level and the bend-over portion that is long enough to accurately establish the slope. Nevertheless, the majority of slopes that were measured exceeded 2.5, and many, especially those recorded from the basal turn, were equal to 3. The conclusion then appears to be valid that the rate of rise of the CM combination tone input–output functions, including the function for the $2f_1 - f_2$ component, conforms to the polynomial nonlinearity model.

The final demonstration of combination-tone-related CM behavior concerns the contrast between the components $2f_1 - f_2$ and $2f_1 + f_2$. There is apparently a vast difference between these two combination tones (in detectability and prominence) when investigated by psychoacoustic means or by the single-fiber neural recording method. Such differences do not exist

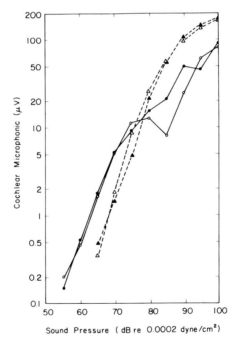

Fig. 6.22. Comparison of the CM input–output functions of four combination components: $f_2 - f_1$ (○), $f_2 + f_1$ (●), $2f_1 - f_2$ (△), and $2f_1 + f_2$ (▲). The intensities of the primaries ($f_1 = 500$ Hz, $f_2 = 760$ Hz) are the same and are shown on the abscissa. Recording is from the basal turn of a guinea pig.

in microphonic recordings. Figure 6.22 shows CM input–output functions for $2f_1 - f_2$ and $2f_1 + f_2$ components, and it is self-evident that the two functions are practically identical. In this figure we have also included input–output functions for $f_2 - f_1$ and $f_2 + f_1$ for the same primaries. It is notable that these two functions are again highly similar and that the simple difference and summation components appear at lower SPL than the two higher-order distortion products. The first observation, combined with the similarity of the $2f_1 - f_2$ and $2f_1 + f_2$ functions, reaffirms our earlier contention that CM distortion components of similar order tend to have similar input–output functions. The second observation also supports the notion that combination tones in CM are the result of a nonlinear process that can be expressed as a polynomial. In such a scheme the lower order components would be expected to occur at lower stimulus levels.

The principal finding highlighted in the above discussion is that combination tones of the type $2f_1 - f_2$ as recorded from CM potentials do not in any respect behave contrary to the expectations based on a simple polynomial nonlinearity model. This finding is highly significant when one considers that Goldstein (1967) and Goldstein and Kiang (1968) arrived at diametrically opposed conclusions concerning the behavior of this difference tone on the basis of psychoacoustic experiments with human observers and physiological studies of single-unit responses in the cat auditory nerve. Quite clearly the behavioral and neural data on the one hand and the microphonic data on the other do not seem to correlate.

The results pertaining to the $2f_1 - f_2$ content of CM are in complete accord with some of our previous findings (Sweetman and Dallos, 1969; Dallos and Sweetman, 1969; Dallos, 1969b) concerning the spatial distribution and mode of generation of cochlear distortion components. It appears from our various experiments that distortion products measured in the CM originate in at least a two-stage process. At low and moderate intensity levels (up to approximately 70–80 dB SPL), all orders of distortion components are relatively well localized in the cochlea to the region of significant excitation by the primary stimuli. These distortion components appear to originate in the nonlinearity of the mechanoelectrical transduction process, and they do not seem to be accompanied by traveling waves of their own. At high intensity levels, the recordable distortion components are much better behaved, in that they become most prominent in the region that is most appropriate as determined by their own frequency and the spectral filtering properties of the cochlea. These high-level distortion products are evidently distributed by traveling waves. It is not resolved whether the high-level distortion products originate in the nonlinearities of the middle ear or if they arise primarily from nonlinear hydromechanical causes within the cochlea. It is conceivable that both sources contribute to some extent.

It appears to us that audible psychoacoustically measurable nonlinear components are most likely to arise from two probably unrelated sources. The first of these is tied to the high-level second stage of peripheral distortion, while the second process produces the $(n + 1)f_1 - nf_2$ components that were studied by Zwicker (1955) and Goldstein (1967). It is to be emphasized again that the low-level distortion, so apparent in CM, that can be well described by a classic polynomial nonlinearity evidently does not have an audible correlate. Conversely, the peculiar distortion components of order $(n + 1)$ $f_1 - nf_2$, and particularly the $2f_1 - f_2$ cubic product, do not seem to have a microphonic correlate that would match their properties. It is conceivable that a particular mechanical or hydromechanical distortion in the cochlea, such as that associated with the production of $(n + 1)f_1 - nf_2$, might not produce such a deformation of the hair cell that is conducive to CM production, while it could still be an effective stimulus to the auditory nerve. Clearly a great deal of speculation is possible, but it would not be particularly valuable without further experimental evidence.

III. Subharmonics and Fractional Harmonics

As we have seen, one of the most important properties of a harmonically driven nonlinear system is its ability to generate frequency components that are totally absent in the forcing signal. The most common such distortion components are the harmonics of the input sinusoid. Depending on the symmetry properties of the nonlinearity, even, odd, or both types of harmonics can be generated by the system. If the driving function consists of more than one pure sinusoid, the interaction of the input components in the nonlinearity results in the phenomenon of intermodulation distortion.

The generation of harmonics and intermodulation components can occur in any nonlinear system without significant restrictions about initial and boundary conditions. In contradistinction only fairly restricted conditions allow the maintenance of the nonlinear phenomenon known as subharmonic generation. Subharmonics are integral submultiples of the fundamental (driving) frequency, or they can occur as powers of such a submultiple. In either case, the period of the nonlinear oscillation is longer than that of the fundamental. The most prevalent subharmonic in a given system is dependent on the order of the nonlinearity (if expressible as a polynomial). Thus in a system where the nonlinearity is cubic, the subharmonic most easy to elicit is the $\frac{1}{3}$-order subharmonic. Other orders, however, can also be excited under appropriate driving conditions. In fact, the general comment that one can make about subharmonic oscillations is that these vibrations can be initiated and sustained only under rather specific conditions. Namely, there are frequency and intensity bands within which certain subharmonics are excitable and outside of which they cannot be sustained. Appropriate initial conditions are also required if subharmonic oscillation is to be started. The frequency and intensity regions in which subharmonics are permissible of course depend on the type of nonlinearity and on the frequency response characteristics of the associated linear part of the system (assuming for simplicity that the nonlinearity can be separated conceptually from the rest of the system).

We have noted that the output of a nonlinear system can contain both multiples and submultiples of the driving frequency. One can state that if the stimulus frequency is f_0 and n and m are integers then the possible harmonic and subharmonic frequencies are mf_0 and f_0/n. One can include both harmonic and subharmonic distortion in a general class of fractional-harmonic distortion, with the resulting frequencies expressible as mf_0/n. A response that contains a fractional harmonic mf_0/n is periodic with a period of n/f_0. A further generalization of the fractional-harmonic distortion obtains for the case when $m/n = p$, where p is an irrational number. Under such a condition the response of the nonlinear system is not periodic. Nonperiodic oscillations in response to periodic excitation are obtained in some peculiar systems under stringent restrictions on the parameters of the system and of the excitation. The systems can usually be characterized as nonlinear, parametrically excited systems. In such a system one of the parameters (for example, the value of damping or stiffness) is a periodic function of time. One of the most common findings in systems that produce nonperiodic responses is that the resulting frequencies appear in pairs that have the following property:

$$f^U + f^L = f_0 \tag{6.18}$$

where f^U and f^L are the two fractional harmonics with $f^U > f^L$. This type of distortion was apparently first seen by Korpel and Adler (1965) in an ultrasonically excited acoustic interferometer and by Dallos and Linnell (1966b) in the CM of the chinchilla cochlea. Since these first reports, fractional harmonics have been observed in a variety of liquid-filled cavities, in the form of fractional-harmonic phonons in solids, and in the oscillations of two coupled electrical circuits (Bamberg and Cook, 1967; Adler and Breazeale, 1970; Mahon *et al.*, 1967; Eller, 1969).

In acoustical systems harmonics are often called overtones, intermodulation distortion components are termed combination tones, and subharmonics can be named undertones. The presence of overtones and combination tones in the auditory system has been known for at least two centuries. A formidable volume of research has accumulated on these phenomena and, while the subject is certainly not considered to be closed, at least the nature (if not necessarily the cause) of these distortion processes is adequately described. In contrast to the copious number of investigations that dealt with harmonics or combination tones, subharmonics were not discovered in the auditory system until 1949, and even after their discovery they were not studied in detail until 1966.

In 1949, Davis and his associates were the first to observe the presence of undertones at one-half of the stimulus frequency in potentials recorded from the apex of guinea pig cochleae. They found the subharmonics to be evident primarily above 2500 Hz at high intensity levels. A unique characteristic of these potentials was their sudden appearance with very slight increments in the driving stimulus. Later, von Gierke (1950) described the presence in both humans and animals of undertones at one-half of the driving frequency at intense sound levels. Von Gierke detected these harmonics that were radiated back by the eardrum from the guinea pig ears in the frequency range of 3500–23,000 Hz. Eldredge (1950) exposed human subjects to intense (140–146 dB SPL) pure tones at 9200 Hz and observed that his subjects heard subharmonics of this tone well enough to match them to pure tones presented to the opposite ear. The experimenter could also detect the first subharmonic ($f_0/2$) radiated from the subject's eardrum at a level of 60–80 dB below that of the exposure tone.

The middle ear has been generally assumed to be the site of generation of undertones. Davis and his colleagues (1949) speculated that the appearance of subharmonics is coincident with the change in the mode of vibration of the stapes at intense sound levels, as was described by von Békésy (1960). Pong and Marcaccio (1963) attributed the subharmonics to the asymmetric restoring force of the eardrum and ossicles that was described by Kobrak (1948) and developed a mathematical model from which certain characteristics of subharmonic vibrations could be predicted. Their predictions are stated to be in reasonable agreement with von Gierke's unpublished data.

In 1966 Dallos and Linnell (1966a,b) reexamined the even-order undertones. Their general properties and their site of generation were described. A completely novel subharmonic vibration was also discovered and studied in detail (Dallos, 1966). These latter, fractional subharmonics possess a number of fascinating properties, and are of more importance, for these distortion components were shown to originate in the inner ear.

A. EVEN-ORDER SUBHARMONICS

Subharmonic potentials are normally observed in cochlear microphonics when the ear is stimulated by sustained tones of sufficient intensity. We have been able to elicit this nonlinear phenomenon in all species tried; the results that follow are based on recordings from guinea pig and chinchilla.

When the cochlear potentials are viewed on the oscilloscope screen, the subharmonic distortion appears quite dramatically and its presence or absence is easy to discern. The two photographs in Fig. 6.23 illustrate the appearance of undertones. These pictures were taken from the oscilloscope screen. In both, the top traces are the microphonic potentials, while the lower traces show the sound monitored at the eardrum. In the top photograph, both sound and microphonic appear relatively pure. As the stimulus intensity is increased by a small increment, the microphonic undergoes a radical change. Every second peak of the waveform becomes accentuated, at the expense of the interspersed peaks. The picture clearly indicates that the waveform can be

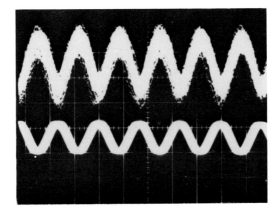

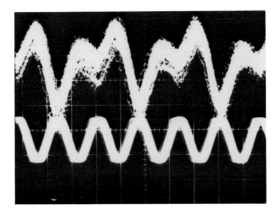

Fig. 6.23. Cochlear microphonic (top traces) and sound at the eardrum (bottom traces) recorded from a guinea pig cochlea at two sound levels of a 3000-Hz pure tone stimulus. The levels are from top to bottom 116.5 and 119.5 dB SPL. (Modified from Dallos and Linnell, 1966a, p. 7.)

made up as the sum of two voltages, one having the same frequency as the driving signal and a second at one-half of the stimulus frequency. Note that the sound monitored at the eardrum seems undistorted in both pictures. The pattern shown in this figure is the general one: As the sound pressure is increased, one sees the undistorted cochlear microphonic response (or potentials containing gradually increasing amounts of overtones) until a particular critical intensity is reached. When this intensity is surpassed, the response pattern changes abruptly as one or more subharmonic components appear.

The most common subharmonic component is the one at one-half the fundamental frequency. The one-quarter-frequency component is also quite frequent, and can best be observed with high-frequency fundamentals during recordings from the more apical turns. On very rare occasions, we recognized distortion components at 1/6, 1/8, and 1/16 of the fundamental. In all cases, the appearance of the basic one-half-frequency component precedes that of the lower-order components. That is to say, we did not see one-quarter- or lower-frequency components appearing unless the one-half-frequency product was already present at a lesser sound intensity.

Unlike cochlear microphonic and its overtones, the subharmonic potentials possess a true threshold. It was seen in previous photographs that a small change in stimulus intensity produces the abrupt appearance of subharmonics at relatively large amplitudes. Even-order subharmonics appear above 110 dB SPL; they are rarely seen at lesser intensities. If the threshold depends on the frequency of the fundamental at all, this dependence is slight. The general tendency appears to be a lowering of the threshold for high frequencies (above 5000 Hz). Below 2000 Hz the threshold sound pressure is also somewhat lower than in the midfrequency range. As a rule subharmonics can be elicited only above approximately 600 Hz; below this frequency they are an exception at any intensity level.

The pattern of response above the level at which subharmonic distortion appears can best be studied from input–output functions. Such functions are shown in Fig. 6.24, where the relationship between signal magnitude and sound pressure level is shown for one fundamental and the two associated subharmonic components. The general feature of the undertones is quite prominent in this plot, namely, the narrow dynamic range that they possess. One sees that, after the rapid initial rise, the undertone climbs some more, but rapidly reaches a peak beyond which it decreases, and quite often completely disappears again. All this usually takes place within a 10- to 15-dB range. In this picture, another common occurrence is also shown. Observe that several decibels beyond the threshold for the one-half-frequency component, the one-quarter undertone occurs. This component exhibits the same general behavior as the first subharmonic, with the exception of higher threshold, and generally even narrower dynamic range. To show visually how the transformation occurs from undistorted waveform to predominant one-half subharmonics, and from those to predominant one-quarter subharmonics, a series of photographs is also included in this composite figure.

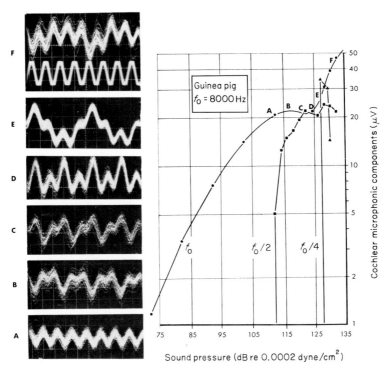

Fig. 6.24. Cochlear microphonic waveforms and input–output functions recorded from the first turn of a guinea pig cochlea with a pure tone stimulus of 8000 Hz. Three input–output functions are shown, one for the fundamental (f_0) CM component, one for the one-half subharmonic ($f_0/2$), and one for the one-fourth subharmonic ($f_0/4$). The letters A to F next to the input–output functions indicate the location of the corresponding waveforms. The bottom trace in photo F depicts the waveform of the sound at the eardrum. (From Dallos and Linnell, 1966a, p. 10.)

The letters indicate the points on the fundamental where the individual pictures belong.

The approach in delimiting the site of origin of even-order undertones was based on the observation that when subharmonic distortion is present in the cochlear microphonic it can also be measured in the sound field in the external meatus. The presence of sound energy at the frequency of the subharmonic is undoubtedly due to the radiation of the eardrum, since the sound produced by the equipment does not contain any measurable subharmonic distortion when measured in a rigid coupler at maximum output level. The subharmonic radiated by the eardrum was found to be from 54 to 95 dB below the strength of the eliciting fundamental. The fact that undertones are radiated by the tympanic membrane definitely indicates that mechanical factors play an important role in the generation of this nonlinear distortion; however, this observation alone does not place the site of generation in the middle ear in a decisive manner.

In seeking the site of undertone generation our approach was to measure subharmonics in the sound field in front of the eardrum while various portions of the cochlea and middle ear were systematically destroyed. The effects of these alterations on the excitability of various modes of subharmonic oscillation were studied. The following steps were generally used in an experiment. First, with intact inner and middle ear the sound pressures at which undertones could be first detected in the sound field were measured for a wide range of frequencies. The magnitude of the subharmonic component at threshold was also recorded. Subsequently, the cochlea was removed while great care was taken not to interfere with the middle ear structures, including the annular ligament and the stapes footplate. The measures of subharmonic excitability were then repeated. Next, the stapes was disarticulated and removed, while the drum and malleus–incus were kept intact. Our sound field measures were again repeated. Finally, as a control, the drum itself was removed and the measures were again carried out.

When the cochlea was removed and an attempt was made to excite subharmonic vibrations, it was observed that the fractional subharmonics could no longer be obtained. It was found, however, that the one-half-frequency undertones were present in the sound field at the frequencies where they could be seen when the cochlea was intact. In general a slight elevation (2–3 dB) in subharmonic threshold accompanied the destruction of the cochlea, but the general properties of these even-order undertones remained unaltered. When the stapes was disarticulated and removed, the one-half-frequency subharmonics continued to persist without significant change in threshold or magnitude.

Thus even-order subharmonics can be detected in the sound field in front of the experimental animal's eardrum as long as the tympanic membrane is intact. The cochlea itself or the stapes does not seem to exert any effect on the excitability of this vibratory mode. It can be surmised that at higher frequencies the eardrum itself can sustain subharmonic vibrations, probably due to its nonlinear elastic properties.

B. FRACTIONAL SUBHARMONICS

1. Properties of Fractional Subharmonics

In chinchilla between the approximate frequency limits of 750 and 3000 Hz, instead of the simple one-half-frequency undertone, a much more complex subharmonic pattern can be observed. In most cases at the threshold of their appearance the undertones have frequencies that are rational fractions of the fundamental. The frequencies of these subharmonics are always in the vicinity of one-half of the fundamental and, specifically, they are always between 1/3 and 2/3 times the fundamental. In the majority of cases, no one-half-frequency subharmonic coexists with the fractional undertones. These subharmonics are normally measured in CM, but they can equally well be demonstrated in the sound field in front of the tympanic membrane. They appear abruptly with a real threshold, just as the even-order subharmonics do.

Most often at threshold, the odd subharmonics appear at certain "permissible" frequency pairs. If the frequency of the fundamental is denoted by f_0 and that of the undertone by f_s, then the following two relationships can be shown to describe the experimental data:

$$f_s^L = f_0 \frac{n}{2n+1} \quad \text{and} \quad f_s^U = f_0 \frac{n+1}{2n+1} \tag{6.19}$$

where n can be any integer, 1, 2, 3, ... Thus at threshold the subharmonic frequency obeys the above relationships, with some n in any particular case. The most commonly seen permissible ratios are 2/5, 3/5; 4/9, 5/9; 7/15, 8/15; and 3/7, 4/7 in order of their frequency of occurrence. A systematic relationship between fundamental frequency and the order of the associated subharmonic has not been discovered. In other words, $(4/9)f_0$ is as likely to occur at 1000 Hz as at 2500 Hz,

In most cases at the threshold of their appearance only the above-described rational fractions are seen. In some cases at threshold, and in all cases above threshold, however, the f_s/f_0 ratio becomes irrational. When this happens, the total response (fundamental plus subharmonics) ceases to be periodic. The irrational fractional subharmonics also appear in pairs; their frequencies fall in the same range as those of the rational ones. One can define a deviation frequency, f_D, as the difference between the subharmonic frequency and $\frac{1}{2}f_0$; $f_D = f_s^U - \frac{1}{2}f_0 = \frac{1}{2}f_0 - f_s^L$. The deviation frequency changes smoothly when the intensity of the fundamental is changed, or when the fundamental frequency is changed at constant intensity. These changes in the deviation frequency are relatively unsystematic. At one time (Dallos, 1966) it appeared that above threshold the deviation frequency always increased, pretty much as a linear function of intensity, but we have now seen exceptions

(Boston, 1971). It is notable that above threshold the fractional subharmonics exist over a limited range only. This range generally does not exceed 10–15 dB. At the high end of the range the fractional-harmonic frequencies become unmeasurable. Instead of clearly defined discrete frequency components, the undertones assume a noiselike character; bands of frequencies appear.

Several interesting observations on the behavior of the fractional subharmonics can be made with the aid of Fig. 6.25, in which the deviation

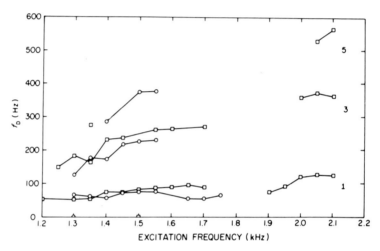

Fig. 6.25. Deviation frequency versus excitation frequency for one chinchilla. Data obtained by keeping the sound amplitude constant. The components having the basic deviation frequency (f_D) are represented by the data points denoted by 1. The higher-order deviation frequencies, usually $3f_D$ and $5f_D$, are denoted by 3 and 5. Legend: $\bigcirc$, 110 dB SPL; $\square$, 115 dB SPL. (From Boston, 1971, p. 82.)

frequency is plotted as the function of fundamental frequency at two levels of SPL. At many frequencies more than a single pair of fractional subharmonics appear. It seems that pairs of frequencies with frequency deviation of rf_D (where $r = 1, 3, 5$ in most cases) can coexist above the subharmonic threshold. At the lower SPL the fractional distortion is confined in this case to the band between 1.3 and 1.75 kHz, while at 5 dB higher two bands appear. In both situations more than one pair of frequencies exist around $\frac{1}{2}f_0$, and at two frequencies even a pure $\frac{1}{2}f_0$ subharmonic is present. Not only frequency components at $f_s = \frac{1}{2}f_0 \pm rf_D$ are common, but also frequencies at $q \cdot \frac{1}{2}f_0 \pm f_D$ (where $q = 1, 3, 5, \ldots$). One could construe the two groups of frequencies as if the first arose from harmonics of the deviation frequency and as if the second were generated around the harmonics of the fundamental. It should be pointed out quickly that this is merely a conceptual framework since very diligent search failed to demonstrate a frequency component at f_D in the composite signal.

Boston (1971) made the important observation that the fractional distortion components are intimately tied to transient processes in the cochlea. It has been seen quite often that just below the threshold of stable fractional subharmonics the characteristic subharmonic pattern can be detected on the oscilloscope screen but that this pattern rapidly extinguishes and gives way to the picture of the simple fundamental. In other words, one often sees brief transient subharmonics below the intensity at which they can be observed over lengthy time periods. It now appears that even above threshold of sustained subharmonic presence, the frequencies of these distortion components are often unsteady. Upon a change in excitation (intensity or frequency) the deviation frequency moves toward a new steady value relatively slowly. During such frequency transients the subharmonic magnitude generally remains relatively constant. The exact nature of the transient apparently is dependent on both stimulus parameters and the immediate past history of the preparation.

At one time we were convinced that fractional distortion was very strongly species specific, and it appeared that it was confined to chinchillas. The work of Robbins (1971) has demonstrated that this type of distortion can be elicited in all species for which an attempt is made. There is, however, an apparent species dependence in threshold intensitities, in the range of frequencies where fractional distortion can exist, and in the stability of the distortion components. In Figs. 6.26 and 6.27 the median, the interquartile range, and the full range of fundamental intensities and frequencies at subharmonic threshold are given for five species of rodents. The species were chosen to sample all major suborders of the order Rodentia. It is apparent from the two figures that chinchillas are able to generate fractional distortion with the least intensity requirement and at the lowest frequencies. The other species not only require more intensity to elicit subharmonics but the incidence of unstable, transient, and noiselike components is also increased over that seen in the chinchilla.

2. Origin of Fractional Subharmonics

It was mentioned before that when subharmonics are monitored in the sound field in front of the tympanic membrane, the fractional subharmonics invariably disappear with the destruction of the cochlea while the one-half-frequency undertone persists as long as the tympanic-membrane–malleus complex is intact. It would be hazardous, on the basis of this evidence alone, to attribute the generation of fractional subharmonics to the cochlea, for these components could be generated by the eardrum, just as the half-frequency components were shown to be. Conceivably, however, the acoustic loading by the cochlea could be necessary for their establishment. In order to test the hypothesis that fractional distortion is excited in the cochlea, the middle ear mechanism was bypassed in the elicitation of cochlear response of chinchillas. With either intracochlear or round-window electrodes placed, a two-step process was carried out (Dallos, 1966). First, the fundamental CM pseudothresholds and subharmonic thresholds were measured for several frequencies. The eardrum and the fused malleus–incus were then removed, and a vibrating needle was carefully introduced and brought into contact with and cemented to the neck of the stapes. With this direct actuation, the CM pseudothresholds were obtained at all the previously measured

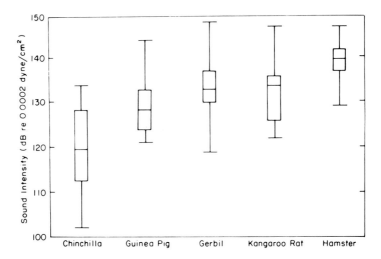

Fig. 6.26. Medians, interquartile and total ranges of intensity requirements for the elicitation of fractional subharmonics in five different species. (From Robbins, 1971, p. 64a.)

frequencies (this is, of course, a relative measure expressed in decibels re an arbitrary voltage across the vibrator), and then an attempt was made to elicit subharmonics. The following should be considered. First, with such direct excitation of the stapes, subharmonics could be elicited in the approximate frequency range 750–3000 Hz. At higher frequencies, the vibrator was not generally capable of supplying sufficient power to exceed the would-be subharmonic thresholds. Second, the subharmonics that were obtained under the direct drive condition were overwhelmingly of the fractional variety, although, occasionally, half-frequency components were also seen. The order of the fractional subharmonics at any frequency was not maintained, as a rule, when transition was made from air elicitation to direct drive. Finally, at any frequency where undertones were successfully excited with both air conduction and direct stapes drive, there was generally good agreement between the relative subharmonic thresholds (i.e., subharmonic threshold minus the CM pseudothreshold) observed under the two conditions.

One can conclude that the evidence seems quite clear-cut in supporting the statement that fractional subharmonics are not generated in the middle ear but that the site of their origin is beyond the stapes. The following results should be considered in support of this contention. First, the fractional subharmonics recorded in the sound field invariably disappear when the cochlea is destroyed. Second, these subharmonics can be elicited without the mediation of the middle ear, as was shown in the experiments where the

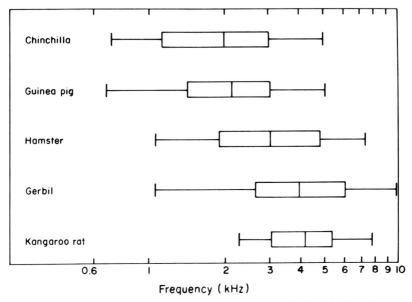

Fig. 6.27. Medians, interquartile and total ranges of effective stimulus frequencies that can elicit fractional subharmonics in five different species. (From Robbins, 1971, p. 64b.)

stimulus was delivered directly to the stapes in the form of mechanical vibrations.

The fact that the fractional subharmonics that are shown to be generated in the inner ear can also be detected in the sound indicates that the distortion occurs in the mechanical processes within the inner ear and not in the mechanoelectrical conversion process. One should envision the situation where the distortion originates, say, in the hydrodynamic processes in the cochlea. Since the cochlear fluids, the ossicular chain, and the eardrum form a coupled system for which certain degrees of reciprocity should be applicable, a transmission in the reverse direction takes place with the end result that the tympanic membrane acts as the cone of a loudspeaker in radiating vibratory energy.

Boston (1971) in a theoretical analysis considered the feasible mechanism of fractional-distortion production. He considered the stability problem of an acoustic flow over a flexible boundary. It was shown that small disturbances to the primary flow can lead to fractional-distortion pairs. These pairs exist within a narrow range of excitation intensity. In a real viscous fluid the sequence of events upon increasing stimulation appears to be as follows. At relatively intense stimulus levels small disturbances to the flow have the potential to develop into fractional pairs. Because of the frictional losses in both fluid and the flexible boundary, these fractional pairs are rapidly dissipated; in other words, they are transients. At higher levels the frictional forces can be overcome and the fractional pairs can exist as stable components. When the excitation exceeds a critical level the flow becomes unstable. It appears that in theory the instability is manifested in the appearance of an exponentially growing half-frequency subharmonic. This sequence of events agrees quite well with the experimental observations. The initial fractional transients, the stable subharmonics, and final instability were all observed. The instability of the flow in the inner ear was manifested in the appearance of noise in place of the stable undertones. Noise in the flow spectrum is usually associated with turbulence, which is an instability. In the animal cochleae the turbulent component always remained bounded; its magnitude was considerably smaller than the primary flow.

3. The Subharmonic Squelch Effect

When a stable fractional subharmonic f_s is elicited by a primary tone f_0, and another tone $f_{pr} = f_s + \Delta f$ is introduced and the intensity of this second, probe tone is increased, it is seen that the existence of the subharmonic is influenced. In general, if the probe tone is made intense enough it can completely obliterate the fractional subharmonic. This phenomenon, subharmonic squelch effect, is discussed below on the basis of its original description (Dallos, 1966).

The degree of squelching of an undertone by an interfering tone depends on both the separation in frequency between the two tones and the intensity of the latter. The relationships between squelching, frequency separation, and intensity can be studied with the aid of Figs. 6.28 and 6.29. In Fig. 6.28 the magnitude of the CM potential of one component of a fractional subharmonic is shown. The fundamental frequency in this case is 2000 Hz, and the undertones appear at 860 and 1140 Hz. This figure presents data on the upper undertone. The SPL of the probe (squelching) tone is plotted on the abscissa, while the separation in frequency between the undertone and

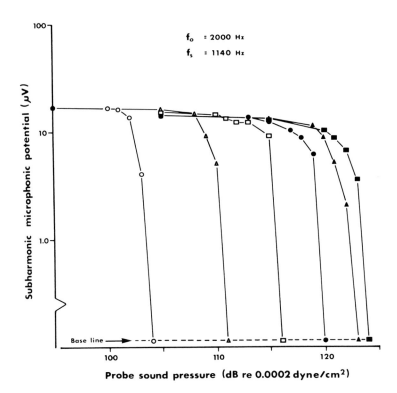

Fig. 6.28. Subharmonic squelch effect. The subharmonic CM component ($f_s = 1140$ Hz) is plotted as the function of the sound pressure of the squelching tone (f_{pr}). The frequency difference between the subharmonic and the squelching tone is the parameter ($f_s - f_{pr}$). The SPL of the stimulus pure tone ($f_0 = 2000$ Hz) is kept constant during all measurements. Parameter: ○, 20; △, 40; □, 60; ●, 80; ▲, 100; ■, 120 Hz. (From Dallos, 1966, p. 1387.)

the probe tone is the parameter. It is seen, for all interfering tones, that the squelch effect is quite abrupt in that up to a certain intensity there is no significant diminution of the undertone, but above the critical intensity the undertone disappears with great rapidity. The critical intensity is smaller for probe tones that are close in frequency to the subharmonics, and it increases with frequency separation. An important observation is made when the subharmonics are monitored in the sound field in front of the eardrum. When probe tones of sufficient intensity are introduced, the fractional-subharmonic components in the sound are squelched just as are those in the microphonic potentials. The intensity and frequency dependence of the squelch effect for undertones in the sound is the same for cochlear potentials.

Some ramifications of frequency dependence are seen in Fig. 6.29. Here, the fundamental frequency is 1000 Hz and the undertone being studied is at 400 Hz. The probe tones are introduced 20 Hz away from the undertone, 10 and 30 Hz away from $\frac{3}{2}f_0 - f_D$, and at two frequencies (755 and 2169 Hz) that are in no way related to the undertone or to any of the higher-order components. In order to compare the effects of interfering tones widely separated in frequency, the squelch effect is plotted as the function of the sound pressure of the probe tone relative to the sound pressure required for that particular frequency tone to elicit a 10-μV microphonic response when

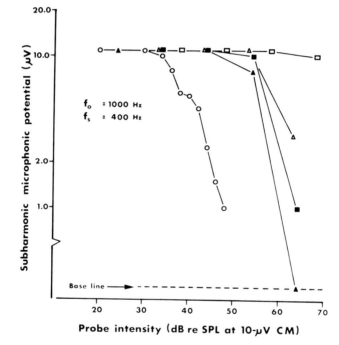

Fig. 6.29. Subharmonic squelch effect. The subharmonic CM ($f_s = 400$ Hz) is plotted as the function of the relative magnitude of the squelching tone expressed in reference to the 10-μV pseudothreshold. The frequency of the squelching tone (f_{pr}) is the parameter ($\bigcirc$, 420; $\blacktriangle$, 1410; $\blacksquare$, 1430; $\triangle$, 755; $\square$, 2169 Hz).

presented alone. The curve obtained with the 420-Hz probe tone can be construed as a reference to which all other curves can be compared. For this curve, the frequency difference between the subharmonic and the interfering tone is only 20 Hz; thus, this curve represents a very high level of squelch. In contrast, the function plotted for the 2169-Hz probe tone represents a very small degree of squelch, for the frequency difference is large (1769 Hz). An intermediate function is obtained with a probe at 755 Hz.

Here, the frequency separation is sizable (355 Hz) but not so large as to preclude any influence on the subharmonic by the probe tone. Note that neither probe frequency (755 or 1769 Hz) is close to any higher component. Two additional squelch functions are shown in Fig. 6.29. These functions are obtained with the probe tone at 1410 and 1430 Hz. These frequencies are 10 and 30 Hz removed from 1400 Hz, which is the frequency of the first higher-order distortion component expressible as $\frac{3}{2}f_0 - f_D$. The reader will recall that, concomitant with fractional-subharmonic generation, energy appears at certain higher frequencies. It is a significant fact that, as is seen

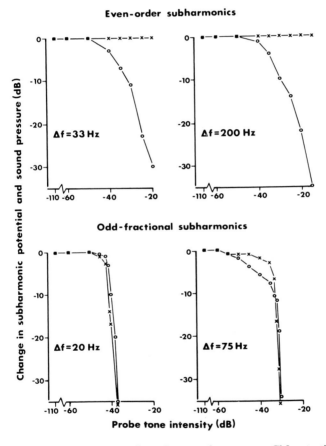

Fig. 6.30. Comparison of the effect of a secondary tone on CM potential and sound pressure (measured at the drum) of both even and fractional subharmonics. Both ordinate and abscissa are expressed in arbitrary logarithmic units; parameter is frequency separation $(f_s - f_{pr} = \triangle f)$ between the subharmonic component and the interfering (squelching) tone. Circles denote CM, and crosses denote sound pressure. (From Dallos, 1966, p. 1388.)

in Fig. 6.29, when the interfering probe tone is in the vicinity of one of the higher distortion components, then the amount of squelch is greater than would be expected from the frequency separation between the subharmonic and the probe. It is clear that, in the case presented, the probes at frequencies of 1410 and 1430 Hz (1010 and 1030 Hz removed from f_s^1) precipitated a more pronounced squelch effect than did the probe at 755 that is only 355 Hz away from the undertone. Thus, it appears that interaction between an interfering tone and a subharmonic component can be most effectively achieved if the frequency of the interfering tone is close to that of the subharmonic or to a higher-order component of the subharmonic.

Even- and fractional-order subharmonics can be contrasted very effectively when their respective behavior is studied in the presence of intense interfering tones. Two squelch functions for fractional undertones are plotted in Fig. 6.30 and contrasted with two functions that are based on even-subharmonic data. There are two major differences between the effects of interfering tones on even or fractional subharmonics. First, while fractional undertones are squelched equally, both in CM potentials and in the sound field, an interfering tone has no effect on the even-order subharmonic components recorded in the sound even though the microphonic potentials are diminished. This is shown very dramatically in Fig. 6.30. Second, the squelch effect on fractional subharmonics is a very abrupt phenomenon in that, after some diminution of undertones is observed, a relatively slight increase in probe intensity causes complete disruption of the undertone pattern. A different situation is in evidence for the even-order subharmonic. The diminution of this distortion potential is quite gradual with the increase in intensity of the interfering tone. This effect is very much like the interference phenomenon described by Wever et al. (1940d).

It can be concluded that the squelch effect seen with fractional undertones is an actual disruption of the subharmonic vibratory pattern, while the effect of a probe tone on the even subharmonic can be explained with the interference phenomenon.

CHAPTER 7

Feedback Mechanisms

Regulatory and control processes permeate all living organisms and they form an essential part of sensory systems as well. The hearing organ is quite well endowed with subsystems that can be considered as feedback mechanisms. Among these are the orienting pinna reflex, the middle ear muscle reflex, the efferent innervation of the organ of Corti, and the adrenergic innervation of the 8th nerve. The first of these reflexes is relatively trivial, while virtually nothing is known of the last system. Much information is available on the second two, even though their exact function is still obscure. This book would not be complete without some information on these feedback systems, and in this chapter an attempt is made to summarize some of the available knowledge on the middle ear muscle reflex and on the efferent system. Before presenting experimental data on these mechanisms, however, we shall briefly examine the properties of feedback systems in general. The aim is to give a very brief account of the capabilities of systems that are equipped with feedback and to emphasize some of the unique advantages that accrue when feedback is introduced into a process.

I. Definition and General Properties of Feedback Systems*

Feedback is a physical as opposed to a mathematical concept. This means that it is the configuration of the system and not its mathematical description

* Grodins (1963), Jones (1969).

465

that determines whether it is a system incorporating feedback. The same mathematical expression (transfer function) can belong to systems with or without feedback. Jones (1969) gave the following requirements for a feedback system. (a) It should be made up of component processes (subsystems) that can be characterized by input and output quantities. (b) It is necessary that these subsystems interrelate in a cyclical manner. That is, if there are n such component systems and if the ith system is described by $x_{i+1} = f_i(x_i)$, where x_i is the input and x_{i+1} is the output of the ith element, then one should have the series of relationships $x_2 = f_1(x_1)$, $x_3 = f_2(x_2)$, ..., $x_n = f_{n-1}(x_{n-1})$, and finally $x_1 = f_n(x_n)$. (c) At least one of the $x_{i+1} = f_i(x_i)$ elements should be unidirectional; in other words, whatever happens at the output of that element should not be felt as its input. (d) If a so-called negative feedback system is of interest then a fourth requirement must be included: There should be an odd number of sign inversions in the chain of subsystems.

These concepts can be crystallized, and the general configuration of a feedback system can be elucidated, with the aid of Fig. 7.1. For simplicity, only

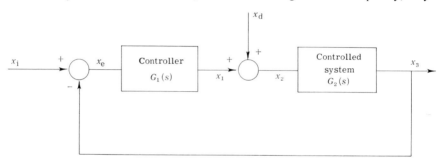

Fig. 7.1. Block diagram representation of a feedback system.

two subsystems are included in this feedback loop; they are characterized by their transfer functions $G_1(s)$ and $G_2(s)$. It is remembered from our discussion in Chapter 3 that the transfer function is alternately defined as the Laplace transform of the system's impulse response or as the ratio of the Laplace transforms of its output and input. Thus in our example if the Laplace transform of x_i is X_i, if that of x_d is X_d, and so forth, then $G_1(s) = X_1(s)/X_e(s)$ and $G_2(s) = X_3(s)/X_2(s)$. The variable s is remembered to be the complex generalized frequency. The most common independent variable of the various x functions is time, but a space variable is equally conceivable. To make the discussion more general, we shall label $G_2(s)$ as the controlled system and $G_1(s)$ as the controller. In other words, with this designation we assume that some property of the system G_2 must be controlled and that G_1 and the feedback are included to facilitate this control. In this context x_3 is considered as the output of the system and the controlled quantity, while x_i is the system input. The variable x_d is construed as an unwanted disturbance that enters the system beyond the controller. The difference between the input and the feedback signals, $x_i - x_3$, is commonly designated as the error signal, x_e. The circles represent so-called summing points; these are locations in the system where variables are added or subtracted. A plus or minus sign placed next to the input lead to the summing point indicates the operation that is performed on the input quantity, namely, addition or subtraction. In Fig. 7.1 we have drawn the system so that its output and feedback signals are the same. In some systems operations are performed on the output signal before it is fed back to the input summing point. The type of system shown here is designated as a unity feedback system; this simply means that the transfer function of the feedback path is $G(s) = 1$.

Depending on the value of the input quantity x_i one can classify feedback systems into two major categories. When $x_i = 0$, that is, when there is no external input to the system, it is commonly called a *regulator*. In this case the function of the feedback system is to maintain the output quantity x_3 at a constant level. When $x_i = x_i(t)$, a variable, the system is designated as a *servomechanism*. Its function is to provide an output that is a replica of the input. One can ask why it is necessary to use these complex feedback systems to obtain either constant output or an output that simply follows the input. Why not use simple forward elements? The answer is that the inherent property of a feedback system, and its claim for legitimacy, is its resistance to changes caused by external disturbing factors. For example, let us assume that we want to operate the system in Fig. 7.1 as a regulator; that is, we take $x_i = 0$. Now as long as x_d is also zero and as long as the system parameters of $G_2(s)$ remain unchanged, the system output will remain constant, which is the desired condition. When $x_d \neq 0$, however, or if something within the controlled system changes then the output will follow these variations. This of course is undesirable. As we shall see below, with the introduction of appropriate feedback, the system can be made quite impervious to disturbing input or to internal parameter variations. Thus the most general function of feedback is to reduce unwanted disturbances and to stabilize the operation of the system. It is not generally possible to achieve these goals without feedback.

In biological systems both regulators and servos are common. The first, so-called homeostatic mechanisms, are typified by the various control systems that stabilize blood chemistry. For example, if an animal's environment changes so that he breathes a larger than normal concentration of CO_2 in the air then the arterial CO_2 pressure, pCO_2, increases. The effect of this is to stimulate ventilation, which in turn causes the reduction of arterial pCO_2 and brings this variable back to normal. We are clearly dealing with a feedback regulator whose function is to keep arterial pCO_2 constant. An example of the biological servomechanism is the accommodation reflex of the eye. As visual targets move toward and away from the eye, the image formed on the retina by the crystalline lens becomes blurred. The blurring of the image activates a control process whose end result is a change in the focal length of the lens and the consequent refocusing of the image on the retina.

We can now begin a more formal analysis of feedback systems, which will help us to understand how disturbances are eliminated and how other advantageous properties are gained by the incorporation of feedback. Let us first express the output of the system shown in Fig. 7.1 in terms of the input (x_i), the disturbance (x_d) and the transfer functions G_1 and G_2. The following series of relationships hold: $X_e = X_i - X_3$, $X_1 = G_1 X_e$, $X_2 = X_1 + X_d$, and $X_3 = G_2 X_2$. After eliminating the internal variables X_e, X_1, and X_2 one obtains the relationship

$$X_3 = X_i \frac{G_1 G_2}{1 + G_1 G_2} + X_d \frac{G_2}{1 + G_1 G_2} \tag{7.1}$$

Let us first examine the special case of operation of the system when it functions as a regulator, that is, when $X_i = 0$. Under this condition,

$$X_3 = X_d \frac{G_2}{1 + G_1 G_2} \tag{7.2}$$

In the steady state the gains of the two transfer functions G_1 and G_2 can be symbolized by k_1 and k_2. In other words, in the steady state, $x_1 = k_1 x_e$ and $x_3 = k_2 x_2$. The usual and desirable case is when $k_1 \gg k_2$. Under such conditions we can write the steady-state equation

$$x_3 = x_d \frac{k_2}{1 + k_1 k_2} \approx x_d \frac{1}{k_1} \tag{7.3}$$

It is immediately clear that since $k_1 \gg 1$, the output of the system due to the disturbance x_d is significantly attenuated. Thus as a consequence of the feedback the influence of the disturbance on the system output is reduced. One should consider that without the feedback the steady-state output of the controlled system in response to the disturbance would be $k_2 x_d$. Clearly unless one makes k_2 very small, which would really destroy the system, there is a significant output component due to the disturbance.

One disturbance of great importance would be a change in a parameter of the controlled system itself. For simplicity, let us assume that the steady-state gain of this system changes for any of a number of undesirable reasons. It is apparent that Eq. (7.3) is not sensitive to variations in k_2, and thus such internal parameter changes are attenuated by the feedback process just as external disturbances are. It is of some interest to obtain a quantitative measure of the sensitivity of a feedback system to such disturbances as parameter variations in the controlled system. Let us assume again that k_2 changes and let us compute the fractional change in x_3 in response to a given percent change in k_2. One notes that

$$\frac{dx_3}{dk_2} = x_d \frac{1}{(1+k_1k_2)^2} = \frac{x_3}{k_2(1+k_1k_2)} \tag{7.4}$$

Consequently

$$\frac{dx_3}{x_3} = \frac{dk_2}{k_2} \frac{1}{1+k_1k_2} \tag{7.5}$$

It is notable that in the general case when $k_1k_2 \gg 1$ the sensitivity of the output to a small disturbance in the system gain is reduced by a factor of $(1+k_1k_2) \gg 1$. Thus the sensitivity to disturbances is small and perturbations in the steady-state output are suppressed.

If the system functions as a servo, that is, if $x_i \neq 0$, then the output in the steady state can be written as

$$x_3 = x_i \frac{k_1k_2}{1+k_1k_2} + x_d \frac{k_2}{1+k_1k_2} \tag{7.6}$$

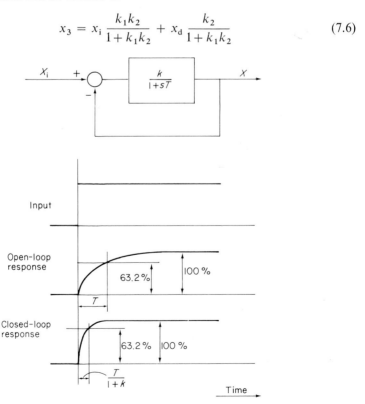

Fig. 7.2. Transient responses of a simple feedback system in both the open- and closed-loop conditions; T is the time constant of the controlled system.

If we again assume that $k_1 \gg k_2$ and that $k_1 \gg 1$ then the above relationship can be approximated as follows:

$$x_3 \approx x_i + x_d \frac{1}{k_1} \approx x_i \tag{7.7}$$

In other words, the disturbance is again suppressed and the output follows the input. This is exactly what is desired from a good servo or follower. It should provide an output that replicates the input and it should do this in the presence of unwanted disturbances or parameter shifts.

It is clear that the presence of negative feedback around a system can have highly beneficial results, one of which, as we have seen, is the reduction in the effect of unwanted disturbances or parameter fluctuations. There are some other significant benefits that accrue from negative feedback, such as increased system bandwidth with a concomitant increase in the speed of the response to input changes, increased input impedance of the system, and the reduction in nonlinear distortion that originates in the controlled system. It might be instructive to consider some of these properties. The simple feedback system shown in Fig. 7.2 incorporates a controlled system having a transfer function $G(s) = k/(1 + sT)$. This system corresponds to a low-pass filter; its open-loop response can be expressed as $X = X_i k/(1 + sT)$. Let us assume that the input to the open-loop system is a step function of magnitude x_i. Under such conditions the Laplace transform of the output is

$$X(s) = \frac{x_i}{s} \frac{k}{1 + sT} \tag{7.8}$$

and the output time function is expressible as

$$x(t) = x_i k(1 - e^{-t/T}) \tag{7.9}$$

This response of the open-loop system is an exponential rise with a time constant of T; it is depicted in the first insert of Fig. 7.2. When the feedback loop is established, the system transfer function becomes

$$X = X_i \frac{G}{1 + G} = X_i \frac{k/(1 + sT)}{1 + [k/(1 + sT)]} = X_i \frac{k}{1 + k} \frac{1}{1 + [sT/(1 + k)]} \tag{7.10}$$

If the input is again a step of magnitude x_i, then the transform of the output time function is written as

$$X = \frac{x_i}{s} \frac{k}{1 + k} \frac{1}{1 + [sT/(1 + k)]} \tag{7.11}$$

with the corresponding inverse transform,

$$x(t) = x_i \frac{k}{1 + k} (1 - e^{-t/[T/(k+1)]}) \tag{7.12}$$

It is apparent that with the introduction of the feedback the system response remained an exponential rise, but its time constant decreased from a value of T to the potentially much smaller value of $T/(1+k)$. The new output response is also shown in the first insert of Fig. 7.2. It is clear that, when fast response speed is of importance in the operation of a system but, when the basic system is inherently slow, the introduction of feedback and the resulting servo operation can improve the response function. It is notable that faster time response and wider bandwidth go hand in hand. Thus in the open-loop case the bandwidth is $1/T$ radians/second, while in the closed-loop case it increases to $(1+k)/T$ radians/second.

One more item is worth mentioning here—the reduction in harmonic distortion that originates in the controlled system. Let us assume that in G_2 of the system depicted in Fig. 7.1 harmonic components of the input x_i are generated, with the magnitude of an nth harmonic being x_n. Clearly there is no reason why the treatment of these internally generated components should be different than that of the disturbance x_d. Thus in the steady state one can write for the system output

$$x_{\text{out}} = x_i \frac{k_1 k_2}{1 + k_1 k_2} + \sum_n x_n \frac{k_2}{1 + k_1 k_2} \tag{7.13}$$

In the case where the controller gain k_1 is significantly greater than the system gain k_2, the above expression simplifies to yield $x_{\text{out}} \cong x_i$. In other words, the internally generated harmonic distortion components are attenuated by the feedback process. Of course if the input contained two sinusoidal components, the internally generated intermodulation distortion components would suffer the same fate as the harmonics that result from a single input; namely, these would be reduced as well. The actual reduction in the distortion content of the output signal due to the feedback is by a factor of $(1 + k_1)$.

II. The Middle Ear Muscle Reflex

A. GENERAL CONSIDERATIONS

The two middle ear muscles, stapedius and tensor tympani, serve as the final effector elements in one of the most conspicuous peripheral auditory control systems. The descending path of this system consists of neural connections between the superior olivary complex and the motor nuclei of the two muscles, primary innervation of the tensor via a branch of the trigeminal nerve and of the stapedius via a branch of the facial nerve. Both muscles apparently receive secondary innervation from several sources (Lawrence, 1962; Blevins, 1963, 1964), the most important of which is probably the fibers reaching the stapedius from the vagus nerve. Apparently both muscles possess sensory endings, muscle spindles, or free arborization of sensory fibers, which provide proprioceptive self-control and probably cross control of the muscles. The latter might take place in that the contractions of the stapedius could initiate contractions of the tensor via the auricular branch of the vagus nerve (Starr and Solomon, 1965).

From the structural viewpoint both muscles can be classified as primarily pennate types; that is, they consist of large numbers of parallel fibers that can provide considerable tension with minimal displacement during contraction. From a functional viewpoint it is possible that two types of fibers constitute these muscles, one group providing tonic and another group tetanic contractions (Erulkar *et al.*, 1964). This notion is now disputed (Candiollo, 1967). The tendons of both muscles are rich in elastic tissue. The ability of a muscle to perform finely graded contractions is ususally determined by its innervation ratio, that is, the ratio of efferent nerve fibers and motor fibers. By this criterion the middle ear muscles should be able to deliver very finely graded contractions inasmuch as the innervation ratio of the tensor is approximately 1:7 and that of the stapedius is between 1:5.6 and 1:3.5. These are unusually high ratios. There is a distinct possibility that there are two types of motor units in the middle ear muscles (nerve fiber plus the muscle fibers that are innervated by it), tonic and phasic (Okamoto *et al.*, 1954).

The middle ear muscles can be activated by a variety of auditory and nonauditory stimuli. When the chain of events that culminates in the contraction of either or both muscles is initiated by an acoustic stimulus, the overall process is described as the *acoustic reflex*. This reflex will receive our primary attention in the pages that follow. The muscles can be activated by nonacoustic sensory stimuli, such as tactile stimulation of various regions of the face and the earcanal, and by various somatic functions, such as mastication and vocalization. The acoustically elicited reflex is bilateral; that is, stimulation of either ear results in muscle activity in both ears.

Owing to the relative physical arrangement between the two muscles and the ossicular chain, when the muscles contract they exert opposing effects on the middle ear bones. The tensor is inserted at the manubrium of the malleus, and when it is activated it pulls the malleus inward. This results in an inward motion of the eardrum. The stapedius is attached at the neck of the stapes and its contraction pulls this bone outward from the oval window and also at a right angle to the major plane of the entire ossicular chain. As a consequence of these differing directions of pull, the simultaneous contraction of both muscles results in an increased rigidity, or stiffening, of the ossicular chain and also in a rocking motion of the stapes. The latter could produce a functional partial disarticulation of the incudostapedial joint and also some motion of the incus. The direction of motion of the eardrum (if any) due to a stapedius contraction is difficult to predict. The end result of the various movements and effects within the middle ear mechanism that follow from cocontraction of the two muscles is an overall reduction of sound transmission by the ossicular chain and thus a decrease in energy that reaches the cochlea. One can thus state that anatomically the two muscles are antagonists but physiologically they are synergists. Their opposing displacement results in the more effective reduction of middle ear transmission.

A block diagram depicting the various way stations of the middle ear muscle reflex is shown in Fig. 7.3. It is apparent from this figure that active

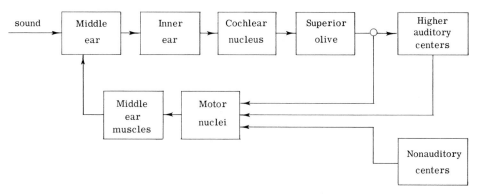

Fig. 7.3. Simplified block diagram of the middle ear muscle reflex as a multipath feedback mechanism.

muscle function can represent two different types of operation. When the initial stimulus that activates the reflex is sound, it is clear that the various structures in the system constitute a feedback process. Specifically, the primary stimulus, sound, initiates activity in the motor nuclei of the stapedius and tensor. This causes the muscles to contract, and this alters the middle ear transmission, which in turn changes the input to the motor nuclei. A clear-cut feedback operation is in evidence. When the information that initiates muscle contraction is derived from nonauditory centers of the brain, however, the various active structures align themselves in a straight forward path of action; there is no feedback involved in the operation. In other words, the muscle reflex influences the middle ear transmission, but itself is not directly influenced by the auditory input.

The role of the middle ear muscle reflex has been endlessly debated. Many theories of function have been advanced but none has gained clear favor with the scientific consensus. It appears today that these muscles fulfill several roles and consequently more than one of the proposed theories can be considered correct. The most persistent suggestion is based on the observation that in the presence of loud sounds the muscles reflexively contract and reduce transmission through the middle ear. In doing so the reflex limits the acoustic input that reaches the inner ear and consequently it protects the cochlea from excessive stimulation. This observed chain of events led to the assumption that the role of the reflex is protection. According to another proposal, known as the accommodation theory, the function of the muscle reflex is to "tune" the middle ear for optimal absorption of sound energy by changing its transmission characteristics. The fixation theory supposes that the muscles provide needed rigidity for the ossicular chain and that they prevent changes in the articulation between the ossicles during high acceleration. Other, more exotic theories have also surfaced but they do not require discussion here.

Simmons (1964) brought some order and considerable light to the jungle of conflicting middle ear muscle reflex theories. He made simple observations on awake cats in which he permanently implanted round-window electrodes for the measurement of CM, and EMG electrodes for the measurement of muscle electromyograms. Simmons' first question was aimed at the most popular protection theory. He asked where in nature sounds are loud enough to have necessitated the evolution of a protective mechanism to guard against them. The answer to this is of course nowhere, and thus one must be careful in assigning a purely protective role to the muscle reflex. It should be emphasized that even though the reflex probably did not evolve as a protective device against loud environmental sounds, it undoubtedly functions as such under appropriate conditions. This we shall see in detail below. It is thus likely that the protection given by the reflex against certain loud sounds is actually a bonus and not the primary function.

Simmons noted that there are three main modes of muscle activity. The first is a simple change in muscle tonus, that is, spontaneous activity, which is clearly observable in awake and alert animals. This fluctuation in tonus must of necessity induce changes in the transmission characteristics of the middle ear. One possible result is the reduction in the size of the antiresonant peak in the transfer function that we discussed in detail in Chapter 3. The reduction in this peak yields a smoother transfer function, which in turn provides for higher-fidelity transmission. We have already presented Simmons' experimental evidence supporting this claim. In Fig. 3.19 the CM response obtained at constant SPL was shown in situations of awake and anesthetized cats, as well as for cases of intact and severed middle ear muscles. In all situations where the muscles were inactive (cut or anesthetized) a deep notch was evident around 4000 Hz, whereas in the normal awake cat the transmission function was quite smooth. It appears then that the normally fluctuating muscle tonus might be sufficient to produce a variable detuning of the middle ear antiresonance and thus to "average out" its effect. A second proposed function of fluctuating middle ear transmission brought about by changing muscle tonus is to provide a variable auditory background which, in analogy with the operation of the visual system, would enhance the maintenance of auditory attention. This attractive suggestion is yet to receive experimental verification.

Simmons demonstrated that the muscle reflex can become active at sound levels considerably lower than those called for by the protection theory. It appears that as part of the animal's common orienting response to a novel environmental sound, middle ear muscle contractions take place along with the more obvious head and body movements. In this context the reflex could serve to attenuate inborne sounds of the organism and could thus help it to zero in on the external stimulus. It is now clear that middle ear muscle contractions can take place in connection with a variety of skeletal muscle action such as head movement, vocalization, chewing, and swallowing. In these situations the middle ear muscle reflex is not sound elicited; in fact it begins considerably before the commencement of the major skeletal muscle activity. Thus, for example, the middle ear muscles begin to contract about 100 mseconds prior to the onset of vocalization and their activity is sustained during sound production. The type of muscle activity that was mentioned above as being efficient in eliciting the middle ear muscle reflex is inherently noisy. In other words, chewing, for example, does create a great deal of internal noise within the organism. Such noises are capable of effectively masking environmental sounds. An extreme example of self-noise is provided by certain bats that emit intense cries and listen to the returning echo for spatial localization. Clearly the outgoing sound is much more intense than the returning echo, and thus the former could mask the latter. In order to avoid this, bats contract their stapedius prior to the emission of the cry and they thus reduce the acoustic energy reaching the cochlea. The muscle then relaxes and allows the full intensity of the returning echo to be utilized. It is apparent that great evolutionary gains can be made by animals that are able to reduce their self-generated, internal noises and thus can improve the signal-to-noise ratio of the external sounds of the environment. Simmons proposed that this function of the middle ear muscles, namely, the anticipatory contraction during noise-producing skeletal muscle activity, might be their most important contribution.

B. The Acoustic Reflex

1. Problems of Measurement

While, in light of the above discussion, the sound-elicited, acoustic reflex might not be the sole or even most important facet of middle ear muscle function, it is the one that lends itself to experimental observation and quantification. Moreover, whatever is learned about the acoustic reflex can be translated to delineate the properties of nonacoustically evoked reflex action. Because of these considerations we shall devote some space to the description of the properties of the reflex and a considerable segment of the discussion will be presented on the basis of acoustically elicited operation. There is a sizable body of literature on the properties of the muscle reflex that is based on animal experiments (e.g., Wiggers, 1937; Wever and Bray, 1942; Wever and Vernon, 1955; Wersäll, 1958; Galambos and Rupert, 1959; Simmons, 1959; Møller, 1964, 1965; Starr, 1969), but much of our knowledge on this subject comes from work with human beings. While the former body of information is emphasized in the discussion to follow, some selected data are also drawn from the latter.

Several methods have been utilized for assessing the effects of muscle activity on middle ear sound transmission. Among these are electromyography, measurement of CM, determination of changes in the acoustic input impedance of the ear, and measurement of pressure changes in the sealed earcanal due to movements of the tympanic membrane (tympanic manometry). The last of these methods is difficult to interpret and the first three have produced the greatest bulk of data on the subject. Impedance measurement has been particularly useful in studies on the human acoustic reflex, where other methods of course cannot easily be utilized. The most direct information about changes in middle ear transmission can be derived from CM data, while myography supplies relatively indirect data on the input to the muscles. Acoustic impedance measurements give an indirect indication of changes in transmission properties; they actually provide a view of the system from the outside. Under particular conditions the input impedance and transmission measures are very closely related and thus one can infer from the former to the latter. Møller (1965) addressed himself to the problem of clarifying these conditions, and he measured both input impedance and CM in cats and rabbits under a variety of conditions. First he noted that the magnitudes of static impedance at the drum and the CM sensitivity curve are very similar over the most significant portion of the frequency range. In Fig. 7.4 the impedance and the reciprocal of the CM magnitude when measured at a constant SPL are shown for one cat. It is impressive that between 400 and 4000 Hz the two curves can be made virtually to superimpose. In this frequency band the velocity of the eardrum is apparently proportional to the velocity of the stapes, $v_d \approx v_s$, and the CM at the round window is proportional to the pressure at the oval window, $CM \approx p_s = v_s Z_c$. If the cochlear input impedance is resistive and constant then from the above relations it follows that $CM \approx v_s \approx v_d$. It is clear, however, that the input impedance of the ear, Z_d, is equal to the ratio of the pressure at the drum and its velocity. Thus at a constant SPL, $Z_d \approx 1/v_d$, and thus finally $CM \approx v_d \approx 1/Z_d$. These relations and Møller's findings imply that the input admittance is a good measure of the middle ear transmission characteristics at the mid-frequencies. We now know that the low-frequency discrepancy is due to the high-pass filter effect of the helicotrema (see Chapter 4, Section II,E) and thus it is fair to say that the input admittance is a good measure of the output of the middle ear of the cat at all frequencies up to about 4000 Hz.

Møller demonstrated that the correspondence between input admittance and CM holds in the presence of various manipulations of the middle ear.

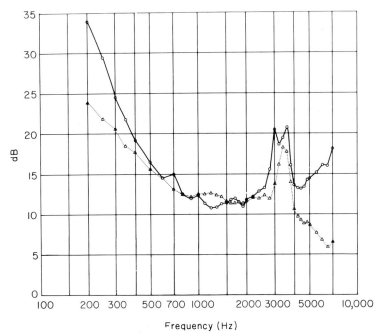

Fig. 7.4. The numerical value of the acoustic impedance (dotted line) at the eardrum and inverse cochlear microphonic (solid line) at constant SPL at the eardrum in an anesthetized cat. Bulla intact; acoustic impedance given in logarithmic measures relative to 100 cgs units. Reference for the CM is arbitrary. (From Møller, 1965, p. 133.)

For example, the opening of the bulla changes both measures significantly and quite similarly. The deviation between the two measures (CM and $1/Z_d$) in fact is less than about 5 dB between 200 and 4000 Hz. Similarly good agreement was found between the two measures when Møller increased the static air pressure of the middle ear by 10 cm H_2O. Interestingly, the agreement was rather poor in the situation when the middle ear pressure was reduced by 10 cm H_2O. In this latter case the CM measure indicated a loss in transmission about 10 dB greater than what one would have surmised from the impedance data. Since the reactive part of the impedance tended to change the same amount with equal positive and negative pressure, while the resistive part changed very asymmetrically (resistance virtually disappeared with increasing negative pressure), and since the latter component is due primarily to the cochlear load on the ossicular chain, one can deduce that during negative pressure conditions the cochlea becomes effectively decoupled from the middle ear. Thus, while under such conditions the impedance change at the eardrum is not more radical than when positive pressure is used, the transmission is greatly impaired.

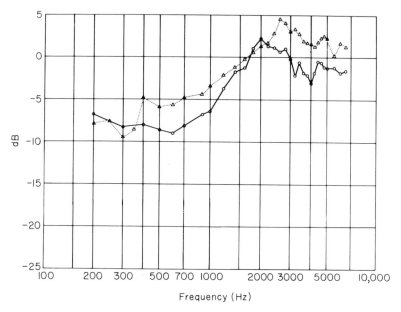

Fig. 7.5. The change in transmission (solid line) compared with the inverse change in the acoustic impedance (dotted line) at the eardrum during stapedius muscle contraction. (From Møller, 1965, p. 145.)

We are discussing these fine points because interestingly during middle ear muscle contraction the change in impedance is again different from the change in transmission (CM). An example of the effect of stapedius contraction on both measures is shown in Fig. 7.5. It is notable that at the low frequencies more reduction is shown by the CM than by the impedance. Above 2000 Hz these relations reverse, but at no frequency are the differences greater than about 5 dB in cat. In rabbit, Møller found similar discrepancies. While the absolute magnitude of the change in transmission might not be predicted with perfect accuracy from input impedance changes, the alterations in these two quantities do seem to show similar time courses during muscle contraction. These considerations indicate that one is probably justified in studying the effects of the middle ear muscle reflex by recording changes in the ear input impedance. This is a happy conclusion because the vast bulk of quantitative information that is available on the muscle reflex has been obtained with the impedance method. Let us now examine some of the salient properties of the middle ear muscle reflex, and more specifically those of the acoustic reflex.

2. Properties of the Reflex

a. Static Characteristics. The excitability of the acoustic reflex as a function of the frequency of the stimulus sound has been measured in man, cat, and rabbit (Lorente de Nó and Harris, 1933; Wever and Vernon, 1955; Price, 1963; Møller, 1962; Borg and Møller, 1968). Most experimenters agree that the threshold function of the reflex largely parallels the CM sensitivity function, which in turn fairly closely reflects the behavioral sensitivity curve. In general, low frequencies are less efficient in eliciting the acoustic reflex; the threshold improves up to approximately 1000–3000 Hz, beyond which it stays relatively constant. The general trend can be illustrated with some of Price's findings (1963). In Fig. 7.6 the sound pressure required to produce a CM of 10 μV and that needed for obtaining the first sign of CM depression due to muscle contraction are shown for a group of rabbits. Apparently between 200 and about 2000 Hz both functions decrease at a rate of 12 dB/octave; they level off at higher frequencies. The difference between the two curves is a relatively constant 50–55 dB. The absolute value of this difference is of course immaterial since the CM criterion measure is arbitrary. In human beings Møller (1962) noted that the audibility curve and a curve depicting 10% impedance change due to the reflex (elicited by contralateral stimulation) paralleled one another with approximately 80 dB separation. It thus appears that the reflex is activated at any given frequency when the output of the cochlea reaches a certain threshold level. It has been observed that band-pass-filtered noise is a more effective stimulus in initiating the acoustic reflex than are pure tones. If the energy content of a tone and a noise band centered around the same frequency as that of the tone are compared, then the noise stimulus can elicit reflex action about 5 dB below the level of the tone (Møller, 1962). Once the reflex threshold is surpassed, the strength of muscle contraction, as expressed by the concomitant impedance change, increases roughly in proportion with the magnitude of the stimulus. As Fig. 7.7 demonstrates, the response increases over an approximately 30-dB range, above which it levels off. Thus the acoustic reflex is active over a relatively narrow dynamic range between its threshold and level of saturation. Within its range of operation the reflex is certainly effective

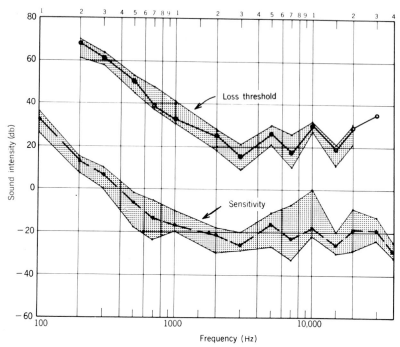

Fig. 7.6. The median threshold of the acoustic reflex (labeled "loss threshold") and the median 10-μV sensitivity curve for the rabbit. The acoustic reflex threshold was established by noting the first evidence of decrease in round-window CM. The shaded area represents the interquartile range. Sound pressure is shown in dB with respect to 1 dyne/cm². (From Price, 1963, p. 226.)

in altering middle ear transmission. The characteristics of this alteration will now be examined.

There is universal agreement that the effects of muscle contraction on the transmission characteristics of the middle ear are strongly frequency dependent. From the earliest experiments it became clear that the primary influence of the reflex is on low-frequency transmission. Wever and Bray (1937, 1942) stretched the tensor and the stapedius with known tension and measured the SPL required to produce standard CM responses at various frequencies in the cat. Møller (1965) elicited the reflex acoustically and measured the changes in CM in both cat and rabbit as the function of frequency. Starr (1969) used electrical stimulation of the muscles, and again he measured their effects on CM at various frequencies. For comparison with Møller's results on the cat (Fig. 7.5) Starr's data are given in Fig. 7.8. It is notable how similar the results of these two divergent experiments are. At low frequencies the attenuating effect of the contraction of either muscle (stapedius in Møller's and tensor in Starr's experiment) is maximal, it diminishes around 1500 Hz, and in a narrow frequency range there is actually an increase in transmission, which is once again followed by a modest attenuation at higher frequencies. The two muscles are approximately equal in their ability to attenuate the acoustic input to the cochlea, and they summate their effects during cocontraction. Maximally active muscles can produce reductions in middle ear transmission up to 20–30 dB. These large effects are of course observed only at low frequencies.

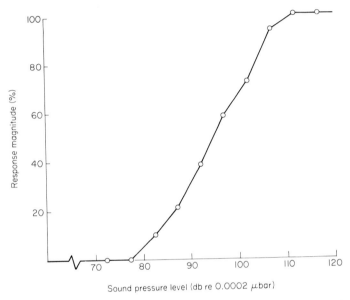

Fig. 7.7. Median input–output function of the acoustic reflex. Ordinate is expressed as the percentage of maximum response (input impedance change) while the abscissa shows the level of the stimulating wide-band noise. (From Dallos, 1964b, p. 2179.)

One could summarize the results discussed on the last few pages by noting that any sound can elicit the acoustic reflex but that the primary effect of the active reflex is on the low-frequency transmission of the middle ear. We can now recall some of Simmons' ideas and realize that most self-noises that an organism generates are low-frequency noises. These sounds are most effectively attenuated by the middle ear muscle reflex and thus the value of the reflex in improving the signal-to-noise ratio of environmental sounds can be quite significant.

Since much of the information on the reflex has been gathered by the impedance method, it would be valuable to briefly mention how the active middle ear muscles alter the input impedance of the ear. During stimulation (reflex active) the magnitude of the input impedance generally increases, and in most cases the increase is less than 500 dynes second/cm^5. Along with the increase in magnitude the phase also changes to a moderate degree, and the change is toward a decreased phase lag. One can translate these results and note that the primary effect of the reflex is an increase in the reactive component of the input impedance (increased stiffness); the resistive component has been seen to either increase or decrease. These changes reflect

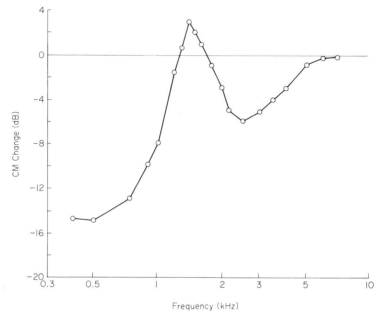

Fig. 7.8. Effect of tensor tympani contractions on acoustic transmission of the middle ear. The data are derived from a single experiment. Change in round-window CM is plotted on the ordinate of the graph and the frequency of the CM-eliciting tone on the abscissa. Stimulation is with tetanic electrical shocks to the body of the tensor muscle. (From Starr, 1969, p. 103.)

the result that during muscle contraction the sound absorption by the middle ear is decreased and the reflected sound energy from the eardrum is increased (Dallos, 1964b).

We have mentioned that the primary effect of middle ear muscle contraction is the reduction of low-frequency input to the cochlea. One can easily construe this operation as that of a feedback regulator whose task is to maintain a relatively constant output level once the input exceeds a certain preset value. A theoretical (and of course grossly simplified) analog of this type of regulator is shown in Fig. 7.9a. Here the input signal x_i symbolizes

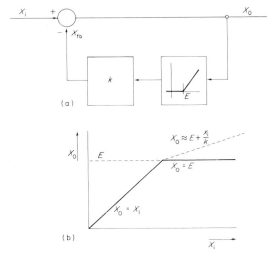

Fig. 7.9. (a) Schematic representation of a feedback system with unity-gain forward path, a feedback gain of k, and a threshold element in the feedback path. (b) Input–output function of this feedback system. Below threshold the output follows the input; above threshold the system gain is reduced. If $k \to \infty$ then the output is clamped at the threshold level, and if k is large the output gain is reduced (dashed line).

the input to the middle ear; x_o is the output. The feedback path contains two elements. The first is a threshold device whose output is zero if its input is less than the threshold, and it is proportional to the excess input over the threshold when the latter is exceeded. The second feedback element simply signifies a gain of magnitude k, as in Section I; here, as well, we assume that k is large. The following relationship can be written on the basis of the block diagram:

When $\quad x_i < E \quad$ then $\quad x_o = x_i$

When $\quad x_i \geq E \quad$ then $\quad x_o = x_i - x_{fb} \quad x_{fb} = k(x_o - E)$ $\qquad$ (7.14)

From the last two relations one can solve for x_o in the $x_i > E$ condition.

$$x_o = \frac{x_i}{1+k} + \frac{kE}{1+k} \approx E \qquad (7.15)$$

We note that for the case in which the gain is high, the system output is held constant at the threshold level, no matter how high the input becomes. The graphical representation of this input–output relationship is shown with heavy lines in Fig. 7.9b. If we do not insist that k should be extremely large, while we still maintain its value so that $k \gg 1$, then the output is not clamped at the value of E above threshold, but it slowly increases at an approximate rate of x_i/k. This more realistic input–output relationship is depicted with the broken line in Fig. 7.9b. One can summarize these theoretical considerations by saying that this feedback system operates as a unity-gain open-loop system below threshold and that it operates as a system having a gain of $1/k$ above threshold. Thus the influence of the input on the output is greatly diminished above the threshold and it approaches zero as the system gain approaches infinity.

The question that naturally arises is, how well is the acoustic reflex represented by a theoretical regulator such as the one that we have just discussed? Moreover, how good is the regulation or, to put it in a different light, how large is k? There have been some attempts to answer these questions, and we shall review some of them below. An interesting approach was used by Borg (1968), who compared the rate of rise of the magnitude of the impedance change due to the acoustic reflex in a group of patients during stapedius paralysis and after the alleviation of the disease. He stimulated on the paralyzed side and measured on the other side.* Consequently during the active stage of the disease the stapedius could not contract on the stimulated side and could not reduce the input to the cochlea. As a result muscle contraction (and impedance change) on the contralateral side, which was assumed to reflect the cochlear output from the ipsilateral side, was proportional to the *unregulated* cochlear output. When the disease was checked, the ipsilateral reflex was active, and consequently the contralateral muscle contraction (impedance change) represented the *regulated* cochlear output.

Two of Borg's plots are reproduced in Fig. 7.10. With a stimulus of 500 Hz, the unregulated (diseased) impedance change rises at a rate of 11.1% per decibel above reflex threshold, while in the regulated (normal) case the rate of rise is reduced to 5.0% per decibel. It appears that the system gain changes by a factor of 2.2 as a consequence of the presence of the feedback provided by stapedius contractions. In other cases greater discrepancies were noted. An interesting additional comparison between open- and closed-loop operations obtains if one realizes that the acoustic reflex is effective only at low frequencies. Consequently, when elicited by high-frequency sounds, the muscle reflex should not affect the cochlear input, which means that in such cases the reflex cannot produce regulatory action. This can be rephrased by stating that at high frequencies our feedback system operates in open loop. If this is indeed the case then stapedius paralysis should not affect the rate of rise of the contralateral reflex. We see in the 1450-Hz plot of Borg, which is also reproduced in Fig. 7.10, that this is indeed the case. The functions rise at the same rate in both the normal and

* We have already noted that the reflex is bilateral; when elicited, muscle contractions occur on both sides. We shall discuss this topic in more detail in the pages that follow.

paralyzed state. Moreover their rate of rise is approximately 10% per decibel, which is virtually the same as was seen in this individual for the open-loop (paralyzed) case at 500 Hz. The results indicate that as a consequence of the stapedius reflex the rate of increase of the cochlear input is cut at least by a factor of 2 compared to that below the reflex threshold. This reduction in gain is significant, but it certainly does not approach "perfect regulation," which would imply a clamping of the output to a constant value.

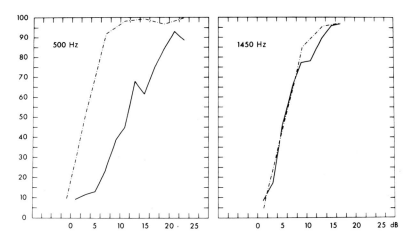

Fig. 7.10. Impedance change in percentage of maximum obtainable as a function of sound level in decibels re ipsilateral reflex threshold. The interrupted line shows the contralateral reflex during ipsilateral stapedial paralysis and the solid line relates to the reflex after recovery. Data at two frequencies are shown. (From Borg, 1968, p. 465.)

Some fine animal experiments of Wever and Vernon (1955) produced evidence indicating that near-perfect regulation of the cochlear input by the acoustic reflex can be achieved over a limited intensity range. They measured CM in decerebrated (unanesthetized) cats in response to a steady test tone, which was delivered to the same ear. Stimuli used to elicit the acoustic reflex were led to the other ear. The reduction in the CM response to the test tone in the contralateral ear was taken as a measure of the change in the cochlear input during acoustic reflex action. They noted the functional relation between reflex action and middle ear transmission that is now quite familiar: Low frequencies were the most severely attenuated, there was a narrow midfrequency region of enhancement, and this was followed by further moderate attenuation at the higher frequencies. They showed a curve of CM change versus frequency that was obtained 2 dB above the reflex threshold. The shape of this curve is quite similar to what we have demonstrated in Fig. 7.8. When the intensity of the contralateral stimulus was increased above the reflex threshold an orderly decrease in the CM response to the test tone was seen.

In Fig. 7.11 we have reproduced their results that apply to the case in which both muscles were actively contracting to produce the overall attenuation effect. It is quite apparent that in a range of about 20 dB above the reflex threshold the CM is proportionally decreased from its prereflex value. The decrease is almost a perfect 20 dB for the 20-dB increases in the stimulus. This indicates that in the intensity region just above the reflex threshold the mechanism is capable of performing as a virtually perfect regulator. This implies that in the stimulated ear the output from the middle ear was held constant over the 20-dB span of stimulus increase. Beyond this intensity range the CM in the contralateral ear levels off, and this signifies that at such high levels the reflex is no longer capable of providing additional attenuation. This observation is very much in line with our previous comments concerning the narrow dynamic range of the reflex. The mechanism quite apparently saturates 20–30 dB above its threshold, probably as a consequence of the muscles reaching their maximal tension.

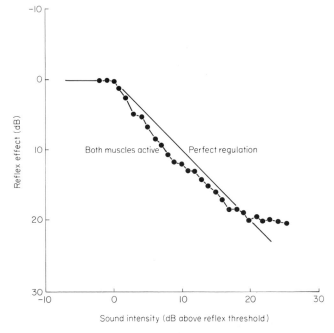

Fig. 7.11. Effects on ipsilateral CM of varying the strength of contralateral stimulation. The curve shows results when both muscles are active, as seen in the decrease of cochlear potential response to a 300-Hz tone. (From Wever and Vernon, 1955, p. 437.)

The bilaterality of the acoustic reflex was mentioned before. It has been noted in both animals and man that when one ear is adequately stimulated, muscle contractions are observable in both ears. This fact has permitted most experiments that utilize the impedance technique to be performed; usually stimulation is done in one ear while the other is used as an indicator ear for measuring purposes. While the reflex is apparently bilateral, it now appears that neither the reflex threshold nor the strength of muscle contractions is completely symmetrical for ipsilateral and contralateral elicitation. This can be explained by some impedance data of Møller (1962). He measured the change in acoustic impedance of a human subject in both ears under three conditions: ipsilateral, contralateral, and bilateral stimulation. It was observed that the reflex threshold is approximately 5–10 dB poorer with contralateral as opposed to ipsilateral stimulation. Moreover, at any intensity above reflex threshold the impedance change is less in the contralateral case. It is interesting that, when both ears are stimulated, the reflex threshold is improved over the ipsilateral elicitation, and the impedance change at a given SPL is also greater. Above reflex threshold the impedance changes at approximately the same rate, no matter how the reflex is initiated. At least as a first approximation the differences among the three modes of elicitation can be considered as mere threshold discrepancies.

b. Dynamic Characteristics. The middle ear muscle reflex modifies the input to the cochlea. Since the acoustic environment, and thus the input to the inner ear, as a rule changes rapidly in time, if its modification by the reflex is to be effective then the latter must respond with commensurate speed. Thus in discussing the properties of the acoustic reflex it behooves us to pay at least as much attention to its dynamic characteristics as to the static behavior. In order to assess the dynamic properties of the reflex one must examine stimulus–response relationships when the input signal is some sort of acoustic transient. The most informative data have been obtained by using tone and noise bursts, impulsive sounds, and amplitude-modulated sinusoidal signals as stimuli.

When a tone is turned on rapidly and the muscle reaction is measured by some suitable means, it is a universal observation that there is a characteristic silent interval between the onset of the stimulus and the onset of the response. This silent interval—variously designated as response latency, dead time, time lag, or latent period—elapses before the muscles actually begin to contract after the stimulus is received by the organism. The magnitude of the latent period is found to be inversely proportional to the strength of the acoustic stimulus. We have observed a range of latencies between 40 and 160 mseconds in human subjects when the stimulus was wide-band noise. Other investigators have reported both shorter and longer dead times. While the average latencies show a very definite relationship with intensity, individual response latencies may vary widely. Such variability exists not only among subjects, but for the same subject from trial to trial as well. While there is this general inverse relationship between stimulus strength and latency at the onset of the stimulus, no similar characteristic dependence on intensity can be generally noted at the cessation of the response. One can estimate that the off latency ranges between 75 and 100 mseconds and is largely independent from stimulus strength in human subjects. The existence of the latent period has important practical and theoretical consequences in relation to the functioning and effectiveness of the acoustic reflex. As an example, one should simply consider that due to the latency the reflex is unable to perform its postulated protective role when elicited by a very brief stimulus, no matter how intense this might be. Obviously, if the stimulus is over before the muscles are even beginning to contract, the attenuation effect cannot influence the cochlear input.

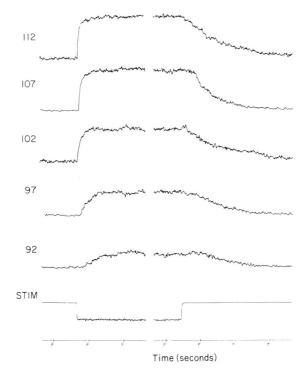

Time (seconds)

Fig. 7.12. Recordings of impedance changes for one subject. The top traces show the response to the onset and cessation of the stimulating noise burst; the bottom two traces give the duration of the stimulus and 1-second time marks, respectively. Parameter is the stimulus SPL. The scale factors are the same for the top three traces, and they are increased 1.2- and 1.5-fold in the fourth and fifth trace. (From Dallos, 1964b, p. 2179.)

After the initial dead time the middle ear muscles achieve their final state of contraction with a particular time course, which can be shown to depend on both the intensity and the frequency content of the stimulus. The peculiarities of this time course are reflected in the pattern of input impedance change, and most information pertaining to the quantitative features of reflex dynamics were gathered by recording the input impedance to the ear. Let us first focus our attention on the most conspicuous feature of the on and off responses: their asymmetry. In Fig. 7.12 a series of recordings of impedance changes is shown at a series of intensities of a wide-band noise burst stimulus. Both the onset and cessation responses are shown. It is apparent that at every stimulus level the on response is considerably faster than the corresponding off response. In physiological terms this observation implies that the contraction process is much more rapid than the relaxation process in the middle ear muscles, and it is in line with experimental results obtained with many other skeletal muscles. In terms of system description the asymmetry alerts us that the middle ear muscle reflex is a nonlinear system whose characteristics depend on the direction (that is, increase or decrease) of the input.

Beyond the basic asymmetry of the on and off responses, other interesting features can also be discerned. In order to make these more apparent, the on and off portions of the responses shown in Fig. 7.12 are replotted on an amplitude-normalized basis in Fig. 7.13. This is done by taking the steady-state response magnitude as 100% at each intensity and plotting the relative size of the responses at any given instant of time beyond the latent period. Remember that these are responses to wide-band random noise stimuli,

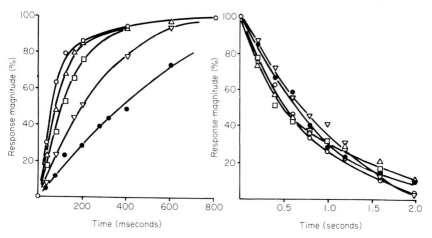

Fig. 7.13. Normalized on and off responses of one subject computed from the type of traces shown in Fig. 7.12. Parameter is stimulus SPL. Left panel: ○, 112; △, 107; □, 102; ▽, 97; ●, 92 dB. Right panel: ●, 112; ○, 107; △, 102; □, 97; ▽, 92 dB.

and thus whatever frequency dependence the acoustic reflex possesses is effectively eliminated by having all important frequencies represented in the acoustic input. The stimulus strength has a dramatic effect on the on response, while it apparently does not influence the normalized off response. In the normalized on responses an orderly progression of the curves is seen. The higher the stimulus intensity, the more rapid is the response. This phenomenon appears to be quite general from one subject to another. The fact that the response curves corresponding to various signal intensities do not overlap for the onset response, but do so for the cessation response, attests to the fact that the former process is itself nonlinear while the latter is linear. To explain these contentions consider once again that, in a linear system when step inputs of varying magnitude are applied, the responses differ by scale factors only. In other words, if the time course of the response can be expressed by the function $x = x(t)$, then the multiplication of the input signal by a factor k will produce a response $y(t)$, where $y(t) = kx(t)$. The implication of this simple mathematical statement is that, irrespective of the shape of the $x(t)$ function (i.e., the response), a change in input magnitude will result in a contraction or expansion of all ordinate values of the function by the same proportion. Thus, when the responses of a linear system to inputs of varying magnitudes are normalized (by, for example, equating the steady-state value, or the maximum of the response, to unity), these normalized responses will be indistinguishable from one another. This process of normalization was applied to typical step responses of the acoustic reflex mechanism, and as we have seen the cessation response met the test of linearity while the onset response did not.

Cursory observation of either the original response traces or the replotted normalized responses suggests that the change in response speed is accomplished without a change in the apparent damping of the system. Specifically, all responses, onset and cessation as well, appear to be overdamped. With noise stimulation, we have never observed overshoots or oscillation in the step response, even though these can occur for the same subject when the stimulus is an intense pure tone of appropriate frequency. In fact, the dependence of the dynamic properties of the response on the frequency content of the stimulus is another fascinating property of the acoustic reflex, equally as interesting as the intensity dependence that we have just discussed. The observation that the steady-state attenuating (regulating) effect of the acoustic reflex is strongly frequency dependent (see, for example, Fig. 7.8) immediately suggests the possibility that the transient properties are frequency dependent as well. To see this possibility, consider our discussion in the introduction to this chapter that pertained to the change of response speed in an open- versus closed-loop system. It is recalled that if the loop gain was high then in a closed-loop situation the system response was considerably faster than in the open-loop case. Since the effect of the acoustic reflex is most pronounced between 200 and 600 Hz, while it becomes very small above approximately 1500 Hz, one can say that the effective feedback gain changes with stimulus frequency, being large at low and small at high frequencies. The best approach to visualizing this is to assume that the gain factor k in the theoretical feedback system of Fig. 7.9 is actually frequency dependent. In the frequency region (high frequencies) where k is small the system response is relatively sluggish, but for frequencies where k is large (low frequencies) the system response is rapid. To see this, consult once again Eq. (7.12), where the effect of gain on the time constant of the system response in the case of a very simple feedback system is considered.

Our discussion clearly indicates that we can anticipate significant changes in the acoustic reflex time response at various stimulus frequencies. Møller (1962) and Hung (1972) studied these effects and noted that in the low-frequency region, where the feedback gain is the highest, the response is strongly oscillatory, while at high frequencies, where the feedback gain is low, the response is overdamped and monotonic. Figure 7.14 can demonstrate these ideas better than any description. Here impedance changes are shown in a human subject at four stimulus frequencies and at a variety of intensities above reflex threshold. At the highest frequency, 1150 Hz, the responses have essentially the same character at all intensities and they are quite like those that we have shown for wide-band noise stimulation (Fig. 7.12). All these responses are overdamped; there is no sign of significant overshoots or oscillations. At the three lower test frequencies the situation is radically different. At the lowest intensities the responses do not show much overshoot and they are not oscillatory. In contrast, at the high stimulus levels all responses possess significant overshoots and they are definitely underdamped, as demonstrated by the multiple oscillations. Note that the least damping (slowest decay of oscillation) is at 650 Hz and the greatest is at 300 Hz. Some of Hung's (1972) results indicate that at the lowest frequencies the response does become overdamped (nonoscillatory). We can summarize these results by noting that the response dynamics depends on both stimulus intensity and frequency. At any given frequency there is apparently a given feedback gain that determines the basic nature of the response. The frequency dependence of this gain factor can probably be likened to a band-pass filter; between 300 and 700 Hz the gain is highest, decreasing at both higher and lower frequencies. In the high-gain region the response tends to be oscillatory, while in the low-gain region it is overdamped. Aside from the frequency dependence, the character of the response is also determined by a magnitude-dependent nonlinearity that has the property of making the response faster as intensity increases. Thus in the high-gain region, as a consequence of the nonlinearity, the response becomes more and more oscillatory as intensity

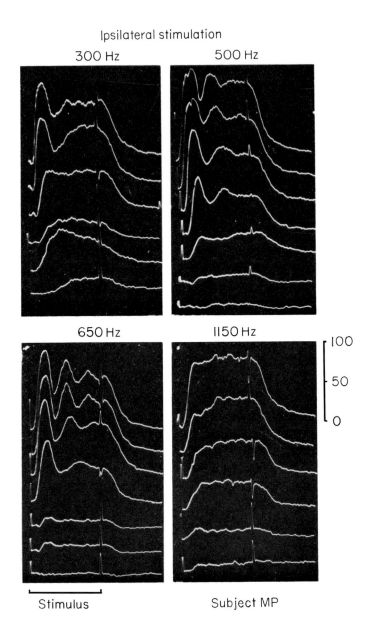

Fig. 7.14. Impedance change versus time for stimulation with sinusoids of four different frequencies. The scale to the right indicates the impedance change in percentage of maximum obtainable change. Stimulus duration was 500 mseconds. (From Møller, 1962, p. 1534.)

increases. In the low-gain region it simply has a decreasing rise time with increased intensity without ever becoming oscillatory. A wide-band noise stimulus behaves as a tonal stimulus in the low-gain region. The cessation response appears to have the same overdamped characteristics independent from the intensity or frequency content of the stimulus. This is then a very simple, apparently linear response whose properties are probably solely determined by the peculiarities of muscle relaxation processes.

3. Modeling of the Acoustic Reflex

Only a relatively moderate amount of effort has been expended on the development of quantitative models of acoustic reflex function. This can probably be attributed to the difficulties in devising appropriate models for such a decidedly nonlinear system as the middle ear muscle reflex. Some of the approaches that have been utilized are discussed in a rather cursory form in this section.

Møller (1962) has provided a number of graphs in which he showed the amplitude and phase characteristics of transfer functions that could be computed from human impedance data. Two of his plots are of particular interest because they point out the frequency-dependent characteristics of the reflex rather well. In Fig. 7.15 the amplitude and phase versus frequency functions are given as obtained from the data of one subject at two frequencies: 525 and 1450 Hz. These plots should be considered to depict the

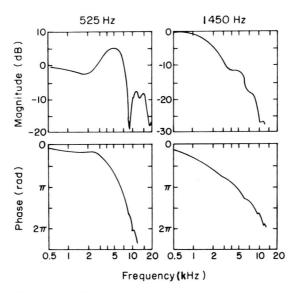

Fig. 7.15. Fourier transform of the muscle reflex response to sinusoidal stimulation at two different frequencies, 525 and 1450 Hz. (Adapted from Møller, 1962, p. 1531.)

frequency response of transfer functions that would provide the experimentally observed step responses at the two carrier frequencies. The differences between the two functions are evident. The transfer function that applies to the 525-Hz carrier has a large gain in the 5-Hz region; this implies that the step response is underdamped and oscillates with an approximate frequency of five per second. The frequency response function that is applicable to the 1450-Hz case does not show positive gain at any frequency, which indicates that its response is overdamped and nonoscillatory. Both of these conditions are borne out by the plots shown in Fig. 7.14. Lest it be misunderstood, the differentiation between carrier frequency and the frequency response of the system to transient disturbances should be emphasized. We have seen that the system itself is sensitive to the carrier frequency in that the feedback gain is dependent on this parameter. At any carrier frequency the system responds to changes in the amplitude of the carrier (i.e., to transient changes) with a certain dynamic characteristic. The latter property is depicted in the plots of Fig. 7.15. To interpret these plots we should note that the faster the carrier amplitude changes the more attenuated the response to this change becomes. For example, with a 1450-Hz carrier if an amplitude change occurs at a rate of 10/second then the response amplitude to this change is about 30 dB less than what it would be to the same size change that would occur at a rate of 0.5/second.

On the basis of on and off step responses to wide-band noise of 100 dB SPL, I have computed transfer functions that represent the impedance change due to the activation and deactivation of the acoustic reflex (Dallos, 1964a). These functions, $G_1(s)$ and $G_2(s)$, are given below.

$$G_1(s) = \frac{K_1 e^{-0.04s}}{s^2 + 43.2s + 324} \qquad G_2(s) = \frac{K_2 e^{-0.04s}}{s^2 + 14.4s + 36} \qquad (7.16)$$

In these expressions K_1 and K_2 are dc gain terms that are not defined by the procedure that yields the functions. The exp $(-0.04s)$ factor represents a dead-time transfer function that provides a phase shift of $2\pi fT$ radians, with $T = 40$ mseconds, which was the experimentally determined value. This same transfer function has unity magnitude, which is appropriate for a pure time delay term. We note that both the on and off transfer functions can be expressed in terms of second-order functions and it is very interesting that the damping factor is approximately the same for both, having a value of 1.2. In contrast with the constancy of the damping, the system's natural frequency changes; it is approximately 3 Hz for the on response and about 1 Hz for the off response. By definition both transfer functions, G_1 and G_2, are linear representations of the system. Combined together they form a so-called piecewise linear description of the acoustic reflex. It is clear on the basis of our previous discussions that such a representation is not generally adequate due to the nonlinear amplitude dependence of the response characteristics and the frequency-dependent feedback gain. A more complete treatment of a reflex model that takes the magnitude dependent effects into consideration is now briefly discussed.

The following set of assumptions enabled us to derive a usable model of the reflex. First, the system to be modeled was assumed to be in the configuration depicted in Fig. 7.16. Since the data on which modeling is based are in

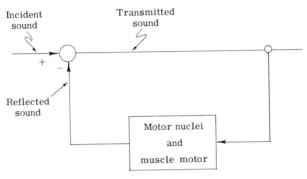

Fig. 7.16. Configuration of the acoustic reflex that is used to derive a mathematical model on the basis of input impedance data. Since the active reflex changes the middle ear transmission, it is assumed that the reflex, whose input is proportional to the transmitted sound, controls the "reflected" sound, that is, the sound energy that does not reach the cochlea on account of the attenuating properties of the active reflex.

the form of impedance changes, the arrangement shown in the figure would provide direct means of comparison. It is assumed that all elements that contribute to the determination of the dynamic response are concentrated in the muscle motors themselves and, further, that these elements can all be placed in the feedback path. These are reasonable assumptions, especially if one considers that the bandwidth of the reflex itself is certainly less than about 10 Hz [recall Fig. 7.15 or Eq. (7.16)] while the middle ear transmission is flat out to about 1000 Hz. Clearly the extremely wide-band middle ear would not influence the slow dynamic changes that are seen during reflex action. For simplicity our model configuration assumes that the signal that activates the acoustic reflex is proportional to the sound transmitted by the middle ear (input to the cochlea) while the effect of the reflex is to increase the sound reflected from the middle ear. To correspond to this configuration, it is assumed that the magnitude of the reflected sound is proportional to the deviation from the quiescent acoustic impedance, which in turn is taken to be proportional to muscle tension.

The final assumption concerns the actual model of the muscle motors. Here the arguments to be advanced closely follow those of Green (1964),

who derived a simple and effective model of skeletal muscle. The development
of the model is illustrated in Fig. 7.17. The two muscles, combined for
simplicity, are represented by a contractile element consisting of elasticity
and friction and a passive series elastic element. The effective mass of the
ossicular chain is represented by m, while additional tendon and ligament
elasticity is shown by the inclusion of the spring with stiffness k_3. In practice
the series muscle elasticity is rather small, and consequently further simplification can be afforded by neglecting it. If the unstretched lengths of the springs

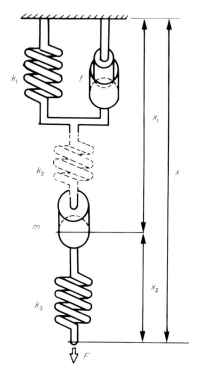

Fig. 7.17. Schematic representation of the middle ear muscle motor. The contractile
element of the muscle is represented by the spring k_1 and dashpot f. These two elements are
under control of innervation. The third muscle element is a passive series spring (k_2) which
is assumed to be very stiff. The equivalent mass of the moving middle ear structure is
modeled by m, while k_3 is the combined series elasticity of the various tendons and ligaments; F is force. The excitation of the muscle is assumed to have a time course $g(t)$, and
thus $k_1 = k_1[g(t)]$ and $f = f[g(t)]$.

are taken as x_1' and x_2', while respective lengths are x_1 and x_2, then the force
equations for this mechanical system can be written as

$$F = (x_2 - x_2')k_3$$
$$F = \ddot{x}_1 m + \dot{x}_1 f + (x_1 - x_1')k_1 \qquad (7.17)$$

One can denote $x = x_1 + x_2$ and $x' = x_1' + x_2'$. The variables x_1 and x_2 and the constants x_1' and x_2' can be eliminated with the resulting equation

$$F = \ddot{x}m - \ddot{F}(m/k_3) + \dot{x}f - \dot{F}(f/k_3) + k_1(x - x' - F/k_3) \qquad (7.18)$$

We mentioned in our early discussion that the middle ear muscles exert great tension without appreciable displacement. This implies that their contraction is semiisometric. Thus it is legitimate to assume for the sake of simplification that the contraction *is* isometric, $x = c$, where c is a constant. With this substitution we obtain

$$\ddot{F} + \dot{F}(f/m) + F(k_1 + k_3)/m - (k_1 k_3/m)(c - x') = 0 \qquad (7.19)$$

Here k_3 can be neglected in comparison with k_1 and if one now assumes that stimulation of this system is mediated by changes in the parameters of the contractile portion of the muscle, that is, in k_1 and f, then an appropriate final equation results in the form.

$$\ddot{F} + A[1 + ag(t)]\dot{F} + Bg(t)F - Cg(t) = 0 \qquad (7.20)$$

where A, B, C, and a are constants and $g(t)$ is the excitation time function. Equation (7.20) can be described as a linear second-order differential equation for the force that is excited in a parametric manner.

As a final step the model of this muscle motor [Eq. (7.20)] is now included in the appropriate feedback loop having the same configuration as was shown in Fig. 7.9. The following substitutions are made to adapt Fig. 7.9 to the present use. The input signal x_i is now $r(t)$, the output signal x_o is now $e(t)$, the feedback signal x_{fb} is now $F(t)$, while the element denoted by the constant k is now the function $F = F(g)$, where $g(t)$ is the input to this block. Here we assume that the reflected sound (the quantity fed back) is directly proportional to muscle tension (F) and for simplicity the proportionality factor is taken as unity. The incident sound is denoted by $r(t)$, where the time function denotes amplitude variations of the carrier. The transmitted sound is signified by $e(t)$, and again the time variation refers to the envelope. To simulate the experimentally observed reflex threshold, such an element is included in the feedback path with a threshold level of E. The operation of the system can be described in two zones with two differential equations. When the transmitted sound is below the reflex threshold, $e < E$, then $g(t) = 0$ and the force (reflected sound) obeys the differential equation

$$\ddot{F} + A\dot{F} = 0 \qquad (7.21)$$

Above the reflex threshold, matters are much more complex. Here $g(t) = r(t) - F(t) - E$ and this substitution yields

$$\ddot{F} + A[1 + a(r - E)]\dot{F} - AaF\dot{F}$$
$$+ [B(r - E) + C]F - BF^2 - C(r - E) = 0 \qquad (7.22)$$

If we denote the quantity $r - E = X$ as the sound pressure above reflex threshold, then we can write our final equation as

$$\ddot{F} + A[1 + aX]\dot{F} - AaF\dot{F} + [BX + C]F - BF^2 - CX = 0 \qquad (7.23)$$

Let us remember again that in Eqs. (7.21) and (7.23) A, B, C, and a are constants, $X = X(t)$ is the envelope of the stimulus sound above reflex threshold, and $F = F(t)$ is the resulting muscle tension that we have taken to be proportional to reflected sound. The simple expression of Eq. (7.21) provides the pattern of force change when the input dips below reflex threshold. The response of this second-order linear differential equation is always overdamped. The active phase of force change that corresponds to operation above threshold is represented by Eq. (7.23), which is a second-order nonlinear differential equation with parametric excitation. The responses generated by this latter equation are clearly complex and depend a great deal on the magnitudes of the excitation. Equation (7.23) was simulated on an analog computer and its step responses were computed. The results were in good agreement with experimentally observed plots. The responses showed overdamped character, decreasing rise time with increasing intensity, and also saturation at high input levels. Thus this model of the middle ear muscle reflex provides a fair representation of the onset step responses of the system, at least those that are elicited by wide-band noise. To simulate the system's response to bursts of tone in the range of 300–700 Hz, where the responses are oscillatory, one would have to increase the feedback gain of the system. It is to be emphasized that the fact that this representation is adequate to describe step responses is no assurance that it would also be appropriate in providing the proper simulation of different types of time-varying responses, such as those generated by amplitude-modulated tones. This of course is a basic property of nonlinear systems.

To demonstrate the power of even the extremely simple piecewise linear model shown in Eq. (7.16) the following experiment was performed (Dallos, 1964a). Briefly, arrangements were made for the introduction of external feedback around the entire reflex arc so that the resulting complex system would be oscillatory. With the knowledge of the external circuit and the piecewise linear reflex model, the characteristics of the ensuing oscillation were predicted and compared to the experimentally obtained behavior. To instrument this experiment the acoustic reflex was measured with the impedance method as a deviation from the static input impedance. The output of the acoustic bridge (which is proportional to the impedance change due to the reflex) was used to turn a wide-band noise stimulus on or off. When the reflex became active and the signal from the bridge exceeded a preset value, it was used to turn the sound stimulus *off*. When the bridge signal fell below another preset value, it turned the sound *on*. Consider what happens in this arrangement. Assume first that the acoustic bridge is balanced to match the input impedance of the ear. Noise is then applied to the contra-lateral ear and it elicits the reflex. The active reflex changes the input impe-dance of the measured ear, the bridge becomes imbalanced, and its output increases. This increased signal when it exceeds a trigger level turns off the stimulus, which results in the relaxation of the reflex. When this happens the bridge signal decreases and when it drops below another trigger level it turns the stimulus back on. This results in a renewed reflex contraction and so on. Clearly a cyclic operation results.

The bridge here serves as a detector of the error signal, which is considered to be the deviation from the static impedance. The controlling trigger and switching circuits can be represented as a relay with hysteresis. If the error signal is small then the "relay" is active, and its output is a large constant signal (stimulus noise). If the error is large than the "relay" is open and there is no signal passed by it to the ear. Hysteresis is included in this represen-tation simply because it was found that the circuitry turned the stimulus *on* if the decreasing error signal fell below 37.5 acoustic ohms, while it turned the signal *off* when the increasing error signal exceeded 87.5 acoustic ohms. The magnitude of the stimulus was so chosen that the applied step change of noise caused an impedance change of 125 dynes second/cm^5. This value was commensurate with the magnitude of the step response from which Eq. (7.16) was derived. Thus if the output of the relay (stimulus) is denoted by $E(t)$ and the error signal (change in impedance) by $c(t)$, and if the time delay $T = 0.04$, then the following set of equations represents the system:

$$\ddot{c} + 14.4\dot{c} + 36c = E(t - T) \qquad \dot{c}(t) < 0$$

$$\ddot{c} + 43.2\dot{c} + 324c = E(t - T) \qquad \dot{c}(t) > 0$$

$$E(t) = 125 \qquad \left| c(t) \right| < 37.5$$

$$E(t) = 0 \qquad \left| c(t) \right| > 87.5 \qquad (7.24)$$

The characteristics of this system were analyzed in the phase plane (Dallos, 1964a) and the analysis predicted an oscillatory response of a period of approximately 0.8 second and having a very asymmetrical waveform in which increasing rates of impedance change (corresponding to muscle contractions) are much higher than decreasing rates. The gratifying finding of the theoretical considerations was that the predicted oscillation matched the time pattern of the experimental oscillation extremely well. To demon-strate this, in Fig. 7.18 the theoretical phase portrait of the oscillation is compared with one derived from experimental observations. In other words, a graphical solution of the equation system, Eq. (7.24), yielded a closed trajectory in the phase plane. Such a trajectory describing the oscillatory

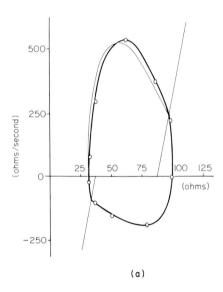

(a)

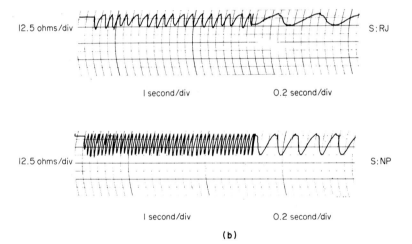

(b)

Fig. 7.18. (a) Comparison between the theoretical response characteristics of the self-oscillating reflex (thin line) and experimentally obtained pairs of impedance magnitude and rate of change of impedance values in one subject during reflex oscillation. The results are given in the form of a phase portrait in which a closed path indicates a self-sustaining oscillation. Such a path is called a limit cycle. (From Dallos, 1964a, p. 7.) (b) Time course of self-oscillations of the reflex in two subjects. The limit cycle shown in (a) can be constructed from this type of data.

behavior of a nonlinear system is called a limit cycle because no matter from what condition the system starts, its response eventually reaches the stabile oscillation that is represented by the limit cycle. The actual time response of the combined system was graphically differentiated and pairs of impedance and rate of change of impedance values were also graphed. The thin line in Fig. 7.18a is the theoretical limit cycle that is based on the solution of Eq. (7.24), while the data points connected by the heavy line are the actual values read off from graphical records of impedance change that were obtained during the experiment. Two examples of such a time record are included in Fig. 7.18b to demonstrate the appearance of the raw data. These oscillations are very interesting; they are of course completely involuntary, and their time characteristics are largely determined by the properties of the reflex mechanism. Of course if the magnitude of the stimulating signal or its frequency content is altered then the behavior (waveform and period) of the oscillation changes also. One can also alter the oscillation by modifying the external feedback circuit. Thus, for example, a change in gain or the elimination of the hysteresis or introduction of additional time delay can all affect the character of the resulting oscillation. This method of rendering the acoustic reflex oscillatory by positive feedback around it could become a powerful tool in investigating its dynamic properties.

III. The Efferent System

The classic anatomical experiments of Rasmussen that began in 1942 and the electrophysiological observations of Galambos (1956) initiated one of the busiest periods of auditory research. This era of investigation is still very much in progress, and the search for the definitive description of the function of the efferent auditory system is still on. The present treatment is very sketchy, and of course it is confined to the manifestations of the action of the efferent system on the inner ear. A very complete treatment of the subject has appeared (Rossi, 1967) and the reader is referred to it for details.

In Chapter 1 the basic anatomical facts were presented on the efferent system. A brief review of the salient facts should enable us to zero in on some of the key issues that will concern us in the present discussion. The final paths of the efferent innervation are comprised of three important branches. These are the crossed olivocochlear bundle (COCB) that leads from the contralateral superior olivary complex to the cochlea, the uncrossed olivocochlear bundle (OCB) that courses from the homolateral superior olive, and the reticulocochlear (RC) bundle that leads from the reticular formation to the cochlea. All three pathways come together to form Rasmussen's bundle (RB), which joins the 8th nerve to form the final neural pathway of the efferent system. There is some indication that the COCB innervates the outer hair cells exclusively and that the OCB supplies the inner hair cells primarily (Iurato, 1965). There is a very striking and significant difference in the mode of innervation by the efferent system of the two hair cell groups. The sketch of Fig. 7.19 should help to demonstrate these

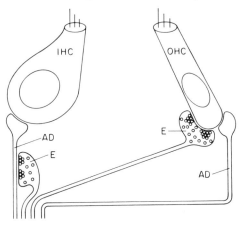

Fig. 7.19. Schematic representation of efferent synaptic connections in the organ of Corti of the cat. At the outer hair cells (OHC) synaptic contacts are almost exclusively with the sensory cell and at the inner hair cells (IHC) only with the afferent dendrites (AD); E, efferent ending. (Adapted from Spoendlin, 1970, p. 21.)

differences. Fibers running to the inner hair cells make contact only with the afferent dendrites from these cells, not with the cell bodies. These connections are thus classed as axodendritic, and the effect on the output of the hair cells by the efferents is thus postsynaptic. In contrast, the outer hair cells receive their primary (and possibly exclusive) innervation by nerve endings that act directly on the cell body. These are axosomatic contacts, and their effect on the hair cells is presynaptic as far as the hair cell–afferent synapse is concerned. About three-fourths of the fibers in the RB are COCB fibers. In addition the total number of efferent fibers is astonishingly small, only about 500, but these ramify very extensively, providing a truly impressive number of nerve endings (about 40,000). These endings are not only numerous but quite voluminous as well. The most extensive innervation of the outer hair cells takes place in the basal turn, and there is a gradual thinning out of these efferent nerve endings as the apex is approached. These bits and pieces of anatomical facts do have, as we shall see, a marked effect on the electrophysiological findings concerning the effect of the efferent system on the cochlea.

A very large segment of the pertinent electrophysiological literature is based on the study of the effect of efferent activity on single-unit discharges in the 8th nerve. This portion of the literature is certainly beyond the scope of the present work and thus it is not treated in any detail. It is also apparent that there is no direct effect on the cochlear output by the axodendritic connections of the OCB, since these connections do not influence the hair cells themselves. This being the case, we shall confine ourselves to the demonstration of these facts by describing the lack of influence of OCB action on cochlear potentials. The operation and effects of the reticulo-cochlear fibers are largely obscure and thus we will not dwell on these efferents. Clearly, most of our concern here is with the function and electro-physiological manifestations of COCB activity.

The most productive method of activating the COCB is to deliver trains of electrical shocks to the bundle at the point where it crosses the midline at the floor of the fourth ventricle. The most effective stimulus consists of shocks at a rate of about 400 per second. None of the various effects on the cochlear output that are brought about by the electrical stimulation of the COCB can be duplicated by contralateral sound stimulation. This is the more remarkable if one considers that single fibers in the COCB do respond to sound that is delivered to the animal's ear (Fex, 1962). Consequently, we cannot provide a description of COCB action on cochlear responses when this action is elicited by "natural" stimulation.

In 1956, Galambos first demonstrated that electric shocks applied to the COCB result in the decrease of the magnitude of the compound action potential in response to acoustic clicks that could be recorded from the contralateral round window. This depression in the N_1-N_2 complex could be counteracted by the administration of relatively small doses of strychnine or brucine (Desmedt and Monaco, 1960). These drugs counteract inhibitory effects in the central nervous system, and thus it can be said that the action of the COCB comprises a true inhibitory effect in which hyperpolarizing transmitter substances that inhibit afferent neural function are released. The series of photographs in Fig. 7.20 depicts the typical effect of COCB activity. The click-evoked N_1-N_2 complex is shown in the upper traces at five different intensities spaced 10 dB apart. The traces below are obtained when the COCB is stimulated by trains of electric shocks. It is notable that at the -60-dB intensity the COCB is capable of completely eliminating the AP. At -50 dB the AP is reduced to a size that is normally obtained by a -70-dB stimulus. In other words, the active COCB under the optimal condition represented here is capable of an inhibitory effect that is equivalent to a 20-dB reduction in the stimulus strength. The same magnitude of reduction is evident at the -30-dB stimulus level, where the inhibited response is about the same size as the uninfluenced -50-dB response. This titration method, as Desmedt denoted the equating of a COCB effect to the reduction

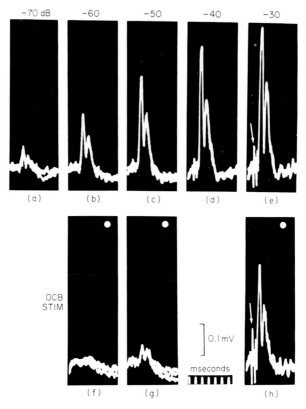

Fig. 7.20. Titration of COCB efferent effects on N_1 in terms of equivalent decibel change. (a)–(e) Responses from the round window evoked by clicks whose intensity is indicated in decibels below arbitrary reference level (same for all experiments). The arrow in (e) points to the cochlear microphonic potential appearing in the stronger clicks. (f)–(h) Responses of corresponding intensity, but preceded by COCB stimulation (40 shocks at 400/second, with train-click interval of 9 mseconds). The frames involving COCB stimulation are marked with a white dot in the upper right-hand corner. Three to four sweeps are superimposed in each frame to show consistency. (Cat, chloralose anesthesia, flaxedil, middle ear muscles cut.) (From Desmedt, 1962, p. 1483.)

in sound intensity, reveals that the maximal effect that one can expect from the COCB on the compound AP is about 25 dB. Sohmer (1965) compared the percent reduction in AP with the titrated equivalent SPL change and some of his results, along with those of Desmedt (1962), tend to show that the latter measure is more independent (even though by no means constant) from the absolute stimulus level than is the former. Thus in Sohmer's results the percent changes in AP magnitude ranged from about 63 % at low intensity to about 18 % at high SPL, while the equivalent sound pressure change ranged between 11 and 17 dB, in a seemingly unsystematic manner.

All indications point to the fact that the COCB is much more effective at low sound pressure levels. Just how much so can best be appreciated from some AP input–output functions obtained with and without COCB stimulation. In Fig. 7.21 some of the results of Konishi and Slepian (1971) are shown for COCB effects on various cochlear potentials. We shall refer to this figure in further discussions, but now let us concern ourselves with the AP results shown in panel (a). The curve composed of filled triangles depicts a now-familiar AP input–output function in which two segments can clearly be discriminated. It is remembered that we associated the low-intensity segment with outer hair cell function, while the high-intensity portion is commonly thought to reflect inner hair cell elicitation. Under electrical shocks to the COCB the low-intensity portion of the function is altered while the high-level segment is quite evidently unmodified. The change in the low-level response is roughly equivalent to a reduction in SPL by 20 dB. Note that approximately 25 dB above the crossover point between the two segments of the AP function (that is, at an estimated 100–110 dB SPL) the effect of the COCB disappears. These results go along with the anatomical evidence that the COCB primarily innervates the outer hair cells in an exemplary fashion. Since this innervation is the most prominent in the basal half of the cochlea, and since this very segment is responsible for the generation of the whole-nerve action potential, it is reasonable that COCB action should be optimally manifested in that portion of the AP that is mediated by the outer hair cells. It apparently is, as panel (a) of Fig. 7.21 testifies.

Aside from the inhibition of the AP, an apparent potentiation of the CM has also been shown to result from COCB activation (Fex, 1959). In contrast with the relatively sizable effect on the AP, this potentiation is quite small; it never amounts to more than about 3 dB equivalent change in SPL. There seems to be some discrepancy in the literature concerning the relative magnitude of CM augmentation as a function of stimulus strength. Sohmer (1965) found that the augmentation is slightly greater at low SPL's, while Konishi and Slepian (1971) assert that there is no augmentation in the linear portion of the CM input–output function. In the view of the latter authors the potentiation of the CM is observable only at levels where the function has already entered its saturation zone. Their plots for the CM that are included in Fig. 7.21 indicate this situation.

A great deal of effort has been expended by various students of the efferent system to reconcile what they considered a paradoxical increase of the CM in the face of the AP inhibition. It appeared difficult for some to accept that these two potentials (which they consider causally related) could be pushed in different directions by a physiological modification of the system. Among the various explanations of CM augmentation, I favor that proposed by Fex (1967a) and it is presented here in a somewhat expanded form. It is recalled that the nerve endings of the COCB fibers innervate the

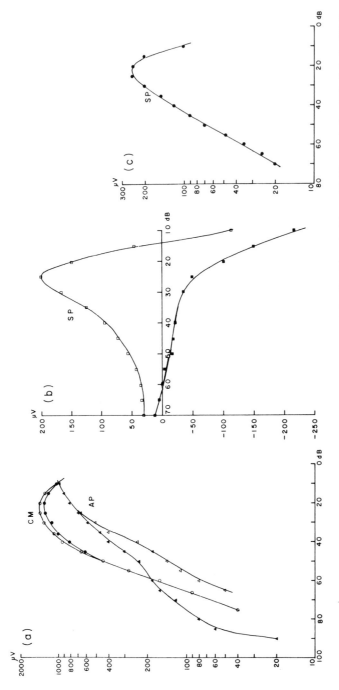

Fig. 7.21. One example of the input–output function of CM, AP (a), and SP (b) with and without COCB stimulation. Filled circles (CM), filled triangles (AP), and filled squares (SP) represent without, and open symbols represent with, COCB stimulation. The abscissa shows the readings of attenuator (100 dB corresponds to approximately 36 dB SPL). The ordinate indicates the magnitude of CM or AP in (a) and SP in (b). Acoustic stimuli, 6-kHz tone bursts. (c) Differences in magnitude of SP with COCB stimulation as a function of sound intensity. The ordinate indicates vertical deviation between control and COCB stimulation in (b). (From Konishi and Slepian, 1971, p. 484.)

outer hair cells directly; that is, the connection is axosomatic. It appears that the action of these nerve endings is a hyperpolarization of the post-synaptic membrane (hair cell membrane). This is in accord with Eccles' (1964) description of synaptic inhibition. The hyperpolarization of the outer hair cells results in an increased intracellular negativity, which of course raises the potential gradient across the reticular lamina. Since the most likely source of the CM is a modulation of the resting current that flows across the apical pole of the hair cells, and since the resting current is directly related to the potential gradient, it follows that a hyperpolarization of the cell membrane should result in an increased CM. Clearly the CM augmentation is not at all paradoxical but a direct consequence of the action of the COCB on the outer hair cells. The very same mechanism of hyperpolarization of the postsynaptic (from the viewpoint of the efferent flow) membrane of course results in the decreased ability of the presynaptic (from the viewpoint of the afferent flow) structures to release transmitter substances. Consequently the inhibition of afferent impulses and the augmentation of CM are both the consequence of the hyperpolarizing effect of COCB on the hair cell membrane.

There is a dearth of information on the effect of COCB activation on the summating potential. Fex (1967a) did not note any significant change of either the negative or the positive SP recorded from scala media of the first turn of the cat cochlea in response to high- or low-frequency, high-intensity stimuli. In contrast, Konishi and Slepian (1971) described significant changes in the SP. They recorded these potentials from the first turn of guinea pig cochleae with differential electrodes and noted a systematic alteration of the input–output function of SP that was obtained with 6000-Hz tone burst stimuli. Their results are included in panels (b) and (c) of Fig. 7.21. In panel (b) the closed squares depict the reference function. This has the expected intensity dependence; namely, it is positive at low levels and turns increasingly negative at higher SPL's. With activated COCB the function shifts quite radically toward the positive direction. The absolute change in voltage between the two functions is plotted in panel (c). There appears to be a contradiction between Fex's preliminary results and the findings of Konishi and Slepian. This might be simply due to the difference in stimulus frequency (above 8000 and below 2800 Hz in the former case and 6000 Hz in the latter case) since the DIF and SM components of the SP are in a transitional stage at the middle test frequency, while a relatively pure SP⁻ and SP⁺ can be studied at the flanking frequencies. Another possibility is that the data of Konishi and Slepian are somewhat confounded by transient effects since they used an ac-coupled system (6-msecond time constant) and measured their SP 2 mseconds after the CM onset. This procedure is not free from danger; it would be desirable to repeat these experiments utilizing a system with considerably longer coupling time constant, longer stimulus duration, and measurements of the SP in the quasi-steady-state, which means at least 20 msecond after the onset of the CM. Until such measurements are obtained we must consider the results on SP as provocative and must await their confirmation.

One of the most interesting aspects of COCB function is the presence of a slow potential, COCB potential or COCP, that can be recorded from within the cochlea during and immediately after electrical stimulation of the COCB. This COCP was described by Fex (·1967b). When recorded in scala tympani or from the organ of Corti this potential is positive with respect to the animal's body. In contrast the potential is negative within the scala media and about 4–10 times as large as it is outside the cochlear partition. The time course of the potential is the same no matter at which recording location it is obtained; there simply is a polarity reversal at the level of the reticular lamina. The potential rises to its maximum value relatively slowly after the initiation of a shock train to the COCB and it dissipates even slower after the discontinuation of the electrical stimulus. In fact the COCP can outlast the stimulation by about 200 mseconds. Between the onset of the stimulus and the COCP one can observe a significant latent period that might range between 12 and 40 mseconds. The magnitude of the potential can reach 3 mV in the scala media.

It is a reasonable assumption that the COCP is simply a manifestation of the changes in the operating properties of the outer hair cells during COCB activation. To explain, we again invoke the hypothesis (Fex, 1967a) that the COCB influences the outer hair cells by hyperpolarizing their cell membranes. We noted that such hyperpolarization should result in an increase of the dc potential gradient across the reticular lamina and consequently an increased current flow though the hair cell. This increased current flow is measured as a potential drop on any of the resistive elements of the cochlear network. In other words, the mechanism of COCP production is essentially the same as CM production in the sense that both of these potentials are the manifestations of *current changes* through the hair cells. While the latter is brought about by mechanical stimulation of the cell, the former is produced by synaptic hyperpolarization of the cell membrane. Just as the sound-evoked cochlear potentials (CM and DIF SP) the COCP is also seen in opposite polarity on two sides of the reticular lamina and is also larger (by about the same factor) in SM than in the perilymphatic space. The latter fact is most likely the simple consequence of the peculiarities of cochlear electroanatomy, namely, that the insulating properties of the SM are better than those of the outer scalae. It is probably prudent to carry our line of thought to its logical conclusion and to consider the COCP as a simple manifestation of the hyperpolarizing activity of the efferent system and *not* as the agent that would be responsible for the inhibitory (on AP) or potentiating (on CM) effect of the active COCB. To put this suggestion in different words, the generation of COCP, the inhibition of AP, and the potentiation of CM are all the consequence of the hyperpolarization of the outer hair cell membrane by inhibitory transmitters released from the nerve endings of the COCB. This is in contrast with the possibility that the direct effect of COCB action would be the generation of the COCP within the outer hair cell, and that this potential in turn would act as the mediating agent in the decrease of the AP and increase of the CM.

A discussion of the efferent system would not be complete without mentioning the known effects of the active uncrossed OCB. Electrical stimulation of the OCB (Desmedt and LaGrutta, 1963; Fex, 1967a) results in the inhibition of the AP as recorded from the round window. These effects are extremely similar to those obtained with COCB stimulation. One significant difference, not concerning the AP, is that no effect on the CM has ever been observed with OCB stimulation. Apparently, no "OCP" is generated either; in other words, the electrical stimulation of the OCB has no comparable cochlear potential associated with it as is present in the COCP during the activation of the COCB. These findings underscore the anatomical results that the dominant OCB innervation goes to the inner hair cells but that synaptic contact is not made with the cell bodies, only with the afferent dendrites. Clearly this anatomical arrangement is suitable for producing postsynaptic inhibition of the neural response, but in no way is it appropriate to modify the electrical conditions of the organ of Corti via the hair cells.

A very sizable literature has accumulated on the pharmacological mechanisms that operate during the activation of the efferent system. The specific question to which most investigators have addressed themselves concerns the identification of the chemical transmitter substance that is secreted in the large vesiculated endings of the efferent fibers. It is probably correct to say that this problem is not yet resolved with certainty, even though it appears that acetylcholine (ACh) is the most likely transmitter (Fex, 1968). The early experiments of Schuknecht *et al.* (1959), in which they investigate the presence of acetylcholinesterase (AChE) in the cochlea in normal situations and after the cutting of the olivocochlear bundle, indicated that when the COCB was intact there was a more marked AChE activity. Gisselson (1960b) noted an augmentation of the CM during the electrophoretic application of ACh to the organ of Corti, and he suggested that ACh is the transmitter for the COCB fibers. The findings of Desmedt and Monaco (1960) that strychnine blocks COCB inhibition mediated against the argument that ACh is the transmitter substance but did not rule it out as a possibility. Fex (1967b) applied *d*-tubocurarine to the perilymph and noted a decrease in the COCP. On this basis he made a strong argument in favor of ACh as the transmitter substance (Fex, 1968). Others, notably B. Johnstone [see discussion in Fex's paper (Fex, 1968)], feel that the blocking of inhibitory effects by strychnine and brucine but not by picrotoxin is very strong evidence against the possibility of cholinergic synaptic mechanisms. Clearly the issue is not yet resolved.

Just as the biochemistry of the efferent system, the function of this mechanism is also intensely debated and unresolved. The only clearly demonstrated physiological effect is a moderate inhibition, but it does not appear likely that such a well-developed and complex system as the efferent innervation of the cochlea would have only a marginal inhibitory function. This is especially unlikely when one considers that fibers in the RB exhibit tonotopic relationships just as afferent fibers of the 8th nerve do. In fact, Fex (1962) demonstrated that both OCB and COCB fibers possess well-defined excitatory and inhibitory areas (certain frequencies increase, others inhibit, the resting discharge in these fibers). Aside from the frequency discrimination ability, the very large number of efferent endings in the cochlea is also impressive, and this suggests a relatively significant function as well. On the credit side of the ledger is the very small number of efferent fibers (some 500) which makes it unlikely that very precise control could be exerted on the cochlea by the efferent system. It is also disturbing that thus far no electrophysiological effect has been demonstrated with a *sound*-activated efferent mechanism. There is a plethora of suggestions concerning possible functions of the system, but we do not see the solution as yet. (For an interesting discussion of some of these possibilities see de Reuck and Knight, 1968.)

CHAPTER 8

Summary

A vast amount of material was heaped upon the reader in the previous seven chapters. It is probably difficult to ferret out the truly significant features of the operation of the peripheral auditory system from the necessary, but often confusing, tangle of detail. In order to put matters into better focus, this brief chapter attempts to highlight only the essential contributions of the auditory periphery to the hearing process. In other words, on the basis of our previously developed understanding of the various subsystems of the auditory periphery, let us now integrate the available information and construct a unified description of the auditory periphery and its influence on hearing.

It is apparent that the truly astounding abilities of the hearing organ are largely determined by the capabilities of its peripheral apparatus. Thus all auditory information that the central nervous system can utilize must be transmitted and transduced by the sense organ, and the limits of performance of the overall system are certainly set by the latter. This of course implies that it is the end organ that must be capable of resolving threshold energies in the neighborhood of 10^{-16} W/cm^2, it is the end organ that must function over a frequency range of about 3 decades, and it is the end organ that must preserve timing information to the extent that the central nervous system should be capable of resolving timing irregularities of the order of 1 μsecond (Pollack, 1970). The peripheral auditory system performs these feats by a combination of exquisitely matched mechanical, hydraulic, electrical, and biochemical processes. It is the most complex sense organ in that it has to integrate such a variety of physical processes in order to perform its transducer function.

The middle ear, as we have seen, is essentially a pressure amplifier that is capable of achieving a relatively close match between the acoustic impedance properties of air and the cochlea over a limited frequency range. This frequency band in which the match is good, probably corresponds to the region of frequencies that is the most crucial for the organism to receive with the least attenuation. The amplification is achieved by the mechanical lever action of the ossicular chain and the pressure boost that results from the unequal areas of the eardrum and the stapes footplate. Since the middle ear is a complex mechanoacoustic system, its transmission properties are inherently frequency dependent. The overall effect of the various components —compliance of cavities, ligaments, and drum membrane; the mass of the ossicles; the frictional effect of joints; and the loading of the cochlea—is manifested in the characteristic band-pass filter property of the middle ear. The actual energy transmission into the cochlea is determined by the combined transmission properties of the middle ear and the input impedance of the cochlea. The former can be characterized by a transfer function between sound at the eardrum and stapes velocity. We recall that this function rises at low frequencies at a rate of 6 dB/octave, reaches its peak around 1000 Hz, and then decreases at an approximate rate of 12 dB/octave. The pressure generated by the stapes footplate at the oval window is simply the product of the stapes volume velocity (v_s) and the cochlear input impedance. Thus if the middle ear transfer function is expressed as $H_2(s) = v_s/p_d$ and the cochlear input impedance is $Z_c(s)$, then the pressure at the oval window (p_c) is $p_c = p_d H_2(s) Z_c(s)$. Except at the lowest frequencies, the input impedance of the cochlea is approximately constant and resistive. Thus, since $H_2(s)$ rises at 6 dB/octave below its maximum, the pressure at the oval window, at least as a first approximation, can be considered to replicate the derivative of the pressure at the eardrum. This is an important consideration since the derivative relationship largely determines the temporal properties of the cochlear input for the all-important low-frequency transient signals.

There is considerable evidence that the filter characteristic of the middle ear is the prime determinant of the shape of the behavioral sensitivity contour for a given auditory system. All organisms hear certain frequencies at a least intensity, and the intensity requirements for the elicitation of hearing sensation increase at both lesser and greater frequencies. This band-pass nature of hearing ability is very closely paralleled by the band-pass characteristic of the middle ear transfer function.

The pressure generated at the oval window by the movement of the stapes creates a disequilibrium in pressure on the two sides of the cochlear partition, and it also initiates a pressure wave that propagates away from the stapes in the perilymph of the scala vestibuli. The pressure imbalance equilibrates through the displacement of the cochlear partition. As the result of the movement of the partition there is a consequent increase or decrease (depending on the direction of partition displacement) in pressure on its scala tympani side. The pressure alteration in the scala tympani is made possible by the presence of a flexible pressure release mechanism: the round window. The window communicates with the middle ear cavity; in other words, its outside face is at a zero pressure level. The round-window membrane can move in or out to allow under- or overpressure to develop in the scala tympani. Without this pressure release, the incompressible cochlear fluids trapped in a rigid bony cavity would prevent the movement of the stapes.

The initial displacement of the cochlear partition, and the energy exchange between it and the surrounding fluid, originate a wavelike displacement pattern of the partition which spreads from the basal end toward the apex. The eventual history of this wave depends a great deal on the motion pattern of the driving stapes. If the stapes movement is sinusoidal, the periodic over- and underpressure at the oval window generates a periodic pressure differential across the partition, which results in the periodic displacement of the basal end of the partition. The frequency of all these periodic events is of course the same and is determined by the stimulus alone. At the very basal end of the cochlea, the pressure changes at the oval window; the pressure differential across the partition and the movement of the partition itself are in phase with one another. The driving harmonic pressure change at the oval window initiates a harmonic pressure wave that travels in the perilymph of the scala vestibuli. The amplitude of this wave decreases as it propagates away from the source (the stapes) as a result of the energy exchange between the fluid in the scala vestibuli and the cochlear partition. As the wave travels in the perilymph it creates periodic pressure changes, both in time and space, across the cochlear partition. The partition reacts to these changes by responding with a harmonic motion, by the consumption of energy due to its internal damping, and by transmitting energy to the perilymph in the scala tympani. Periodic pressure changes are thus established in scala tympani also, and of course these set the round-window membrane in periodic vibration. The periodic motion of the cochlear partition takes the form of a traveling wave of displacement. There is a gradually accumulating phase shift from base toward the more apical regions and thus the periodic up and down motion of successive points along the partition form a space–time sequence that can be visualized as a wave that appears to move away from the stapes.

This harmonic traveling wave possesses some extremely characteristic features, all of which are determined by the physical characteristics of the partition itself and by its interaction with the surrounding fluid. The most important property of this traveling wave is the spatial change of its amplitude. For all except the lowest driving frequencies the amplitude of partition displacement gradually increases toward a maximum as the wave travels away from the stapes. Beyond the maximum the amplitude rapidly diminishes, and at a certain distance from the stapes the wave becomes extinguished. Over the same spatial extent that is described by the existence of the partition wave, the pressure waves in the perilymphatic scalae monotonically decrease in amplitude. These waves also tend to zero where the partition wave dies out. This is of course the natural consequence of the fact that the partition and the surrounding fluid form an interrelated system and that the various waves represent an energy exchange between the fluid and partition. The partition wave undergoes a radical change in its wavelength and velocity as it moves away from the basal end of the partition. Both wavelength and velocity decrease with distance and they become infinitesimally small at the point where the amplitude diminishes. Beyond the amplitude maximum the rate of decrease in all three quantities, amplitude, velocity, and wavelength, is very rapid. On the basis of von Békésy's experimental observations of traveling waves in several species, Greenwood (1962) concluded that the distance over which the traveling wave damps out from its maximum to zero amplitude is approximately 12% of the length of the cochlea.

The most impressive property of the traveling wave is the dependence of its spatial properties on the driving frequency. The point of maximum amplitude and the overall extent of the wave are uniquely determined by the frequency of the stimulus. The higher the stimulus the closer the maximum to the base and the more constricted the entire wave pattern. At lower and lower frequencies an increasing segment of the partition is involved in the wave motion, and at the lowest frequencies the wave extends over the entire length of the cochlea. At these extremely low frequencies virtually the entire partition vibrates in phase and there is no clear-cut amplitude maximum. Above approximately 200 Hz the distinct maximum develops at the apex and at higher frequencies the maximum moves toward the base. Clearly, the cochlea performs a mechanical frequency analysis in that a specific location along the cochlear partition is associated with each frequency at which the amplitude of vibration is maximal. At the lowest input frequencies, where the vibration pattern extends over the entire length of the partition, there is actual periodic fluid flow through the helicotrema. This fluid motion constitutes an acoustic shunt to the energy exchange through the cochlear partition, and thus at these lowest frequencies the helicotrema serves as a high-pass filter in reducing the effectiveness of stimuli of extremely low frequency. The main function of the helicotrema is thus to eliminate the effectiveness of infrasonic frequencies as inputs to the auditory system. The size of the helicotrema influences its filtering properties, and depending on the species this high-pass filtering effect can be observed (by a steepening of the low-frequency slope of the sensitivity function) up to a few hundred hertz.

When the vibratory amplitude is observed at a given location while the stimulus frequency is varied, a measure of the frequency selectivity of this vibratory system can be secured. The tuning curves that can be obtained from such observations have characteristic shapes with a relatively shallow (6–24 dB/octave) low-frequency rise and a very steep (~ 100 dB/octave) high-frequency fall. The bandwidth of these curves is probably not constant along the partition, but the tuning might be sharper toward the base and shallower toward the apex. The physical basis of this might follow from the fact that the total volume displacement of the cochlear partition and the volume displacement of the stapes must be equal at any frequency. Consequently, if the stapes volume displacement is kept constant then, since the spatial extent of a traveling wave at high frequencies is smaller than at low frequencies, the amplitudes are constrained to be higher in the former case (Eldredge and Miller, 1971).

The traveling wave obtains its characteristic properties from the physical dimensions and parameters of the cochlear partition. The most crucial property of the partition is its graded stiffness. Because of its wedge shape and because of the change in the dimensions of the supporting cell structure of the organ of Corti that is attached to it, the stiffness of the cochlear partition decreases over a hundredfold from base to apex. This stiffness gradient, plus the facts that the basilar membrane is not under tension in its resting state and that its structure is such that its bending rigidity is greater in the radial than in the longitudinal direction, determine the peculiar spatial characteristics (amplitude and phase pattern) of the traveling wave. The amplitude maximum at a given frequency for a particular location would ordinarily be considered as a resonance phenomenon in which energy is cyclically exchanged between mass and stiffness reactance in the membrane. It is almost certain that the pronounced peaking of the traveling wave is not due to simple resonance of the membrane, but to energy exchange between membrane and fluid. As Zwislocki (1948) has shown, a mathematical model of the cochlea in which the mass component of the membrane impedance is completely neglected can still produce the appropriate description of the traveling wave. It is certain that resonance is not the primary determinant of cochlear phenomena. However, it is conceivable that a resonant component is responsible for the steepening of the basilar membrane tuning curve just below its best frequency, which was found by the Mössbauer measurements and which is not readily predicted by the "nonresonant" cochlear models, such as Zwislocki's.

If one extrapolates from the vibrational amplitudes of the basilar membrane that one can measure at high sound levels down to threshold levels, and if the extrapolation is linear, then the resulting amplitudes are extraordinarily small, about 10^{-3}Å. This extrapolation has been a bone of contention for many years, and a number of authorities profess a disbelief that amplitudes this small could possibly be utilized. Until recently, all experimental evidence indicated, however, that the linear approximation is legitimate, inasmuch as basilar membrane motion appeared to be proportional to the driving sound pressure level. The results of Rhode (1971) are different. He has shown that, in a very narrow frequency range around the best frequency of a given cochlear location, the displacement of the membrane is markedly nonlinear. If confirmed, this important observation could alter the method of extrapolation down to threshold levels with a concomitant increase in the estimate of threshold displacements that could result in a thousandfold increase in the estimated value. Of course, if at the threshold of hearing the basilar membrane moves with an amplitude of 1 Å instead of 0.001 Å, then it is much easier to conceive how this movement is translated into a deformation of the hair cells.

While the overwhelming bulk of the productive experiments on which our knowledge of cochlear functioning is based is comprised of steady-state, harmonic excitation experiments, the sinusoidal test function is an abstraction to which the ear is virtually never subjected in nature. Most natural sounds are transients, and it is these sounds that the cochlea must be capable of efficiently transducing. The stimulus continuum has two extremes. One is a single sinusoid, an event that goes on forever in time, but which has an infinitesimally narrow extent along the frequency scale. The other extreme is an impulse, an infinitesimally short event, but one that encompasses all frequencies.* Frequency and time are thus complementary. When the former is exactly determined the latter is completely indeterminant (as in a sine wave), and conversely when the time is obtained with precision (as in an impulse) the frequency content is smeared out. On the basis of the uncertainty principle of physics, Gabor (1946) formulated a time–frequency uncertainty which simply implies that in any signal the product of effective duration and frequency is greater than a small number, signifying the fact that the precise determination of one precludes the exact knowledge of the other. All signals in nature are somewhere within the continuum between single frequency–– infinite time and extremely brief time—infinite frequency band limits. Thus a

* The Fourier transform of a so-called unit impulse, an infinitely strong and infinitesimally short event, is a continuous spectrum. This is a frequency function in which all frequencies are represented with equal strength.

signal analyzer, such as the cochlea, must by necessity perform a time-frequency analysis. Tonndorf (1962) has emphasized this mode of functioning of the inner ear. He noted that the finite and considerable width of the traveling wave envelope (frequency analysis) is coupled with a finite and considerable decay time (time analysis) of the cochlear partition. It is a realistic assumption that under most conditions the cochlear transducer supplies both frequency (spatial distribution) and timing information to the higher auditory analyzer.

Let us now briefly review the time-analyzing properties of the basilar membrane. The experimental evidence on this subject is largely indirect and is based on the discharge characteristics of single units in the auditory nerve in response to impulsive stimuli (Kiang, 1965; Møller, 1970a). It is now quite evident that, when the stapes is subjected to a rapid transient, an impulse, a large momentary pressure differential is generated across the cochlear partition in the window region of the cochlea. The pressure differential is equilibrated by the motion of the partition. In this sense the partition motion is an after effect; the stimulus has long elapsed when the major motion pattern of the partition is actually in progress. With the impulsive stimulus *all* portions of the basilar membrane are set in vibration, and the vibratory pattern is again in the form of a traveling wave. The mechanism should be considered as follows. At any point along the membrane the vibration is in the form of a decaying oscillation. The frequency of this oscillation is precisely the same as the best frequency (as far as maximum amplitude with sinusoidal stimulation is concerned) of the given site. There are several (5–10) cycles of this oscillation, and thus any point along the partition is in actual vibration for a length of time that is determined by its characteristic frequency. Basal points vibrate for brief durations; apical points vibrate longer. For example, if 10 decaying cycles are assumed to take place at any location, then the basilar membrane point whose traveling wave maximum occurs at 10 kHz would vibrate for 1 msecond, while the point whose best frequency is 100 Hz would vibrate for 0.1 second. It is important to consider that, because of the finite time required for an event to propagate along the basilar membrane, the more apical points commence their decaying oscillation after certain time has elapsed. Thus in the above example the 10-kHz point completely ceases to vibrate before the 100-Hz point even begins to do so, since the travel time between these locations is about 5 mseconds. These time-staggered decaying oscillations form the traveling wave pattern that is generated in response to impulsive stimuli.

When the input signal is relatively simple, for example a harmonic complex consisting of only a few harmonics, such an input is analyzed in the cochlea as if the system were performing a Fourier analysis process. To explain, in such a case the traveling wave pattern is multimodal and the peaks correspond to the appropriate locations of the harmonic input components. In such a simple case Ohm's acoustic law is thus applicable. If two pure tone input signals are brought together in frequency, then below a particular separation a unimodal traveling wave envelope is obtained. The maximum of this envelope corresponds to the average frequency of the two input signals, and the amplitude of the wave waxes and wanes at the rate of the beat between the input frequencies (Tonndorf, 1959). In this situation the cochlea clearly does not perform a Fourier analysis. When the input signals are transients having different time courses, the resulting traveling waves show clear maxima. The location of the maxima can be correlated with the timing characteristics of the input transients. Tonndorf (1962) has shown in cochlear scale models that the locations of the maxima are directly related to the effective duration of these transients.

An interesting situation arises in the analysis of a periodic pulse train input. Those regions of the cochlea whose response period is longer than the repetition period of the input train respond with a sinusoidal motion at the repetition frequency (f_0). The regions whose best frequencies correspond to low-order harmonics of the repetition frequency respond with sinusoidal vibrations at their respective frequencies. This is because the point whose best frequency is, say, three times the repetition frequency ($3f_0$) is excited to perform decaying vibrations with a frequency $3f_0$. Since these vibrations do not decay to zero before the next pulse arrives, the responses from consecutive inputs sum and produce a relatively smooth sinusoidal vibration of frequency $3f_0$. Clearly for those regions of the cochlea whose decaying impulse response is shorter than the pulse train period ($1/f_0$) the essential mode of response is as it would be for individual pulses. In other words, these regions preserve the repetition period. These considerations indicate that a pulse train is analyzed in the cochlea in more than one manner. A partial Fourier analysis is performed by the low-frequency regions of the cochlea that are excited as if the fundamental (f_0) and the lower harmonic frequencies of the pulse train were actually present. A time analysis is also performed, but by the high-frequency region of the cochlea, where the essential timing properties of the pulse train are preserved.

It is apparent from the above examples that under most stimulus conditions the cochlea performs a combined time–frequency analysis, and thus it makes available to the nervous system information that is most suited to a given stimulus pattern.

The movements of the basilar membrane are transmitted to the transducer elements of the cochlea, the hair cells, via the supporting cell structure of the organ of Corti and the tectorial membrane. The cells are supported in a relatively rigid framework consisting of the reticular lamina, the pillar cells, and Deiters' cells. It is quite possible that this framework largely follows the motion of the basilar membrane, on which it rests, at least in the region where the wavelength of the traveling wave is much larger than the height of the organ of Corti. The tectorial membrane sustains the same wave motion as the basilar membrane since it is within the cochlear partition and is surrounded by endolymph. Up to moderately high frequencies the entire partition vibrates in phase. Even though the basilar and tectorial membranes carry the same wave pattern, there is a relative motion between the two resulting from the different points of attachment of these two structures at the osseous spiral lamina and the spiral limbus. The most widely accepted concept in cochlear biophysics is that the relative motion between tectorial membrane and reticular lamina acts as the direct precursor of the stimulation of the transducer cells. This relative motion can take many forms in such a complex three-dimensional vibrating structure as the organ of Corti, and there is no clear-cut agreement on exactly which of the possible modes of relative vibration might be the dominant one.

Parallel movements of the bottom surface of the tectorial membrane and the upper surface of the reticular lamina are considered shearing motions. These movements are probably the most effective in producing stimulation. Because of the interaction between the dimensions of the traveling wave and those of the basilar membrane, the dominant curvature of the membrane, and consequently the primary direction of shear, is radial between the stapes and the peak of the traveling wave envelope, and it is longitudinal on the falling slope of the envelope. The longitudinal shear wave is spatially much more constricted than the traveling wave itself and it is quite possible that this wave is of crucial importance in the initiation of transducer action. If this is indeed the case then the discrepancy between the low-frequency steepness of the mechanical tuning curve of the basilar membrane (which reflects the frequency selectivity of the traveling wave) and that of single-unit tuning curves (which then could reflect the frequency selectivity of the shear wave) can be easily reconciled without any need for formulating complex neural sharpening processes. The problem with assigning a primary role to the longitudinal shear is that the transducer hair cells are morphologically polarized in a *radial* direction. This polarization is dictated by the essentially radial organization of the sterocilia, which is very pronounced on the outer hair cells and less so on the inner hair cells. It then appears that the hair cells (certainly the outer hair cells) are constructed to be primarily receptive to radial shear. We are clearly confronted with a contradiction that is not now resolvable.

One can speculate some on the relative roles of the two hair cell groups— such mental exercises do provide some provocative concepts if not the solutions. One must consider first that, whatever the effective motion differential between reticular and tectorial membranes might be, the resulting stimulation is transmitted to the hair cells via their hairs. The outermost row of stereocilia of the outer hair cells makes contact with the bottom surface of the tectorial membrane, while the other rows of hairs on the outer hair cells, and any hairs of the inner hair cells, make no such contact. It is then apparent that any relative motion between the two parallel membrane surfaces is directly transmitted to, and only to, the outermost row of cilia of the outer hair cells. The inner hair cells do not receive such direct stimulation. The free-standing cilia of both hair cell groups receive their primary stimulation from the streaming of endolymph about them. Because of viscous drag, the streaming fluid exerts a bending force on these cilia. While the bending force that acts on the attached (tallest) cilia is proportional to the relative displacement between the two membrane surfaces and thus eventually to the displacement of the basilar membrane, the viscous force that acts on the free cilia is proportional to the velocity of the basilar membrane. The mode of stimulation of the two groups of hair cells is thus fundamentally different, suggesting the possibility of distinct functional roles. Because of the direct contact of the attached cilia, the outer hair cells can be effectively stimulated at lesser displacements of the basilar membrane than can the inner hair cells. In other words, there is a sensitivity difference between the two groups, as well as a difference in stimulation pattern.

The displacement of the cilia, whether due to direct or viscous force, can transmit a deformation to the apical pole of the hair cells. The actual mode of deformation is unknown; there are at least four possibilities. First, the bending cilia might transmit a force to the cuticular plate and alter the size of the cuticle-free region. Second, the bending force may simply "rock" the cuticular plate in the opening of the reticular lamina. Third, it may be the motion of the cuticular plate, but a transmitted deformation or stress of the long cylindrical boundary of the hair cells, that is the important event. And, fourth, the deformation of any portion of the cell body might not be of importance, but the bending of the cilia themselves could constitute the necessary and sufficient precursor to transducer action.

While there are apparent uncertainties about what the effective deformation of the hair cell (or hair) might be, there are just as many unresolved issues concerning the actual transducer process that commences with the deformation. Of the two most likely possibilities, active membrane permeability change or passive resistance change, the latter has gained the widest acceptance. In this scheme, the effective deformation causes a change in electrical resistance. Depending on which of the four possibilities enumerated above is accepted as the dominant mode of deformation, a different portion of the hair cell is assigned the role of the variable resistance. Thus if the important result of basilar membrane movement is a change in the size of the cuticle-free pore, then it is presumed that the size change is accompanied by a resistance change. Conversely, if only the bending of the hairs is significant, it is the resistance of the cilia themselves that is assumed to change.

No matter what the actual mechanism might be, the resistance change results in an altered current flow through the hair cell, and this so-called receptor current is the first electrical event in the transduction chain. The current itself is maintained by two available voltage sources or biological batteries. The first, and probably more important, of these is the actual intracellular negativity of the hair cells. The second source is the positive polarization of the endolymphatic space, which is maintained by the stria vascularis. These two voltage sources combine in an effective series arrangement to create a potential difference amounting to some 160–180 mV across the cuticular surface of the hair cell. Since the ionic contents of the endolymph and the interior of the hair cell are quite similar, there is no concentration gradient across the reticular lamina for any of the constituent ion species. The existing potential gradient, however, is capable of maintaining a steady current flow from scala media to the inside of the hair cells. This current is most likely to be carried by K^+ ions that are originally secreted by the stria vascularis. These ions are concentrated in the endolymph, they move inside the hair cell along the electrical potential gradient, and they are removed from the hair cell into its surrounding fluid space along the concentration gradient existing there. When the hair cell resistance changes, so does the ionic current through the cell, and this change in current is presumed to be the crucial receptor current that initiates the electrochemical transducer process within the cell.

The cochlear hair cells constitute the sensory receptor cells in the second-order sensory receptor system of the organ of Corti. In such a system the receptor cell is a specialized neuron that has lost its transmission apparatus. It has a receptor pole and a distribution pole. At the receptor pole the cell interacts with its environment via the accessory structure of the sense organ, while at the distribution pole it secretes chemical transmitter agents that activate the following first-order neuron. In the organ of Corti the receptor cells are the hair cells, the first-order neurons are those constituting the afferent portion of the 8th nerve, and the accessory structure is the organ of Corti–basilar membrane complex itself.

In the general scheme of operation of such a complex sensory receptor system, the first electrical event that arises in the sense cell is known as the receptor current (or receptor potential). This electrical signal arises in the cell as a direct response to the absorption of the adequate stimulus that is transmitted to the cell by the accessory structure. This potential (or current) is thought to be responsible for the release of the chemical transmitters at the distribution apparatus of the cell. Between the sense cell and the first-order neuron there generally appears a chemically functioning synapse. The transmitters that are released from the sense cell diffuse through the synapse and initiate a local permeability change in the postsynaptic membrane (receptor pole or dendritic region) of the following neuron. This results in the establishment of a current flow through the dendritic membrane. The current creates a local depolarization, commonly called the generator potential, which is conducted in the dendritic segment by electrotonus to the region of the neuron that is electrically excitable. At this point (initial segment) the generator potential initiates all-or-none discharges that propagate along the transmission apparatus (axon) of the neuron.

The general scheme is quite likely to be an adequate description of the series of events that takes place in the hair cell–synapse–first-order neuron sequence. We do consider the electrical potentials that arise in the hair cells to be receptor potentials; by definition these potentials do *not* initiate neural firing. The junction between the hair cells and dendrites of the auditory nerve bears all morphological signs of a chemically mediated synapse. These signs include the well-defined synaptic cleft and a variety of presynaptic structures, such as synaptic bars and accumulation of vesicles. The afferent transmitter substance is not identified with certainty in the auditory apparatus, and neither has the generator potential been measured directly. As a matter of fact, we do not have a great deal of *direct* information on the receptor potentials either. It is widely conceded that the receptor potential is the cochlear microphonic, and some include the summating potential in this category as well. Of course, we have a completely unmanageable volume of literature on the CM and on the SP, and thus it appears to be a contradiction to say that direct information on the receptor potentials is lacking. Actually, this is not so. The receptor potential is a local potential change of the hair cell membrane. Its true character, time course, and magnitude can be obtained only on the basis of intracellular recordings from the source itself. Such recordings from mammalian cochleae are conspicuously lacking. What we commonly refer to as receptor potentials, CM and SP, are at best a gross extracellular manifestation of the critical intracellular events. As we have seen, the real difficulty in relating the gross CM and SP to the output of an individual generator lies in the complexity of the potential–producing system. In other words, the gross potentials result from the vectorial (for CM) and arithmetic (for SP) summation of the outputs of thousands of generators, each of which is excited with different amplitude and phase, and each of which is seen by the recording electrode through the maze of the electrical network that the three-dimensional cochlea constitutes. Thus only under carefully selected conditions can one assume or hope that the conceptual transition from gross potentials to individual hair cell potentials will yield quantitative information.

The question is often asked, and is receiving renewed attention now, as to whether the CM (and/or SP) is an essential intermediate step in the information transfer at the auditory periphery. We can probably say that the gross CM and SP as we know them are probably not directly involved in the chain of events that lead from the deformation of the hair cell to the initiation of the neural spike. We can also say that chances are extremely good that the "unit CM" (and/or "unit SP"), the receptor potential within the individual cell, is a necessary and significant intermediate step, one that is directly responsible for the liberation of the chemical transmitter. The main purpose of research on the gross potentials is to delimit the conditions under which these can be considered reasonable replicas of the "unit responses." It should also be considered that there is some difficulty in visualizing a role of even the "unit CM" at very high frequencies in mediating transmitter release. These high-frequency ac potentials appear not to be very effective in forcing the ion exchanges that are required in the initiation of the liberation of chemical transmitters. Thus it is reasonable to look toward some component of the "unit SP" as the most significant receptor potential.

The SP itself is a rectification event and a fundamentally nonlinear response of the cochlear analyzer. There are a variety of nonlinearities in the cochlea that could give rise to this dc response to sound. Among these are the fundamental hydrodynamic nonlinearity of basilar membrane displacement at the best-frequency region that was discovered by Rhode, the necessary asymmetry of hair cell stimulation that is due to the geometry of hair arrangement, the nonlinearity of the cochlear electroanatomy, and the nonlinearity of the transducer process in the hair cell itself. It is quite probable that all of these sources contribute some dc response that adds to the overall SP as recorded with gross electrodes. We have noted that this dc response is very complex and that its character is extremely dependent on stimulus conditions.

The gross potentials, CM and SP, are largely the product of the outer hair cells in the normal cochlea. The inner hair cells also produce these potentials but in a much lesser amount. Their contribution can be assessed only after the destruction of a significant portion of the outer hair cells. Under such conditions CM and SP are reduced from 30 to 40 dB, and some significant differences in the characteristics of the remaining potentials from those produced by the outer hair cells can be demonstrated. It should be noted in passing that since in the normal animals the recorded CM and SP are produced by the outer hair cells virtually in their entirety, and since about 90% of the 8th nerve fibers are innervated from inner hair cells, it is clear that it is exceedingly difficult to seek direct correlations between these gross potentials and neural responses.

It is quite apparent that cochlear biophysics and physiology do not constitute a closed chapter, and consequently this book is little more than a glimpse of a field in progress. Rapid development can be expected in the near future in a number of areas that are directly relevant to our subject. Among these are studies of nonlinear processes in the cochlea, which have been shown by a variety of current experimentation to be much more important to the normal functioning of the ear than hitherto assumed. Other areas of active interest are the development of correlations between gross and elementary potentials and the concomitant study of cochlear electroanatomy. The identification and description of the elusive generator potential can also be anticipated to happen in the near future. Much interest will be attached to the delineation of the respective roles and the interaction between inner and outer hair cells. Of great and enduring interest is the mode of functioning of the efferent system with natural sound stimulation. Finally, an important chapter in the investigation of the cochlea has just barely begun with the growing interest in the biochemical mechanisms in hearing. We can all look forward to exciting times.

References

Adler, L., and Breazeale, M. A. (1970). Generation of fractional harmonics in a resonant ultrasonic wave system. *J. Acoust. Soc. Amer.* **48**, 1077–1083.

Adrian, E. D. (1931). The microphonic action of the cochlea in relation to theories of hearing. *In* "Report of a Discussion on Audition," pp. 5–9. Phys. Soc. of London.

Alexander, I. E., and Githler, F. J. (1954). Private communication to E. G. Wever and M. Lawrence. Quoted in "Physiological Acoustics," p. 299. Princeton Univ. Press, Princeton, New Jersey.

Allaire, P. E. (1971). Private communication.

Allaire, P. E. (1972). "Two Dimensional Fluid Waves and Cochlear Partition Stiffness in the Cochlea." Unpublished doctoral dissertation, Northwestern Univ., Evanston, Illinois.

Allen, G., and Habibi, M. (1962). The effect of increasing the cerebrospinal fluid pressure upon the cochlear microphonics. *Laryngoscope* **72**, 423–434.

Allen, G. W., Dallos, P., Sakamoto, S., and Homma, T. (1971). Cochlear microphonic potentials in cats: effects of perilymphatic pressure. *Arch. Otolaryngol.* **93**, 388–398.

Amatniak, E. (1958). Measurement of bioelectric potentials with microelectrodes and neutralized input capacity amplifiers. *IRE Trans. Med. Electron.* **10**, 3–14.

Bamberg, J. A., and Cook, B. D. (1967). Subharmonic generation in an acoustic interferometer. *J. Acoust. Soc. Amer.* **41**, 1584 (A).

Beidler, L. M. (1961). Taste receptor stimulation. *Progr. Biophys. Biophys. Chem.* **12**, 107.

Benson, R. W. (1953). The calibration and use of probe-tube microphones. *J. Acoust. Soc. Amer.* **25**, 128–134.

Beranek, L. L. (1954). "Acoustics," 481 pp. McGraw-Hill, New York.

Billone, M. (1971). Private communication.

Black, L. J., and Covell, W. P. (1936). A quantitative study of the cochlear response. *Proc. Soc. Exp. Biol. Med.* **33**, 509–511.

Blevins, C. E. (1963). Innervation of the tensor tympani muscle of the cat. *Amer. J. Anat.* **113**, 287–301.

Blevins, C. E. (1964). Studies on the innervation of the stapedius muscle of the cat. *Anat. Rec.* **149**, 157–172.

Bode, H. (1945). "Network Analysis and Feedback Amplifier Design." Van Nostrand-Reinhold, Princeton, New Jersey.

Bodian, D. (1962). The generalized vertebrate neuron. *Science* **137**, 323–326.

Borg, E. (1968). A quantitative study of the effect of the acoustic stapedius reflex on sound transmission through the middle ear of man. *Acta Oto-Laryngol.* **66**, 461–472.

Borg, E., and Møller, A. R. (1968). The acoustic middle ear reflex in unanesthetized rabbits. *Acta Oto-Laryngol.* **65**, 575–585.

Bosher, S. K. (1970). Discussion of W. D. Keidel, Biophysics, mechanics, and electrophysiology of the cochlea. *In* "Frequency Analysis and Periodicity Detection in Hearing" (R. Plomp and G. F. Smoorenburg, eds.), p. 79. Sijthoff, Leiden.

Bosher, S. K., and Warren, R. L. (1968). Observations on the electrochemistry of the cochlear endolymph of the rat: a quantitative study of its electrical potential and tonic composition as determined by means of flame spectrophotometry. *Proc. Roy. Soc. Ser. B* **171**, 227–247.

Bosher, S. K., and Warren, R. L. (1971). A study of the electrochemistry and osmotic relationships of the cochlear fluids in the neonatal rat at the time of the development of the endocochlear potential. *J. Physiol. (London)* **212**, 739–761.

Boston, J. R. (1971). "The Origin of Fractional Distortion Components in the Cochlea." Unpublished doctoral dissertation, Northwestern Univ., Evanston, Illinois.

Bredberg, G., Lindeman, H., Ades, H. W., West, R., and Engström, H. (1970). Scanning electron microscopy of the organ of Corti. *Science* **170**, 861–863.

Bredberg, G., Ades, H., and Engström, H. (1972). Scanning electron microscopy of the normal and pathologically altered organ of Corti. *Acta Oto-Laryngol. Suppl.* To be published.

Brödel, M. (1946). "Three Unpublished Drawings of the Anatomy of the Human Ear." Saunders, Philadelphia, Pennsylvania.

Brugge, J., Anderson, D., Hind, J., and Rose, J. (1969). Time structure of discharges in single auditory nerve fibers of the squirrel monkey in response to complex periodic sounds. *J. Neurophysiol.* **32**, 386–401.

Butler, R. A. (1965). Some experimental observations on the DC resting potentials in the guinea pig cochlea. *J. Acoust. Soc. Amer.* **37**, 429–433.

Butler, R. A., and Honrubia, V. (1963). Response of cochlear potentials to changes in hydrostatic pressure. *J. Acoust. Soc. Amer.* **35**, 1188–1192.

Butler, R. A., Konishi, T., and Fernández, C. (1960). Temperature coefficients of cochlear potentials. *Amer. J. Physiol.* **199**, 688–692.

Butler, R. A., Honrubia, V., Johnstone, B. M., and Fernández, C. (1962). Cochlear function under metabolic impairment. *Ann. Otol. Rhinol. Laryngol.* **71**, 648–655.

Candiollo, L. (1967). The control mechanism of the middle ear transmission system: the middle ear muscles. *In* "The Morphology and Function of Auditory Input Control" (J. Tonndorf, ed.), pp. 13–41. Beltone Institute for Hearing Research, Chicago, Illinois.

Christiansen, J. A. (1963). On hyaluronate molecules in the labyrinth as mechano-electrical transducers, and as molecular motors acting as resonators. *Acta. Oto-Laryngol.* **57**, 33–49.

Coats, A. C. (1965). Temperature effects on the peripheral auditory apparatus. *Science* **150**, 1481–1483.

Cole, K. S., and Moore, J. W. (1960). Liquid junction and membrane potentials of the squid giant axon. *J. Gen. Physiol.* **43**, 971–980.

Crane, H. D. (1966). Mechanical impact: A model for auditory excitation and fatigue. *J. Acoust. Soc. Amer.* **40**, 1147–1159.

Crowe, S. J., Guild, S. R., and Polvogt, L. M. (1934). Observations on the pathology of high-tone deafness. *Bull. Johns Hopkins Hosp.* **54**, 315–379.

Dallos, P. (1964a). Study of the acoustic reflex feedback loop. *IEEE Trans. Bio-Med. Eng.* **11**, 2–7.

Dallos, P. (1964b). Dynamics of the acoustic reflex: phenomenological aspects. *J. Acoust. Soc. Amer.* **36**, 2175–2183.

Dallos, P. (1966). On the generation of odd-fractional subharmonics. *J. Acoust. Soc. Amer.* **40**, 1381–1391.

Dallos, P. (1968). On the negative potential within the organ of Corti. *J. Acoust Soc. Amer.* **44**, 818–819.

Dallos, P. (1969a). Comments on the differential electrode technique. *J. Acoust. Soc. Amer.* **45**, 999–1007.

Dallos, P. (1969b). Combination tone $2f_1 - f_h$ in microphonic potentials. *J. Acoust. Soc. Amer.* **46**, 1437–1444.

Dallos, P. (1970). Low-frequency auditory characteristics: species dependence. *J. Acoust. Soc. Amer.* **48**, 489–499.

Dallos, P. (1972). Cochlear potentials: A status report. *Int. Audiol.* **11**, 29–41.

Dallos, P., and Bredberg, G. (1970). Unpublished observations.

Dallos, P., and Cheatham, M. A. (1971). Travel time in the cochlea and its determination from CM data. *J. Acoust. Soc. Amer.* **49**, 1140–1143.

Dallos, P., and Linnell, C. O. (1966a). Subharmonic components in cochlear microphonic potentials. *J. Acoust. Soc. Amer.* **40**, 4–11.

Dallos, P., and Linnell, C. O. (1966b). Even-order subharmonics in the peripheral auditory system. *J. Acoust. Soc. Amer.* **40**, 561–564.

Dallos, P., and Sweetman, R. H. (1969). Distribution pattern of cochlear harmonics. *J. Acoust. Soc. Amer.* **45**, 37–46.

Dallos, P., Schoeny, Z. G., Worthington, D. W., and Cheatham, M. A. (1969a). Cochlear distortion: effect of direct current polarization. *Science* **164**, 449–451.

Dallos, P., Schoeny, Z. G., Worthington, D. W., and Cheatham, M. A. (1969b). Some problems in the measurement of cochlear distortion. *J. Acoust. Soc. Amer.* **46**, 356–361.

Dallos, P., Schoeny, Z. G., and Cheatham, M. A. (1971). On the limitations of cochlear-microphonic measurements. *J. Acoust. Soc. Amer.* **49**, 1144–1154.

Dallos, P., Schoeny, Z. G., and Cheatham, M. A. (1972). Cochlear summating potentials: descriptive aspects. *Acta Oto-Laryng. Suppl.* **302**, 1–46.

Davis, H. (1956). Initiation of nerve impulses in the cochlea and other mechano-receptors. *In* "Physiological Triggers and Discontinuous Rate Processes" (T. H. Bullock, ed.), pp. 60–71. Amer. Physiol. Soc., Washington, D.C.

Davis, H. (1957). Biophysics and physiology of the inner ear. *Physiol. Rev.* **37**, 1–49.

Davis, H. (1958). Transmission and transduction in the cochlea. *Laryngoscope* **68**, 359–382.

Davis, H. (1960). Mechanism of Excitation of Auditory Nerve Impulses. *In* "Neural Mechanisms of the Auditory and Vestibular Systems" (G. L. Rasmussen and W. F. Windle, eds.), pp. 21–39. Thomas, Springfield, Illinois.

Davis, H. (1961a). Some principles of sensory receptor action. *Physiol. Rev.* **41**, 391–416.

Davis, H. (1961b). Peripheral Coding of Auditory Information. *In* "Sensory Communication" (W. A. Rosenblith, ed.), pp. 119–141. Wiley, New York.

Davis, H. (1965). A model for transducer action in the cochlea. *Cold Spring Harbor Symp. Quant. Biol.* **30**, 181–190.

Davis, H. (1968). Mechanisms of the inner ear. *Ann. Otol. Rhinol. Laryngol.* **77**, 644–656.

Davis, H., and Eldredge, D. H. (1959). An interpretation of the mechanical detector action of the cochlea. *Ann. Otol. Rhinol.* **68**, 665–674.

Davis, H., Derbyshire, A., Lurie, M., and Saul, L. (1934). The electric response of the cochlea. *Amer. J. Physiol.* **107**, 311–332.

Davis, H., Gernandt, B. E., Riesco-MacClure, J. S., and Covell, W. P. (1949). Aural microphonics in the cochlea of the guinea pig. *J. Acoust. Soc. Amer.* **21**, 502–510.

Davis, H., Fernández, C., and McAuliffe, D. R. (1950). The excitatory process in the cochlea. *Proc. Nat. Acad. Sci. U.S.* **36**, 580–587.

Davis, H., Tasaki, T., and Goldstein, R. (1952). The peripheral origin of activity, with reference to the ear. *Cold Spring Harbor Symp. Quant. Biol.* **17**, 143–154.

Davis, H., and associates (1953). Acoustic trauma in the guinea pig. *J. Acoust. Soc. Amer.* **25**, 1180–1189.

Davis, H., Deatherage, B. H., Eldredge, D. H., and Smith, C. A. (1958a). Summating potentials of the cochlea. *Amer. J. Physiol.* **195**, 251–261.

Davis, H., Deatherage, B. H., Rosenblut, B., Fernández, C., Kimura, R., and Smith, C. A. (1958b). Modification of cochlear potentials produced by streptomycin poisoning and by extensive venous obstruction. *Laryngoscope* **68**, 596–627.

Deatherage, B. H., Davis, H., and Eldredge, D. H. (1957). Physiological evidence for the masking of low frequencies by high. *J. Acoust. Soc. Amer.* **29**, 132–137.

de Boer, E. (1969). Encoding of frequency information in the discharge patterns of auditory nerve fibers. *Int. Audiol.* **8**, 547–556.

de Boer, E., and Six, P. D. (1960). The cochlear difference tone. *Acta Oto-Laryngol.* **51**, 84–88.

Derbyshire, A. J., and Davis, H. (1935). The action potentials of the auditory nerve. *Amer. J. Physiol.* **113**, 476–504.

de Reuck, A. V. S., and Knight, J., eds. (1968). "Hearing Mechanisms in Vertebrates," pp. 298–309. Churchill, London.

Desmedt, J. E. (1962). Auditory-evoked potentials from cochlea to cortex as influenced by activation of the efferent olivo-cochlear bundle. *J. Acoust. Soc. Amer.* **34**, 1478–1496.

Desmedt, J. E., and LaGrutta, V. (1963). Function of the uncrossed efferent olivo-cochlear fibers in the cat. *Nature (London)* **200**, 472–474.

Desmedt, J. E., and Monaco, P. (1960). Suppression par la strychnine de l'effet inhibiteur centrifuge, exercé par le faisceau olivo-cochléare. *Arch. Intern. Pharmacodynamie.* **129**, 244–248.

de Vries, H. L. (1952). Brownian motion and the transmission of energy in the cochlea. *J. Acoust. Soc. Amer.* **24**, 527–533.

Dohlman, G. (1959). Modern views on vestibular physiology. *J. Laryngol. Otol.* **73**, 154–160.

Dohlman, G. (1960). Der Mechanismus der Haarzellen-Erregung. *Acta. Oto-Laryngol.* **51**, 349–442.

Durrant, J. D., and Dallos, P. (1971). Unpublished data.

Eccles, J. C. (1964). "The Physiology of Synapses." Springer-Verlag, Berlin.

Eldredge, D. H., Jr. (1950). Some responses of the ear to high frequency sound. *Fed. Proc. Fed. Amer. Soc. Exp. Biol.* **9**, 37 (A).

Eldredge, D. H., and Miller, J. D. (1971). Physiology of hearing. *Annu. Rev. Physiol.* **33**, 281–310.

Eldredge, D. H., Smith, C. A., Davis, H., and Gannon, R. P. (1961). The electrical polarization of the semicircular canals (guinea pig). *Ann. Otol. Rhinol. Laryngol.* **70**, 1024–1036.

Eller, A. (1969). The generation of subharmonic frequency pairs in nonlinear systems. *J. Acoust. Soc. Amer.* **46**, 94 (A).

Engebretson, A. M., and Eldredge, D. H. (1968). Model for the nonlinear characteristics of cochlear potentials. *J. Acoust. Soc. Amer.* **44**, 548–554.

Engström, H. (1960). The cortilymph, the third lymph of the inner ear. *Acta Morphol. Neer. Scand.* **3**, 192–204.

Engström, H., and Wersäll, J. (1953). Structure of the organ of Corti. I. Outer hair cells. *Acta Oto-Laryngol.* **43**, 1–10.

Engström, H., Ades, H. W., and Hawkins, J. E., Jr. (1962). Structure and functions of the sensory hairs of the inner ear. *J. Acoust. Soc. Amer.* **34**, 1356–1363.

Engström, H., Ades, H. W., and Hawkins, J. E., Jr. (1965). Cellular pattern, nerve structure, and fluid space of the organ of Corti. *In* "Contributions to Sensory Physiology" (W. D. Neff, ed.), Vol. 1, pp. 1–61. Academic Press, New York.

Engström, H., Ades, H. W., and Andersson, A. (1966). "Structural Pattern of the Organ of Corti," 172 pp. Almqvist & Wiksell, Stockholm.

Erulkar, S. D., Shelanski, M. L., Whitsel, B. L., and Ogle, P. (1964). Studies of muscle fibers of the tensor tympani of the cat. *Anat. Rec.* **149**, 279–298.

Evans, E. F. (1970). Narrow tuning of cochlear nerve fibers. *J. Physiol. (London)* **206**, 14P, 15P.

Fernández, C. (1955). The effect of oxygen lack on cochlear potentials. *Ann. Otol. Rhinol. Laryngol.* **64**, 1193–1203.

Fernández, C., Gernandt, B. E., Davis, H., and McAuliffe, D. R. (1950). Electrical injury of the cochlea of the guinea pig. *Proc. Soc. Exp. Biol. Med.* **75**, 452–455.

Fex, J. (1959). Augmentation of the cochlear microphonics by stimulation of efferent fibers to cochlea. *Acta Oto-Laryngol.* **50**, 540–541.

Fex, J. (1962). Auditory activity in centrifugal and centripetal cochlear fibers in cat. *Acta Physiol. Scand.* **55**, Suppl. 189, 1–68.

Fex, J. (1967a). The olivocochlear feedback systems. *In* "Sensorineural Hearing Processes and Disorders" (A. B. Graham, ed.), pp. 77–90. Little, Brown, Boston, Massachusetts.

Fex, J. (1967b). Efferent inhibition in the cochlea related to hair-cell dc activity: study of postsynaptic activity of the crossed olivo-cochlear fibres in the cat. *J. Acoust. Soc. Amer.* **41**, 666–675.

Fex, J. (1968). Efferent inhibition in the cochlea by the olivo-cochlear bundle. *In* "Hearing Mechanisms in Vertebrates" (A. V. S. de Reuck and J. Knight, eds.), pp. 169–186. Churchill, London.

Fex, J. (1970). Private communication.

Fischler, H., Frei, E. H., Rubinstein, M., and Spira, D. (1964). Measurement of sound transmission in the middle ear. *Med. Electron. Biol. Eng.* **2**, 289–298.

Fischler, H., Frei, E. H., Spira, D., and Rubinstein, M. (1967). Dynamic response of middle ear structures. *J. Acoust. Soc. Amer.* **41**, 1220–1231.

Flanagan, J. L. (1960). Models for approximating basilar membrane displacement. *Bell Syst. Tech. J.* **39**, 1163–1192.

Flanagan, J. L. (1962). Models for approximating basilar membrane displacement—Part II. *Bell Syst. Tech. J.* **41**, 959–1009.

Fletcher, H. (1953). "Speech and Hearing in Communication," 461 pp. Van Nostrand-Reinhold, Princeton, New Jersey.

Flock, Å. (1965). Transducing mechanisms in lateral line canal organ receptors. *Cold Spring Harbor Symp. Quant. Biol.* **30**, 133–145.

Flock, Å., and Wersäll, J. (1962). A study of the orientation of the sensory hairs of the receptor cells in the lateral line organ of fish, with special reference to the function of the receptors. *J. Cell. Biol.* **15**, 19–27.

Flock, Å., Kimura, R., Lundquist, P. G., and Wersäll, J. (1962). Morphological basis of directional sensitivity of the outer hair cells in the organ of Corti. *J. Acoust. Soc. Amer.* **34**, 1351–1355.

Frank, K., and Becker, M. (1964). Microelectrodes for recording and stimulation. *In* "Physical Techniques in Biological Research" (W. L. Nastuk, ed.), Vol. 5, Part I, Chap. 2, pp. 22–87. Academic Press, New York.

Furshpan, E. J., and Potter, D. D. (1959). Transmission at the giant motor synapses of the crayfish. *J. Physiol. (London)* **145**, 289–325.

Gabor, D. (1946). Theory of communication. *J. Inst. Elec. Eng. (London).* **93**, 429–457.

Galambos, R. (1956). Suppression of auditory nerve activity by stimulation of efferent fibers to cochlea. *J. Neurophysiol.* **19**, 424–437.

Galambos, R., and Rupert, A. (1959). Action of the middle ear muscles of normal cats. *J. Acoust. Soc. Amer.* **31**, 349–355.

Geddes, L. A., and Baker, L. E. (1968). "Principles of Applied Biomedical Instrumentation," 479 pp. Wiley, New York.

Gesteland, R. C., Howland, B., Lettvin, J. Y., and Pitts, W. H. (1959). Comments on microelectrodes. *Proc. IRE* **47**, 1856–1862.

Gisselson, L. (1960a). Die Elektrischen Potentiale des Innenohres. *Arch. Ohren- Nasen- Kehlkopfheilk.* **177**, 45–56.

Gisselson, L. (1960b). Effect on microphonics of acetylcholine injected into the endolymphatic space. *Acta Oto-Laryngol.* **51**, 636–638.

Glaesser, E., Caldwell, W. F., and Stewart, J. L. (1963). "An Electrical Analog of the Ear." Technical Documentary Report AMRL-TDR-63-60, Aerospace Medical Division, Air Force Systems Command, Wright-Patterson Air Force Base, Ohio.

Glattke, T. J. (1968). Apical cochlear responses to pulse trains. *J. Acoust. Soc. Amer.* **44**, 819 (L).

Goblick, T., and Pfeiffer, R. R. (1969). Time domain measurements of cochlear nonlinearities using combination click stimuli. *J. Acoust. Soc. Amer.* **46**, 924–938.

Goldman, S. (1949). "Transformation Calculus and Electrical Transients," 439 pp. Prentice-Hall, Englewood Cliffs, New Jersey.

Goldstein, J. L. (1967). Auditory nonlinearity. *J. Acoust. Soc. Amer.* **41**, 676–689.

Goldstein, J. L. (1970). Aural combination tones. *In* "Frequency Analysis and Periodicity Detection in Hearing" (R. Plomp and G. F. Smoorenburg, eds.), pp. 230–247. Sijthoff, Leiden.

Goldstein, J. L., and Kiang, N. Y-S. (1968). Neural correlates of the aural combination tone $2f_1 - f_2$. *Proc. IEEE* **56**, 981–992.

Goldstein, M. H., Jr., and Kiang, N. Y-S. (1958). Synchrony of neural activity in electric response evoked by transient acoustic stimuli. *J. Acoust. Soc. Amer.* **30**, 107–114.

Goldstein, R. (1954). Analysis of summating potential in cochlear responses of guinea pigs. *Amer. J. Physiol.* **178**, 331–337.

Green, D. G. (1964). "An Investigation of the Dynamics of the Pupil Light Reflex." Unpublished doctoral dissertation, Northwestern Univ., Evanston, Illinois.

Greenwood, D. D. (1962). Approximate calculations of the dimensions of traveling-wave envelopes in four species. *J. Acoust. Soc. Amer.* **34**, 1364–1369.

Greenwood, D. D. (1971). Aural combination tones and auditory masking. *J. Acoust. Soc. Amer.* **50**, 502–543.

Grodins, F. S. (1963). "Control Theory and Biological Systems," 205 pp. Columbia Univ. Press, New York.

Grundfest, H. (1961). Excitation by hyperpolarizing potentials. A general theory of receptor activities. *In* "Nervous Inhibition" (E. Florey, ed.), pp. 326–341. Pergamon, Oxford.

Grundfest, H. (1964). Evolution of electrophysiological varieties among sensory receptor systems. *In* "Essays on Physiological Evolution" (J. W. S. Pringle, ed.). Pergamon, Oxford.

Guinan, J., and Peake, W. T. (1967). Middle ear characteristics of anesthetized cats. *J. Acoust. Soc. Amer.* **41,** 1237–1261.

Hagins, W. A. (1965). Electrical signs of information flow in receptors. *Cold Spring Harbor Symp. Quant. Biol.* **30,** 403–418.

Hallpike, C. S., and Rawdon-Smith, A. (1934). The origin of the Wever–Bray phenomenon. *J. Physiol. (London)* **83,** 243–254.

Hallpike, C. S., and Rawdon-Smith, A. F. (1937). The Wever–Bray phenomenon—origin of the cochlear effect. *Ann. Otol. Rhinol. Laryngol.* **46,** 976–990.

Hardy, M. (1934). Observations on the innervation of the macula sacculi in man. *Anat. Rec.* **59,** 403–418.

Harris, G. G. (1968). Brownian motion in the cochlear partition. *J. Acoust. Soc. Amer.* **44,** 176.

Harris, G. G., Frishkopf, L., and Flock, Å. (1970). Receptor potentials from hair cells of the lateral line. *Science* **167,** 76–79.

Hawkins, J. E., Jr. (1959). The ototoxicity of kanamycin. *Ann. Otol. Rhinol. Laryngol.* **68,** 698–715.

Hawkins, J. E., Jr. (1965). Cytoarchitectural basis of the cochlear transducer. *Cold Spring Harbor Symp. Quant. Biol.* **30,** 147–157.

Hind, J., Anderson, D., Brugge, J., and Rose, J. (1967). Coding of information pertaining to paired low-frequency tones in single auditory nerve fibers of the squirrel monkey. *J. Neurophysiol.* **30,** 794–816.

Honrubia, V., and Ward, P. H. (1966). Spatial distribution of the summating potential of the guinea pig cochlea. *J. Acoust. Soc. Amer.* **40,** 1275 (A).

Honrubia, V., and Ward, P. H. (1968). Longitudinal distribution of the cochlear microphonics inside the cochlear duct (guinea pig). *J. Acoust. Soc. Amer.* **44,** 951–958.

Honrubia, V., and Ward, P. H. (1969a). Properties of the summating potential of the guinea pig's cochlea. *J. Acoust. Soc. Amer.* **45,** 1443–1450.

Honrubia, V., and Ward, P. H. (1969b). Dependence of the cochlear microphonics and the summating potential on the endocochlear potential. *J. Acoust. Soc. Amer.* **46,** 388–392.

Howe, H. A., and Guild, S. R. (1933). Absence of the organ of Corti and its possible relation to electric auditory nerve responses. *Anat. Rec.* **55,** Suppl., 20, 21.

Huggins, W. H. (1953). "A Theory of Hearing," 124 pp. Air Force Cambridge Research Center Technical Report 53-14, Cambridge, Massachusetts.

Hung, I. J. S. (1972). "A Study of the Dynamics of the Acoustic Reflex in Human Beings." Unpublished doctoral dissertation, Northwestern Univ., Evanston, Illinois.

Huxley, A. F. (1969). Is resonance possible in the cochlea after all? *Nature (London)* **221,** 935–940.

Iurato, S. (1961). Submicroscopic structure of the membranous labyrinth: II. The epithelium of Corti's organ. *Z. Zellforsch. Mikrosk. Anat.* **53,** 259–298.

Iurato, S. (1962). Functional implications of the nature and submicroscopic structure of the tectorial and basilar membranes. *J. Acoust. Soc. Amer.* **34,** 1386–1395.

Iurato, S. (1965). Private communication to G. Rossi. Quoted in "Morphology and Function of Auditory Input Control" (J. Tonndorf, ed.), p. 63. Beltone Institute for Hearing Research, Chicago, Illinois, 1967.

Jahnke, E., and Emde, F. (1945). "Tables of Functions," 1st ed., 76 pp. Dover, New York.

Jako, G., Hickman, K. E., Maroti, L. A., and Holly, S. (1967). Recording of the movement of the human basilar membrane. *J. Acoust. Soc. Amer.* **41,** 1578 (A).

Jensen, C. E., Koefoed, J., and Vilstrup, T. (1954). Flow potentials in hyaluronate solutions. *Nature (London)* **174,** 110–1102.

Johnstone, B. M. (1968). Private communication.

Johnstone, B. M. (1970). Ion fluxes in the cochlea. *In* "Membranes and Ion Transport" (E. E. Bittar, ed.), Vol. 3, Chap. 5, pp. 167–184. Wiley (Interscience), New York.

Johnstone, B. M., and Boyle, A. J. T. (1967). Basilar membrane vibration examined with the Mössbauer technique. *Science* **158,** 389–390.

Johnstone, B. M., and Taylor, K. (1970). Mechanical aspects of cochlear function. *In* "Frequency Analysis and Periodicity Detection in Hearing" (R. Plomp and G. F. Smoorenburg, eds.), pp. 81–93. Sijthoff, Leiden.

Johnstone, B. M., Johnstone, J. R., and Pugsley, T. D. (1966). Membrane resistance in endolymphatic walls of the first turn in the guinea pig cochlea. *J. Acoust. Soc. Amer.* **40,** 1398–1404.

Johnstone, B. M., Taylor, K. J., and Boyle, A. J. (1970). Mechanics of the guinea pig cochlea. *J. Acoust. Soc. Amer.* **47,** 504–509.

Johnstone, J. R., and Johnstone, B. M. (1966). Origin of summating potential. *J. Acoust. Soc. Amer.* **40,** 1405–1413.

Jones, A. T. (1935). The discovery of difference tones. *Amer. Phys. Teach.* **3,** 49–51.

Jones, R. W. (1969). Biological control mechanisms. *In* "Biological Engineering" (H. P. Schwan, ed.), pp. 87–203. McGraw-Hill, New York.

Katsuki, Y., Yanagisawa, K., and Kanzaki, J. (1966). Tetraethylammonium and tetrodotoxin: effects on cochlear potentials. *Science* **151,** 1544–1545.

Katz, B. (1950). Depolarization of sensory terminals and the initiation of impulses in the muscle spindle. *J. Physiol. (London)* **11,** 261–282.

Khanna, S. M. (1969). Private communication.

Khanna, S. M., and Tonndorf, J. (1969). Middle ear power transfer. *Arch. Klin. Exp. Ohr-, Nas- Kehlik. Keilk.* **193,** 78–88.

Khanna, S. M., Sears, R. E., and Tonndorf, J. (1968a). Some properties of longitudinal shear waves: a study by computer simulation. *J. Acoust. Soc. Amer.* **43,** 1077–1084.

Khanna, S. M., Tonndorf, J., and Walcott, W. (1968b). Laser interferometer for the measurement of submicroscopic displacement amplitudes and their phases in small biological structures. *J. Acoust. Soc. Amer.* **44,** 1555–1565.

Kiang, N. Y.-S. (1965). "Discharge Patterns of Single Fibers in the Cat's Auditory Nerve," Research Monograph 35, 154 pp. MIT Press, Cambridge, Massachusetts.

Kiang, N. Y.-S., and Peake, W. T. (1960). Components of electrical responses recorded from the cochlea. *Ann. Otol. Rhinol. Laryngol.* **69,** 448–459.

Kiang, N. Y.-S., Goldstein, M. H., Jr., and Peake, W. T. (1962). Temporal coding of neural responses to acoustic stimuli. *IRE Trans.* Inform. Theor. **IT-8,** 113–119.

Kimura, R. S. (1966). Hairs of the cochlear sensory cells and their attachment to the tectorial membrane. *Acta Oto-Laryngol.* **61,** 55–72.

Klatt, D. H. (1964). "Theories of Aural Physiology," 142 pp. Communication Sciences Lab. Report 13, Univ. of Michigan, Ann Arbor.

Kobrak, H. (1948). Construction material of the sound conduction system of the human ear. *J. Acoust. Soc. Amer.* **20,** 125–130.

Kohllöffel, L. U. E. (1971). Studies of the distribution of cochlear potentials along the basilar membrane. *Acta. Oto-Laryngol.* Suppl. No. 288, 1–66.

Konishi, T., and Kelsey, E. (1968a). Effect of sodium deficiency on cochlear potentials. *J. Acoust. Soc. Amer.* **43,** 462–470.

Konishi, T., and Kelsey, E. (1968b). Effect of tetrodotoxin and procaine on cochlear potentials. *J. Acoust. Soc. Amer.* **43,** 471–480.

Konishi, T., and Kelsey, E. (1970). Effect of calcium deficiency on cochlear potentials. *J. Acoust. Soc. Amer.* **47**, 1055–1062.

Konishi, T., and Slepian, J. (1971). Summating potential with electrical stimulation of crossed olivocochlear bundles. *Science* **172**, 483–484.

Konishi, T., and Yasuno, T. (1963). Summating potential of the cochlea of the guinea pig. *J. Acoust. Soc. Amer.* **35**, 1448–1452.

Konishi, T., Butler, R. A., and Fernández, C. (1961). Effect of anoxia on cochlear potentials. *J. Acoust. Soc. Amer.* **33**, 349–356.

Konishi, T., Kelsey, E., and Singleton, G. T. (1966). Effects of chemical alteration in the endolymph on the cochlear potentials. *Acta Oto-Laryngol.* **62**, 393–404.

Korpel, A., and Adler, R. (1965). Parametric phenomena observed on ultrasonic waves in water. *Appl. Phys. Lett.* **7**, 106–108.

Kucharski, W. (1930). Schwingunger von Membranen in einer plusierehden Flüssigkeil. *Phys. Z.* **31**, 264–280.

Kupperman, R. (1966). The dynamic DC potential in the cochlea of the guinea pig (summating potential). *Acta Oto-Laryngol.* **62**, 465–480.

Kupperman, R. (1970). The SP in connection with the movements of the basilar membrane. *In* "Frequency Analysis and Periodicity Detection in Hearing" (R. Plomp and G. F. Smoorenburg, eds.), pp. 126–133. Sijthoff, Leiden.

Kurokawa, S. (1965). Experimental study on electrical resistance of basilar membrane in guinea pig. *Jap. J. Oto-Rhino-Laryngol.* **68**, 1177–1195.

Lamb, H. (1945). "Hydrodynamics," 738 pp. Dover, New York.

Laszlo, C. A. (1968). "Measurement, Modeling and Simulation of the Cochlear Potentials." Unpublished doctoral dissertation, McGill Univ., Montreal, Canada.

Lawrence, M. (1962). The double innervation of the tensor tympani. *Ann. Otol. Rhinol. Laryngol.* **71**, 705–718.

Lawrence, M. (1965). Dynamic range of the cochlear transducer. *Cold Spring Harbor Symp. Quant. Biol.* **30**, 159–167.

Lawrence, M. (1967). Electric polarization of the tectorial membrane. *Ann. Otol. Rhinol. Laryngol.* **76**, 287–313.

Lawrence, M., and Clapper, M. (1961). Differential staining of inner ear fluid by Protargol. *Stain Technol.* **36**, 305–308.

Lawrence, M., Wolsk, D., and Burton, R. D. (1959). Stimulation deafness, cochlear patterns, and significance of electrical recording methods. *Ann. Oto-Laryngol.* **68**, 5–34.

Legouix, J. P., and Chocholle, R. (1957). Modification de la distortion du potential microphonique par le polarisation de l'organ de Corti. *C. R. Soc. Biol.* **151**, 1851.

Leibbrandt, C. C. (1966). Periodicity analysis in the guinea pig. *Acta Oto-Laryngol.* **61**, 413–422.

Licklider, J. C. R. (1951). A duplex theory of pitch perception. *Experientia* **7**, 128–134.

Lim, D. J. (1972). Fine morphology of the tectorial membrane; Its relationship to the organ of Corti. *Arch. Otolaryngol.* **96**, 199–215.

Lindsay, R. B. (1960). "Mechanical Radiation," 415 pp. McGraw-Hill, New York.

Loewenstein, W. R. (1965). Facets of a transducer process. *Cold Spring Harbor Symp. Quant. Biol.* **30**, 29–43.

Loewenstein, W. R., Terzuolo, C. A., and Washizu, Y. (1963). Separation of transducer and impulse-generating processes in sensory receptors. *Science* **142**, 1180–1181.

Lorente de Nó, R., and Harris, A. S. (1933). Experimental studies in hearing. *Laryngoscope* **43**, 315–326.

Lurie, M. H., Davis, H., and Derbyshire, J. A. (1934). The electrical activity of the cochlea in certain pathological conditions. *Ann. Otol. Rhinol. Laryngol.* **43**, 321–344.

McElhaney, J. (1966). Dynamic response of bone and muscle tissue. *J. Appl. Physiol.* **21,** 1231–1236.

McLachlan, N. W. (1934). "Bessel Functions for Engineers," 192 pp. Oxford Univ. Press, London.

Mahon, H., Brun, E., Luukkala, M., and Proctor, W. G. (1967). Excitation of fractional phonons in solids. *Phys. Rev. Lett.* **19,** 430–432.

Matsuoka, K., Konishi, T., and Nakamura, T. (1957). Electric impedance of the cochlea and its significance for evaluating cochlear microphonics. *Acta Oto-Laryngol.* **47,** 325–335.

Mellon, D., Jr. (1968). "The Physiology of Sense Organs," 107 pp. Freeman, San Francisco, California.

Metz, O. (1946). The acoustic impedance measured on normal and pathological ears. *Acta Oto-Laryngol. Suppl.* **63,** 1–254.

Miller, H. D., Engebretson, A. M., and Weston, P. B. (1964). Recording the waveforms of periodic acoustic signals at levels near and below 0.0002 μbar. *J. Acoust. Soc. Amer.* **36,** 1591–1593.

Miller, J. D., Watson, C. S., and Covell, W. P. (1963). Deafening effects of noise on the cat. *Acta Oto-Laryngol. Suppl.* **176,** 1–91.

Misrahy, G. A., Shinabarger, E. W., and Hildreth, K. M. (1957). "Studies on Factors Affecting the Summating Potential." WADC Technical Report 57-467, AD-130965. Project 7210.

Misrahy, G. A., Hildreth, K. M., Shinabarger, E. W., and Gannon, W. J. (1958). Electrical properties of wall of endolymphatic space of the cochlea (guinea pig). *Amer. J. Physiol.* **194,** 396–402.

Møller, A. R. (1960). Improved technique for detailed measurements of the middle ear impedance. *J. Acoust. Soc. Amer.* **32,** 250–257.

Møller, A. R. (1962). Acoustic reflex in man. *J. Acoust. Soc. Amer.* **34,** 1524–1534.

Møller, A. R. (1963). Transfer function of the middle ear. *J. Acoust. Soc. Amer.* **35,** 1526–1534.

Møller, A. R. (1964). Effect of tympanic muscle activity on movement of the eardrum, acoustic impedance, and cochlear microphonics. *Acta Oto-Laryngol.* **58,** 525–534.

Møller, A. R. (1965). An experimental study of the acoustic impedance of the middle ear and its transmission properties. *Acta Oto-Laryngol.* **60,** 129–149.

Møller, A. R. (1970a). Unit responses in the cochlear nucleus of the rat to noise and tones. *Acta Physiol. Scand.* **78,** 289–298.

Møller, A. R. (1970b). Studies of the damped oscillatory response of the auditory frequency analyzer. *Acta Physiol. Scand.* **78,** 299–314.

Molnar, C. E., Loeffel, R. G., and Pfeiffer, R. R. (1968). Distortion compensating, condenser-earphone driver for physiological studies. *J. Acoust. Soc. Amer.* **43,** 1177, 1178.

Mountcastle, V. B., and Baldessarini, R. S. (1968). Synaptic transmission. *In* "Medical Physiology" (V. B. Mountcastle, ed.), Vol. II, pp. 1231–1274. Mosby, St. Louis, Missouri.

Mundie, J. R. (1963). The impedance of the ear—a variable quantity. *In* "Middle Ear Function Seminar" (J. L. Fletcher, ed.), pp. 63–85. U.S. Army Medical Research Lab. Department 576, Wright-Patterson Air Force Base, Ohio.

Munson, W. A., and Wiener, F. M. (1952). In search of the missing 6 dB. *J. Acoust. Soc. Amer.* **24,** 498–501.

Naftalin, L. (1965). Some new proposals regarding acoustic transmission and transduction. *Cold Spring Harbor Symp. Quant. Biol.* **30,** 169–180.

Naftalin, L., Spencer Harrison, M., Stephens, A. (1964). The character of the tectorial membrane. *J. Laryngol. Otol.* **78,** 1061–1078.

Newman, E. B., Stevens, S. S., and Davis, H. (1937). Factors in the production of aural harmonics and combination tones. *J. Acoust. Soc. Amer.* **9,** 107–118.

Nieder, P., and Nieder, I. (1968). Some effects of tonal interactions as seen in the cochlear microphonic. *J. Acoust. Soc. Amer.* **43,** 1092–1106.

Niswander, P. (1970). Unpublished results, Northwestern Univ., Evanston, Illinois.

Nordmark, J., Glattke, T. J., and Schubert, E. D. (1969). Waveform preservation in the cochlea. *J. Acoust. Soc. Amer.* **46,** 1587–1588 (L).

Okamoto, M., Sato, M., and Kirikae, T. (1954). Experimental studies on the function of the tensor tympani muscle. *Ann. Otol. Rhinol. Laryngol.* **63,** 950–959.

Olson, H. F. (1943). "Dynamical Analogies," 196 pp. Van Nostrand-Reinhold, Princeton, New Jersey.

Onchi, Y. (1961). Mechanism of the middle ear. *J. Acoust. Soc. Amer.* **33,** 794–805.

Osterhout, W. J. V., and Hill, S. E. (1931). Electrical variations due to mechanical transmission of stimuli. *J. Gen. Physiol.* **14,** 473–485.

Peake, W. T., and Kiang, N. Y-S. (1962). Cochlear responses to condensation and rarefaction clicks. *Biophys. J.* **2,** 23–34.

Peake, W. T., and Weiss, T. F. (1969). Private communication.

Peake, W. T., Goldstein, M. H., Jr., and Kiang, N. Y–S. (1962). Responses of the auditory nerve to repetitive acoustic stimuli. *J. Acoust. Soc. Amer.* **34,** 562–570.

Peake, W. T., Sohmer, H. S., and Weiss, T. F. (1969). Microelectrode recordings of intracochlear potentials. *In* "Quarterly Progress Report," No. 94, pp. 293–304. MIT Research Laboratory of Electronics, Cambridge, Massachusetts.

Perlman, H. B., Kimura, R., and Fernández, C. (1951). Experiments on temporary obstruction of the internal auditory artery. *Laryngoscope* **69,** 591–613.

Pestalozza, G., and Davis, H. (1956). Electric responses of the guinea pig ear to high audio frequencies. *Amer. J. Physiol.* **185,** 595–600.

Peterson, L., and Bogert, B. (1950). A dynamical theory of the cochlea. *J. Acoust. Soc. Amer.* **22,** 369–381.

Pinto, L. H., and Dallos, P. (1968). An acoustic bridge for measuring the static and dynamic impedance of the eardrum. *IEEE Trans. Bio-Med. Eng.* **15,** 10–16.

Plomp, R. (1965). Detectability thresholds for combination tones. *J. Acoust. Soc. Amer.* **37,** 1110–1123.

Pollack, I. (1970). Jitter detection for repeated auditory pulse patterns. *In* "Frequency Analysis and Periodicity Detection in Hearing" (R. Plomp and G. F. Smoorenburg, eds.), pp. 329–338. Sijthoff, Leiden.

Polyak, S. L. (1946). "The Human Ear in Anatomical Transparencies," 136 pp. Sonotone Corp., Elmsford, New York.

Pong, W., and Marcaccio, W. (1963). Nonlinearity of the middle ear as a possible source of subharmonics. *J. Acoust. Soc. Amer.* **35,** 679–681.

Price, G. R. (1963). Middle ear muscle activity in the rabbit. I. The loss threshold. *J. Aud. Res.* **3,** 221–231.

Pumphrey, R. J., and Rawdon-Smith, A. F. (1936). Hearing in insects: the nature of the response of certain receptors to auditory stimuli. *Proc. Roy. Soc. Ser. B* **121,** 18–27.

Ranke, O. F. (1942). Das Masserver-haltnis Zwischen Membran und Flussigkeit in Innenohr. *Akust. Z.* **7,** 1–11.

Ranke, O. F. (1950). Theory of operation of the cochlea: a contribution to the hydrodynamics of the cochlea. *J. Acoust. Soc. Amer.* **22,** 772–777.

Rasmussen, G. L. (1942). An efferent cochlear bundle. *Anat. Rec.* **82,** 441.

Rasmussen, G. L. (1946). The olivary peduncle and other fibre projections of the superior olivary complex. *J. Comp. Neurol.* **83**, 141–219.

Rasmussen, G. L. (1960). Efferent fibers of the cochlear nerve and cochlear nucleus. *In* "Neural Mechanisms of the Auditory and Vestibular Systems" (G. L. Rasmussen and W. F. Windle, eds.). Thomas, Springfield, Illinois.

Reboul, J. A. (1938). Théorie des phénomènes mécaniques se passant dans l'oreille interne. *J. Phys. Radium* **9**, 185–194.

Rhode, W. S. (1971). Observations of the vibration of the basilar membrane in squirrel monkeys using the Mössbauer technique. *J. Acoust. Soc. Amer.* **49**, 1218–1231.

Rhode, W. S., and Geisler, C. D. (1967). Model of displacement between opposing points on tectorial membrane and reticular lamina. *J. Acoust. Soc. Amer.* **42**, 185–190.

Riesco-MacClure, J. S., Davis, H., Gernandt, B. E., and Covell, W. P. (1949). Ante-mortem failure of the aural harmonic in the guinea pig. *Proc. Soc. Exp. Biol. Med.* **71**, 158–160.

Robbins, R. G. (1971). "Anatomical Correlates of the Generation of Odd Fractional Subharmonics." Unpublished doctoral dissertation, Northwestern Univ., Evanston, Illinois.

Rosenblith, W. A., and Rosenzweig, M. R. (1952). Latency of neural components in round window response to pure tones. *Fed. Proc. Fed. Amer. Soc. Exp. Biol.* **11**, 132.

Rossi, G. (1967). The control mechanism at the hair cell/nerve junction, of the central auditory pathways and centers, and the pathways of the cerebral co-ordination. *In* "Morphology and Function of Auditory Input Control" (J. Tonndorf, ed.), pp. 42–116. Beltone Institute for Hearing Research, Chicago, Illinois.

Rubinstein, M., Feldman, B., Fischler, H., Frei, E. H., and Spira, D. (1966). Measurement of stapedial footplate displacements during transmission of sound through the middle ear. *J. Acoust. Soc. Amer.* **40**, 1420–1426.

Saul, L., and Davis, H. (1932). Action currents in the central nervous system: I. Action currents of the auditory tracts. *Arch. Neurol. Psychiat.* **28**, 1104–1116.

Schuknecht, H. F., Churchill, J. A., and Doran, R. (1959). The localization of acetylcho-linesterase in the cochlea. *Arch. Otolaryngol.* **69**, 549–559.

Schwartzkopff, J. (1970). Discussion of W. D. Keidel, Biophysics, mechanics, and electrophysiology of the cochlea, *in* "Frequency Analysis and Periodicity Detection in Hearing" (R. Plomp and G. F. Smoorenburg, eds.), p. 79. Sijthoff, Leiden.

Siebert, W. M. (1962). Models for the dynamic behavior of the cochlear partition. *In* "Quarterly Progress Report," No. 64, pp. 242–258. MIT Research Laboratory of Electronics, Cambridge, Massachusetts.

Simmons, F. B. (1959). Middle ear muscle activity at moderate sound levels. *Ann. Otol. Rhinol. Laryngol.* **68**, 1126–1143.

Simmons, F. B. (1964). Perceptual theories of middle ear muscle function. *Ann. Otol. Rhinol. Laryngol.* **73**, 724–740.

Simmons, F. B., and Beatty, D. L. (1962). The significance of round-window-recorded cochlear potentials in hearing. *Ann. Oto-Laryngol.* **71**, 767–801.

Sivian, L. J., and White, S. D. (1933). On minimum audible sound fields. *J. Acoust. Soc. Amer.* **4**, 288–321.

Smith, C. A. (1968). Ultrastructure of the organ of Corti. *Advan. Sci.* **24**, 419–433.

Smith, C. A., and Sjöstrand, F. S. (1961). Structure of the nerve endings on the external hair cells of the guinea pig cochlea as studied by serial sections. *J. Ultrastruct. Res.* **5**, 523–556.

Smith, C. A., and Takasaka, T. (1971). Auditory receptor organs of reptiles, birds and mammals. *In* "Contributions to Sensory Physiology" (W. D. Neff, ed.), Vol. 5, pp. 129–178. Academic Press, New York.

Smith, C. A., Davis, H., Deatherage, B. H., and Gessert, C. F. (1958). DC potentials of the membranous labyrinth. *Amer. J. Physiol.* **193**, 203–206.

Smith, K. R., and Wever, E. G. (1949). The problem of stimulation deafness. III. The functional and histological effects of a high-frequency stimulus. *J. Exp. Psychol.* **39**, 238–241.

Smoorenburg, G. (1970). Pitch perception of two frequency stimuli. *J. Acoust. Soc. Amer.* **48**, 924–942.

Sohmer, H. S. (1965). The effect of contralateral olivo-cochlear bundle stimulation on the cochlear potentials evoked by acoustic stimuli of various frequencies and intensities. *Acta Oto-Laryngol.* **60**, 59–70.

Sohmer, H. S., Peake, W. T., and Weiss, T. F. (1971). Intracochlear potential recorded with micropipets. I. Correlation with micropipet location. *J. Acoust. Soc. Amer.* **50**, 572–586.

Spoendlin, H. (1966). "The Organization of the Cochlear Receptor," 227 pp. Karger, Basel.

Spoendlin, H. (1967). Innervation of the organ of Corti. *J. Laryngol. Otol.* **81**, 717–738.

Spoendlin, H. (1970). Structural basis of peripheral frequency analysis. *In* "Frequency Analysis and Periodicity Detection in Hearing" (R. Plomp and G. F. Smoorenburg, eds.), pp. 2–40. Sijthoff, Leiden.

Starr, A. (1969). Regulatory mechanisms of the auditory pathway. *In* "Modern Neurology" (S. Locke, ed.), pp. 101–114. Little, Brown, Boston, Massachusetts.

Starr, A., and Solomon, G. (1965). Electromyographic study of the middle ear muscle activity during shock evoked motor activity in cats. *Int. Audiol.* **4**, 28–30.

Stevens, S. S., and Davis, H. (1938). "Hearing," 489 pp. Wiley, New York.

Stevens, S. S., and Newman, E. B. (1936). On the nature of aural harmonics. *Proc. Nat. Acad. Sci. U.S.* **22**, 668–672.

Stopp, P. E., and Whitfield, I. C. (1964). Summating potentials of the avian cochlea. *J. Physiol. (London)* **175**, 45P, 46P.

Sweetman, R. H., and Dallos, P. (1969). Distribution pattern of cochlear combination tones. *J. Acoust. Soc. Amer.* **45**, 58–71.

Tasaki, I. (1954). Nerve impulses in individual auditory nerve fibers of guinea pig. *J. Neurophysiol.* **17**, 97–122.

Tasaki, I. (1957). Hearing. *Annu. Rev. Physiol.* **19**, 417–438.

Tasaki, I. (1960). Afferent impulses in auditory nerve fibers and the mechanism of impulse initiation in the cochlea. *In* "Neural Mechanisms of the Auditory and Vestibular Systems" (G. Rasmussen and W. F. Windle, eds.), pp. 40–47. Thomas, Springfield, Illinois.

Tasaki, I., and Davis, H. (1955). Electric responses of individual nerve elements in cochlear nucleus to sound stimulation (guinea pig). *J. Neurophysiol.* **18**, 151–158.

Tasaki, I., and Fernández, C. (1952). Modification of cochlear microphonics and action potentials by KCl solution and by direct currents. *J. Neurophysiol.* **15**, 497–512.

Tasaki, I., and Spiropoulos, C. S. (1959). Stria vascularis as source of endocochlear potential. *J. Neurophysiol.* **22**, 149–155.

Tasaki, I., Davis, H., and Legouix, J. P. (1952). The space–time pattern of the cochlear microphonics (guinea pig), as recorded by differential electrodes. *J. Acoust. Soc. Amer.* **24**, 502–518.

Tasaki, I., Davis, H., and Eldredge, D. H. (1954). Exploration of cochlear potentials with a microelectrode. *J. Acoust. Soc. Amer.* **26**, 765–773.

Teas, D. C., and Henry, G. B. (1969). Auditory nerve responses as a function of repetition rate and background noise. *Int. Audiol.* **8**, 147–163.

Teas, D. C., Eldredge, D. H., and Davis, H. (1962). Cochlear responses to acoustic transients: an interpretation of whole-nerve action potentials. *J. Acoust. Soc. Amer.* **34**, 1438–1459.

Thurm, U. (1969). General organization of sensory receptors. *In* "Processing of Optical Data by Organisms and by Machines" (W. Reichardt, ed.), pp. 44–68. Academic Press, New York.

Tomita, T. (1965). Electrophysiological study of the mechanisms subserving color coding in the fish retina. *Cold Spring Harbor Symp. Quant. Biol.* **30**, 559–566.

Tonndorf, J. (1958a). Harmonic distortion in cochlear models. *J. Acoust. Soc. Amer.* **30**, 929–937.

Tonndorf, J. (1958b). Localization of aural harmonics along the basilar membrane of guinea pigs. *J. Acoust. Soc. Amer.* **30**, 938–943.

Tonndorf, J. (1959). Beats in cochlear models. *J. Acoust. Soc. Amer.* **31**, 608–619.

Tonndorf, J. (1960). Shearing motion in scala media of cochlear models. *J. Acoust. Soc. Amer.* **32**, 238–244.

Tonndorf, J. (1962). Time/frequency analysis along the partition of cochlear models: a modified place concept. *J. Acoust. Soc. Amer.* **34**, 1337–1350.

Tonndorf, J. (1966). Bone conduction studies in experimental animals. *Acta Oto-Laryngol. Suppl.* **213**, 132 pp.

Tonndorf, J. (1970a). Comments on waveform preservation in the cochlea. *J. Acoust. Soc. Amer.* **48**, 596 (L).

Tonndorf, J. (1970b). Nonlinearities in cochlear hydrodynamics. *J. Acoust. Soc. Amer.* **47**, 574–578.

Tonndorf, J., and Khanna, S. M. (1967). Some properties of sound transmission in the middle and outer ears of cats. *J. Acoust. Soc. Amer.* **41**, 513–521.

Tonndorf, J., and Khanna, S. M. (1968a). Submicroscopic displacement amplitudes of the tympanic membrane (cats) measured by a laser interferometer. *J. Acoust. Soc. Amer.* **44**, 1546–1554.

Tonndorf, J., and Khanna, S. M. (1968b). Displacement pattern of the basilar membrane: a comparison of experimental data. *Science* **160**, 1139–1140.

Vilstrup, T., and Jensen, C. E. (1961). On the displacement potential in acid mucopolysaccharides. *Acta Oto-Laryngol. Suppl.* **163**, 42 pp.

Vinnikov, Y., and Titova, L. K. (1964). "The Organ of Corti—Its Histopathology," 253 pp. Consultants Bureau, New York.

von Békésy, G. (1928). Zur Theorie des Hörens; Die Schwingungsform der Basilarmembran. *Phys. Z.* **29**, 793–810.

von Békésy, G. (1932). Über den Einfluss der durch den Kopf und den Gehörgang bewirkten Schallfeldverzerrungen auf die Hörschwelle. *Ann. Phys. (Leipzig)* **14**, 51–56.

von Békésy, G. (1934). Über die nichtlinearen Verzerrungen des Ohres. *Ann. Phys. (Leipzig)* **20**, 809–827.

von Békésy, G. (1941). Über die Messung der Schwingungsamplitude der Gehörknöchelchen mittels einer kapazitiven Sonde. *Akust. Z.* **6**, 1–16.

von Békésy, G. (1942). Über die Schwingungen der Schneckentrennwand beim Präparat und Ohrenmodell. *Akust. Z.* **7**, 173–186.

von Békésy, G. (1943). Über die Resonanzkurve und die Abklingzeit der verschiedenen der Schneckentrennwand. *Akust. Z.* **8**, 66–76.

von Békésy, G. (1944). Über die mechanische Frequenzanzlyse in der Schnecke verschiedener Tiere. *Akust. Z.* **9**, 3–11.

von Békésy, G. (1947). The variation of phase along the basilar membrane with sinusoidal vibrations. *J. Acoust. Soc. Amer.* **19**, 452–460.

von Békésy, G. (1948). Vibration of the head in a sound field and its role in hearing by bone conduction. *J. Acoust. Soc. Amer.* **20**, 749–760.

von Békésy, G. (1949). The vibration of the cochlear partition in anatomical preparation and in models of the inner ear. *J. Acoust. Soc. Amer.* **21**, 233–245.

von Békésy, G. (1950). DC potentials and energy balance of the cochlear partition. *J. Acoust. Soc. Amer.* **22,** 576–582.

von Békésy, G. (1951). Microphonics produced by touching the cochlear partition with a vibrating electrode. *J. Acoust. Soc. Amer.* **23,** 29–35.

von Békésy, G. (1952). Gross localization of the place of origin of the cochlear microphonics. *J. Acoust. Soc. Amer.* **24,** 399–409.

von Békésy, G. (1953). Shearing microphonics produced by vibrations near the inner and outer hair cells. *J. Acoust. Soc. Amer.* **25,** 786–790.

von Békésy, G. (1960). "Experiments in Hearing," 745 pp. McGraw-Hill, New York.

von Békésy, G. (1966). Pressure and shearing forces as stimuli of labyrinthine epithelium. *Arch. Otolaryngol.* **84,** 122–130.

von Békésy, G., and Rosenblith, W. A. (1951). The mechanical properties of the ear. *In* "Handbook of Experimental Psychology" (S. S. Stevens, ed.), Chap. 27, pp. 1075–1115. Wiley, New York.

von Gierke, H. E. (1950). Subharmonics generated in human and animal ears. *J. Acoust. Soc. Amer.* **22,** 675 (A).

von Helmholtz, H. L. F. (1954). "On the Sensations of Tone as a Physiological Basis for the Theory of Music" (A. J. Ellis, translator). Dover, New York. Translation of the 1863 original.

Wang, C-Y. (1971). "Latency of Action Potentials in Normal and Kanamycin Treated Cochleae." Unpublished doctoral dissertation, Northwestern Univ., Evanston, Illinois.

Wansdronk, C. (1962). "On the Mechanism of Hearing," 140 pp. Philips Research Reports Suppl. No. 1, Philips Research Laboratory, Eindhoven, Netherlands.

Watson, G. N. (1922). "A Treatise on the Theory of Bessel Functions," 804 pp. Cambridge Univ. Press, London and New York.

Weiss, T. F. (1964). "A Model for Firing Patterns of Auditory Nerve Fibers." Technical Report 418, MIT Research Laboratory of Electronics, Cambridge, Massachusetts.

Weiss, T. F., Peake, W. T., and Sohmer, H. S. (1969). Intracochlear responses to tones. *In* "Quarterly Progress Report," No. 94, pp. 305–316. MIT Research Laboratory of Electronics, Cambridge, Massachusetts.

Weiss, T. F., Peake, W. T., and Sohmer, H. S. (1971). Intracochlear potential recorded with micropipets. II. Responses in the cochlear scalae to tones. *J. Acoust. Soc. Amer.* **50,** 587–601.

Wersäll, R. (1958). The tympanic muscles and their reflexes. *Acta Oto-Laryngol. Suppl.* **139,** 112 pp.

Wever, E. G. (1949). "Theory of Hearing," 484 pp. Wiley, New York.

Wever, E. G. (1966). Electrical potentials of the cochlea. *Physiol. Rev.* **46,** 102–127.

Wever, E. G., and Bray, C. (1930). Action currents in the auditory nerve in response to acoustic stimulation. *Proc. Nat. Acad. Sci. U.S.* **16,** 344–350.

Wever, E. G., and Bray, C. W. (1937). The tensor tympani muscle and its relation to sound conduction. *Ann. Otol. Rhinol. Laryngol.* **46,** 947–962.

Wever, E. G., and Bray, C. W. (1938). Distortion in the ear as shown by the electrical responses of the cochlea. *J. Acoust. Soc. Amer.* **9,** 227–233.

Wever, E. G., and Bray, C. W. (1942). The stapedius muscle in relation to sound conduction. *J. Exp. Psychol.* **31,** 35–43.

Wever, E. G., and Lawrence, M. (1954). "Physiological Acoustics," 454 pp. Princeton Univ. Press, Princeton, New Jersey.

Wever, E. G., and Vernon, J. A. (1955). The effects of the tympanic muscle reflexes upon sound transmission. *Acta Oto-Laryngol.* **45,** 433–439.

Wever, E. G., Bray, C. W., and Lawrence, M. (1940a). A quantitative study of combination tones. *J. Exp. Psychol.* **27,** 469–496.

Wever, E. G., Bray, C. W., and Lawrence, M. (1940b). The locus of distortion in the ear. *J. Acoust. Soc. Amer.* **11**, 427–433.

Wever, E. G., Bray, C. W., and Lawrence, M. (1940c). The origin of combination tones. *J. Exp. Psychol.* **27**, 217–226.

Wever, E. G., Bray, C. W., and Lawrence, M. (1940d). The interference of tones in the cochlea. *J. Acoust. Soc. Amer.* **12**, 268–280.

Wever, E. G., Bray, C. W., and Lawrence, M. (1941). The nature of cochlear activity after death. *Ann. Otol. Rhinol. Laryngol.* **50**, 317–329.

Wever, E. G., Lawrence, M., and von Békésy, G. (1954). A note on recent developments in auditory theory. *Proc. Nat. Acad. Sci. U.S.* **40**, 508–512.

Whitfield, I. C. (1967). "The Auditory Pathway," 209 pp. Arnold, London.

Whitfield, I. C., and Ross, H. F. (1965). Cochlear microphonic and summating potentials and the outputs of individual hair cell generators. *J. Acoust. Soc. Amer.* **38**, 126–131.

Wiener, F. M. (1947). Sound diffraction by rigid spheres and circular cylinders. *J. Acoust. Soc. Amer.* **19**, 444–451.

Wiener, F. M., and Ross, D. A. (1946). The pressure distribution in the auditory canal in a progressive sound field. *J. Acoust. Soc. Amer.* **18**, 401–408.

Wiener, F. M., Pfeiffer, R. R., and Backus, A. S. N. (1966). On the pressure transformation by the head and auditory meatus of the cat. *Acta Oto-Laryngol.* **61**, 255–269.

Wiggers, H. C. (1937). The function of the intra-aural muscles. *Amer. J. Physiol.* **120**, 771–780.

Wood, A. (1966). "Acoustics," 594 pp. Dover, New York.

Woodbury, J. W. (1960). Potentials in a volume conductor. *In* "Medical Physiology and Biophysics" (T. C. Ruch and J. F. Fulton, eds.), pp. 83–91. Saunders, Philadelphia, Pennsylvania.

Worthington, D. W. (1970). "Spatial Patterns of Cochlear Difference Tones." Unpublished doctoral dissertation, Northwestern Univ., Evanston, Illinois.

Worthington, D. W., and Dallos, P. (1971). Spatial patterns of cochlear difference tones. *J. Acoust. Soc. Amer.* **49**, 1818–1830.

Zemlin, W. R. (1968). "Speech and Hearing Science—Anatomy and Physiology," 589 pp. Prentice-Hall, Englewood Cliffs, New Jersey.

Zwicker, E. (1955). Der ungewöhnliche Amplitudengang der nichtlinearen Verzerrungen des Ohres. *Acustica* **5**, 67–74.

Zwislocki, J. (1948). Theorie der Schneckenmechanik. *Acta Oto-Laryngol. Suppl.* **72**, 76 pp.

Zwislocki, J. (1950). Theory of the acoustical action of the cochlea. *J. Acoust. Soc. Amer.* **22**, 778–784.

Zwislocki, J. (1953). Review of recent mechanical theories of cochlear dynamics. *J. Acoust. Soc. Amer.* **25**, 743–751.

Zwislocki, J. (1957). Some impedance measurements on normal and pathological ears. *J. Acoust. Soc. Amer.* **29**, 1312–1317.

Zwislocki, J. (1958). Effect of the transmission characteristic of the ear on the threshold of audibility. *J. Acoust. Soc. Amer.* **30**, 430–432.

Zwislocki, J. (1961). Acoustic measurement of the middle ear function. *Ann. Oto. Rhinol. Laryngol.* **70**, 599–606.

Zwislocki, J. (1963). Analysis of middle ear function. II. Guinea pig ear. *J. Acoust. Soc. Amer.* **35**, 1034–1040.

Zwislocki, J. (1965). Analysis of some auditory characteristics. *In* "Handbook of Mathematical Psychology" (R. Luce, R. Bush, and E. Galanter, eds.), Vol. III, pp. 1–97. Wiley, New York.

Zwislocki, J., and Feldman, A. S. (1963). Post-mortem acoustic impedance of human ears. *J. Acoust. Soc. Amer.* **35**, 104–107.

Subject Index

541